A Practical Approach to Operative Dentistry

A Practical Approach to Operative Dentistry

Gordon B. Gray
BDS, MSc, DDS, PGCertEd
Senior Clinical Lecturer in Restorative Dentistry (Retired)
Dental Clinical Dean
Bristol Dental School
Bristol, United Kingdom

Alaa H. Daud
BDS, LDS RCS (Eng.), MFDS RCS (Edin.), MFDS RCS (Eng.), FDTFEd, MSc, PGCertEd, FHEA
Senior Clinical Lecturer in Restorative Dentistry
Bristol Dental School
Bristol, United Kingdom

WILEY Blackwell

This edition first published 2021

Registered Offices
John Wiley & Sons, Inc., 111 River Street, Hoboken, NJ 07030, USA
John Wiley & Sons Ltd, The Atrium, Southern Gate, Chichester, West Sussex, PO19 8SQ, UK

Editorial Office
9600 Garsington Road, Oxford, OX4 2DQ, UK

For details of our global editorial offices, customer services, and more information about Wiley products visit us at www.wiley.com.

Wiley also publishes its books in a variety of electronic formats and by print-on-demand. Some content that appears in standard print versions of this book may not be available in other formats.

Library of Congress Cataloging-in-Publication Data

Names: Gray, Gordon B. (Gordon Brian), author. | Daud, Alaa, author.
Title: A practical approach to operative dentistry / Gordon B. Gray, Alaa Daud.
Description: Hoboken, NJ : Wiley-Blackwell, 2020. | Includes bibliographical references.
Identifiers: LCCN 2020038279 (print) | LCCN 2020038280 (ebook) | ISBN 9781119608424 (paperback) | ISBN 9781119608431 (adobe pdf) | ISBN 9781119608448 (epub)
Subjects: MESH: Dentistry, Operative–methods | Oral Surgical Procedures | Tooth Diseases–surgery | Dental Prosthesis
Classification: LCC RD33.3 (print) | LCC RD33.3 (ebook) | NLM WU 300 | DDC 617/.05–dc23
LC record available at https://lccn.loc.gov/2020038279
LC ebook record available at https://lccn.loc.gov/2020038280

Cover Design: Wiley
Cover Images: Group of dental tools for the treatment of teeth © Sergey Tikhomirov/Getty Images, Teeth Courtesy of Gordon B. Gray

Set in 9.5/12.5pt STIXTwoText by SPi Global, Pondicherry, India
Printed and bound in Singapore by Markono Print Media Pte Ltd

10 9 8 7 6 5 4 3 2 1

Contents

Preface

Problem solving and minimal invasive dentistry must be developed as an innate art, since it is used routinely by clinicians. This art needs to be developed as an undergraduate student, for both clinical practice and diagnostic purposes.

The purpose of this book is to help students reorganise factual knowledge in their mind. Rather than compartmentalising preclinical sciences into subject matter e.g. anatomy, oral biology, biochemistry, pathology and material science, this book aims to integrate knowledge and produce some links between them that can be used in a practical setting.

While this book acts as a core text for teaching clinical skills to dental undergraduate students, it may also be useful for those practicing or teaching dentistry or in preparation for practical professional registration examinations such as Overseas Registration Examination and License in Dental Surgery.

We would like to thank those who have contributed pictures for this book and have reviewed the manuscript and made useful suggestions.

We would like to express our gratitude to Philip Sellen, Joseph Green and Chris Mills for their assistance with the photography and videos in this book.

This book could not have been written without the encouragement of a number of people. Professors Robert Paterson and Andrew Watts for their continued support over many years and for some pictures which are reproduced in this book.

The time involved in writing this book would not have been possible without the understanding and support of family and friends.

Images of any products presented in this book represent examples of dental materials that could be used. The authors declare no conflict of interest or funding from any dental companies.

About the Companion Website

Don't forget to visit the companion website for this book:

www.wiley.com/go/gray/operative-dentistry

There you will find valuable material designed to enhance your learning, including:

- Videos of clinical procedures
- Self-assessment questions

Scan this QR code to visit the companion website

Section I

Restorative Dentistry

1

Instruments

The instruments contained in an operative tray are concerned with the diagnosis of disease and operative management of carious cavities. The dental mirror, straight, and Briault probe are used for diagnosis of cavities. Some kits will also contain periodontal probes.

Diagnosis

Dental mirrors have a number of functions that include not only indirect vision but reflecting light onto tooth surfaces and retracting soft tissues to protect them from sharp burs.

Probes are used for the exploration of tooth surfaces or, more usually, for the exploration of a prepared cavity. This will provide the operator with knowledge of the surface texture and hardness of the dentine surface within a cavity. It should be noted, however, that the use of sharp probes in fissures can break down the surface and accelerate the progress of a carious lesion. The Briault probe is a double ended instrument that is very useful to exploring for cavitation between teeth and under restoration margins. It should be used lightly to avoid iatrogenic damage.

Periodontal probes are used to measure attachment loss, furcation involvement, and bleeding on probing. The WHO probe has coloured bands that correspond to the Basic Periodontal Examination grading system, and this probe has a small ball end to avoid trauma. The Williams probe has markings at 1 mm intervals and is used to make pocket depth measurements around each tooth when completing a periodontal charting.

Operative Management

These instruments include those used in removing carious dentine and refining the margins of a cavity. Excavators come in a variety of shapes and sizes and should be used carefully for paring away soft dentine. Marginal trimmers are excellent in removing unsupported enamel. The instruments have sharp cutting edges and must be kept sharp to be effective. Some marginal trimmers have a tip of tungsten carbide so that they can maintain their sharpness.

A double ended PF10 instrument is used to transfer dental cements to the cavity floor where it can spread the material smoothly and evenly. An amalgam gun is used to transfer the mixed filling material into the cavity, where it can be condensed using a variety of double ended amalgam condensers. Composite resin is used increasingly frequently in the restoration of teeth. Composite

A Practical Approach to Operative Dentistry, First Edition. Gordon B. Gray and Alaa H. Daud.

Companion website: www.wiley.com/go/gray/operative-dentistry

resin sticks to the surface of stainless steel instruments. A range of gold plated stainless steel instruments is available for transferring and shaping this restorative material.

The final shaping of restorations can be achieved using carvers. These double ended instruments have a leaf shaped blade that can be rested on the surrounding tooth structure to help guide the final shape of the restoration.

Instrument Tray

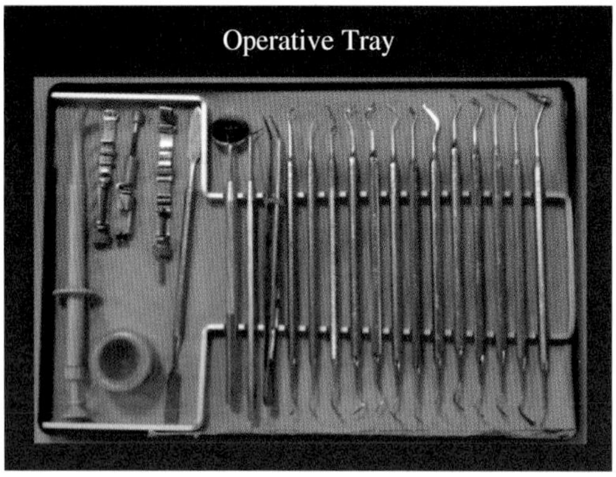

In the accompanying slide a range of diagnostic and operative instruments is shown. There is also a range of matrices for the restoration of class II cavities.
It is important that students learn where each instrument is kept in the tray and that they ensure when an instrument is used it is cleaned on a gauze square before replacing it into its original position.

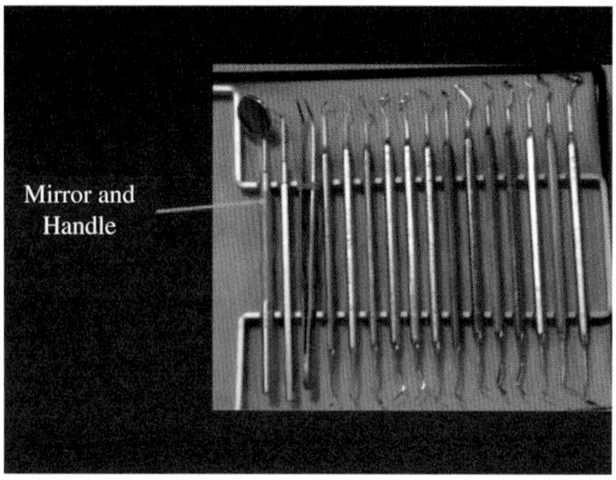

It is important to ensure the dental mirror is securely attached to its handle because these can unscrew for replacement heads to be fitted. Front and rear reflecting mirrors are available as well as magnifying versions.
A front reflecting mirror should be used for endodontic procedures to avoid a double image with close work.

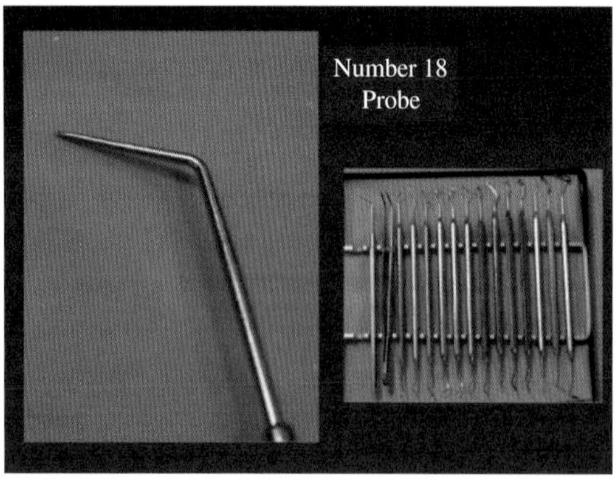

This is a single ended straight probe that should be used to inspect the quality of dentine in cavities. These instruments should be sharp, otherwise they will not accurately convey the information to the operator.
Probes should not be used with force on tooth surfaces because they may break down any demineralised surface zone and enhance the progression of the lesion.

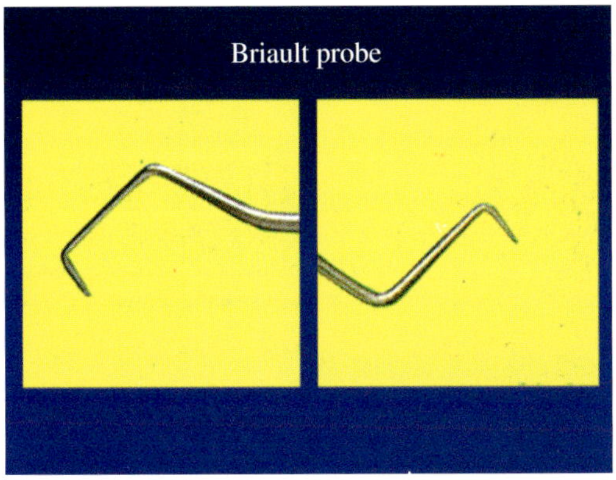

The Briault probe is a double ended instrument that is particularly useful in diagnosing the presence of cavitation or roughness on interproximal tooth surfaces.

It should be used only with light pressure to avoid breaking down any remineralising front to carious lesions and to avoid introducing cariogenic bacteria into lesions.

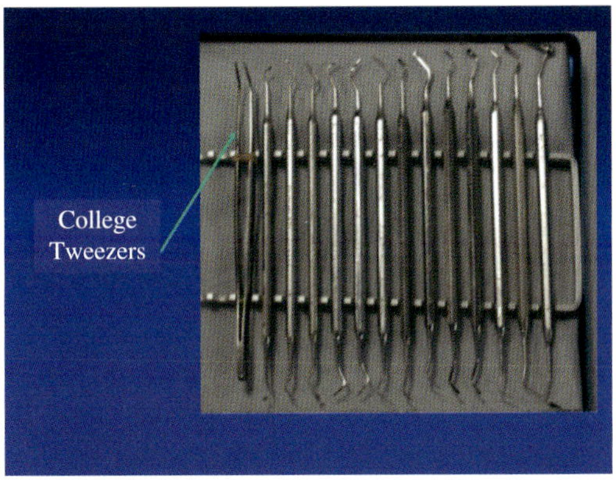

College Tweezers can be used to transfer cotton pellets and cotton wool rolls, etc. to the cavity or mouth.

This instrument is also useful in placing paper points into root canals during endodontic therapy. A locking version is available that is particularly useful for root canal therapy.

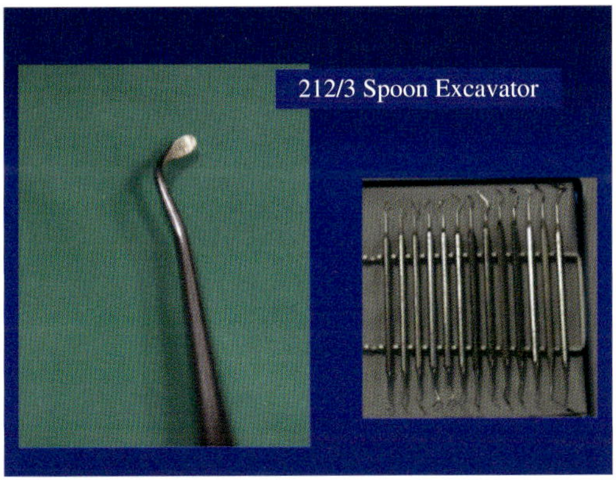

This small excavator has a short neck that can limit the depth to which it can reach into cavities. It is the leading edge of the instrument that is sharp and can cleave carious dentine to allow it to pare away tooth structure.

The instrument shown is a spoon excavator, and its name is derived from the concave upper surface and not from the shape of the overall outline.

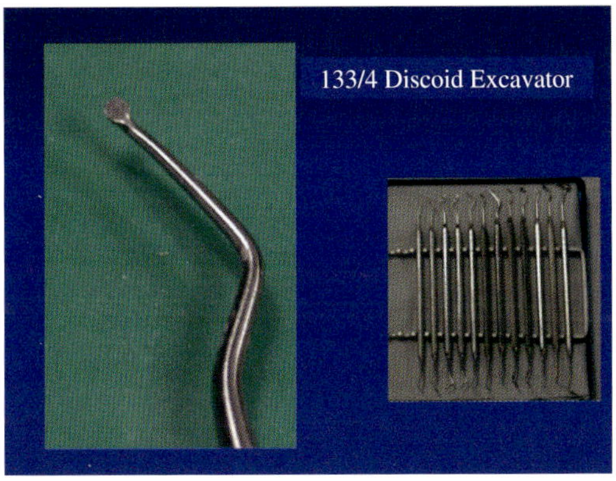

This medium sized excavator has a long neck and allows the instrument to be used into the depth of the cavity.

The instrument shown is a discoid excavator, and its name is derived from the flat upper surface and not from its circular outline.

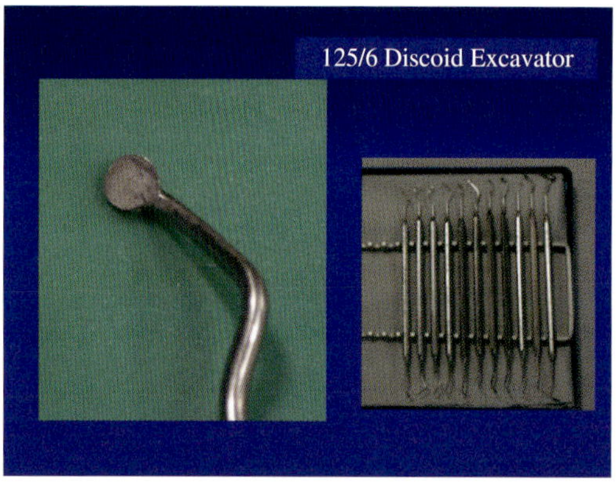

This large excavator is very useful in large carious lesions. It has a sharp leading edge around its outline.
Excavators can be used as an alternative to a round bur for caries removal. They should always be used from a more central area in the cavity towards the periphery, which should have been cleared of caries in an earlier stage of the principles of cavity design.

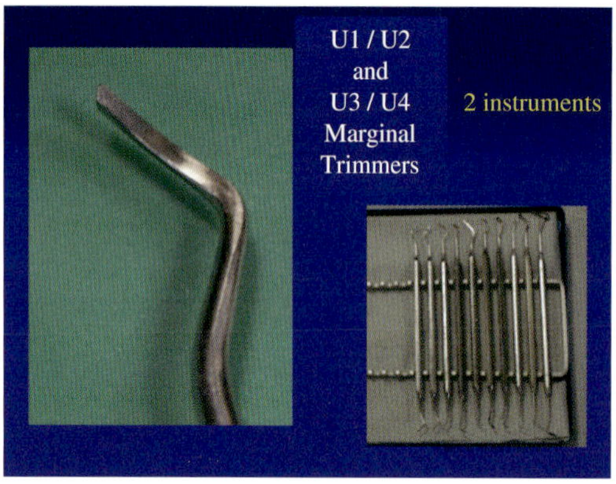

This gingival margin trimmer can be used to pare away unsupported enamel from the floor and walls of a class II box.
The instrument is double ended so that the curved blade can be used to sweep to either the buccal or the lingual aspect of the box.
The sharp leading edge is obliquely cut to remove unsupported tooth structure along the gingival floor of a box preparation or to round internal line angles.
Two of these instruments are required to cover mesial and distal boxes. The difference between the two is the direction of the oblique leading edge.

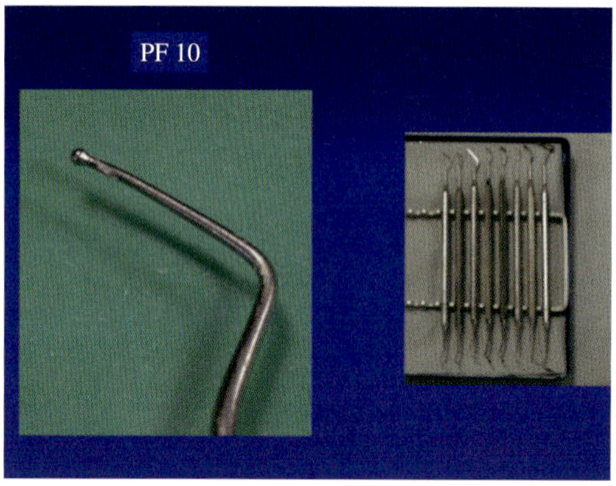

The double ended PF10 instrument is ball ended to collect mixed dental lining cement and smooth it over the cavity floor.
The small size of the ball end allows the material to spread with accuracy.

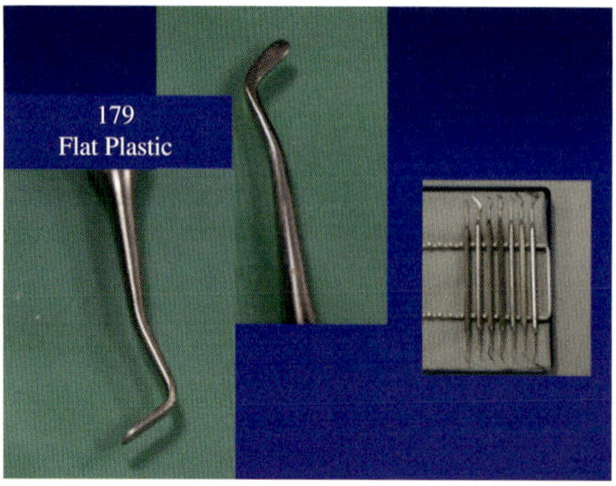

This is a double ended stainless steel instrument that can be used to transfer mixed dental cements into the cavity while still in their putty-like state. One end of the instrument has its blade aligned with the handle, whereas the other end is placed perpendicularly. This allows the base to be applied to the axial wall of a class II cavity.

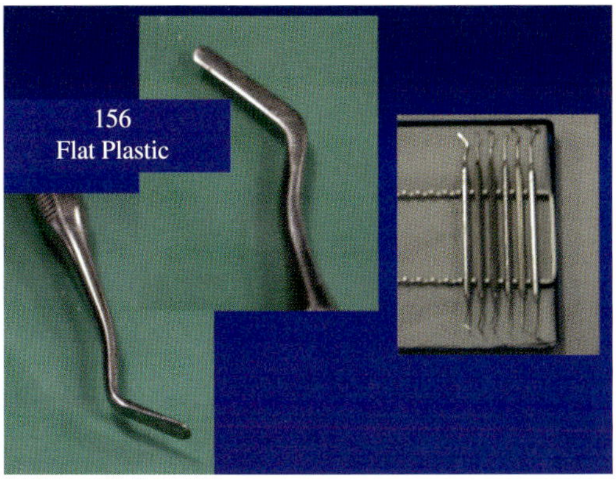

This instrument is similar to the previous one, but the working ends are larger. This makes it particularly useful in transferring a temporary dressing in bulk to the cavity.

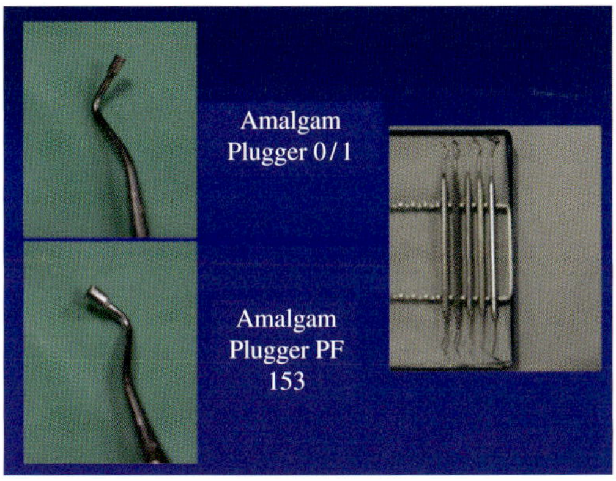

There are a couple of double ended amalgam pluggers in the tray, offering a total of four diameters to condense the filling material into the cavity. The size used will depend on the cavity width.
Smaller instruments will exert greater pressure on the amalgam during the condensation phase and bring a mercury rich layer to the surface.

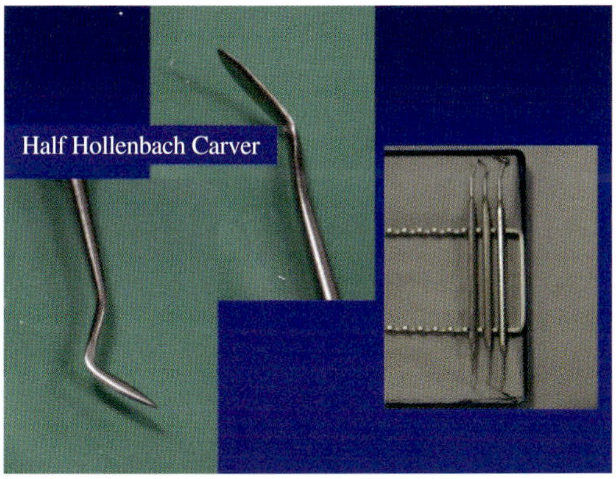

The first of the two carving instruments is the half Hollenbach carver. The leaf shaped blades on either end of the instrument are placed perpendicularly to each other. Part of the blade can be rested on the surrounding cusp slope while the tip of the instrument is held in the mid-line of the tooth. In this way, when the instrument is dragged along the cusp slopes, it carves the correct degree of slope and fissure pattern.

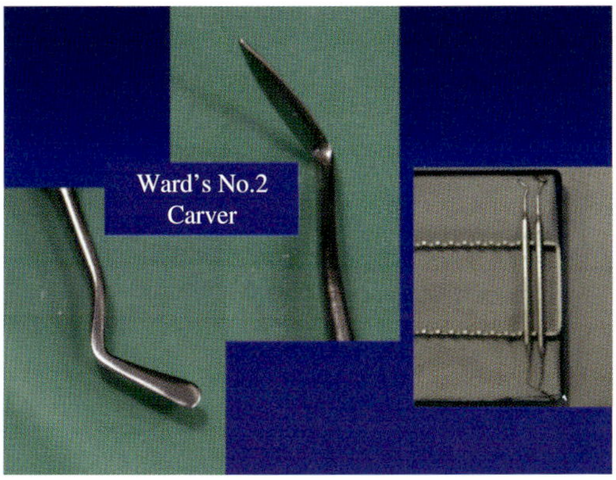

The Ward's carver is similar to the previous carver, but the blade that is in line with the handle is not sharp and can be used to transfer a temporary dressing to the cavity.

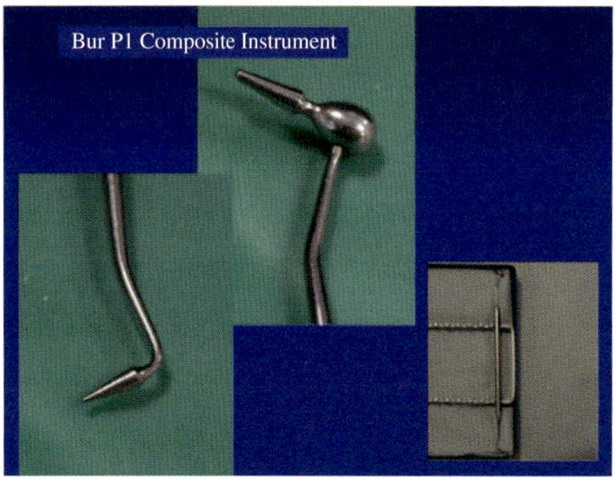

The P1 instrument is one of a range of instruments that can be used to place and shape composite resin. Many similar instruments are gold plated or have tips made from Teflon so the filling material does not adhere.
The cone ends can be used to shape cusp slopes of composite resin, whereas the point makes a fissure pattern.

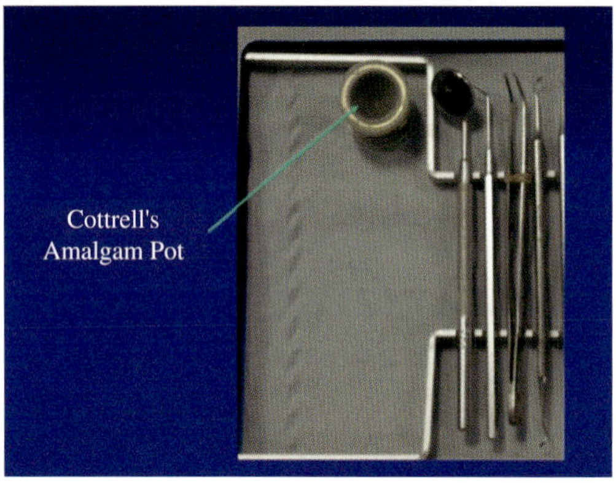

The amalgam pot is dish shaped and receives the mixed or triturated amalgam from a capsule.
The shape of the pot allows the amalgam carrier to be loaded with fresh material.
It is important that the dish is emptied according to Health and Safety recommendations after each use.
The metal ring is autoclavable, and the plastic insert can be replaced.

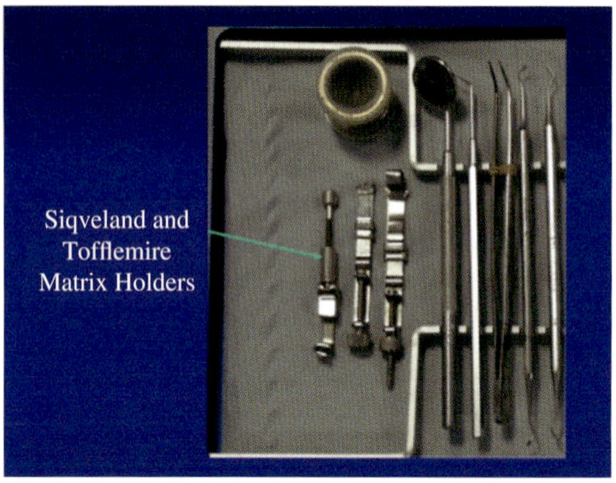

The tray also contains a Tofflemire and two Siqveland matrix bands and holders.
The matrices are used to replace the missing wall of a tooth while filling material is inserted. A matrix allows the filling material to be condensed against it while providing a smooth surface finish.
Single use matrix holders with attached bands can also be used. However, the correct size and shape should be carefully selected.

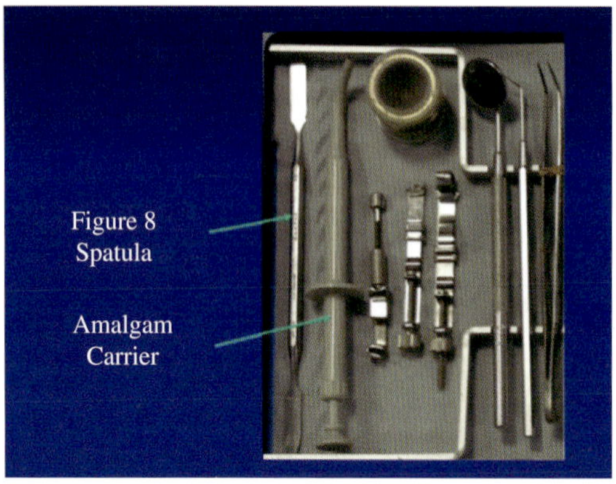

The operative tray also contains a figure 8 spatula with which lining and base cements can be mixed.
This instrument must be cleaned with a gauze square after each use to prevent the dental cement setting on its surface.
The amalgam carrier or gun has an open end into which the amalgam is forced when the tip is pushed into the mixed amalgam mass. The syringe plunger at the other end allows the operator to control the dispensing of the material into the cavity. The gun must be emptied after each use because material left in situ will harden and render the gun unusable.

Handpieces and Burs

Air Turbine

The air turbine or air rotor handpiece is often referred to as the high-speed drill because it rotates at around 400 000–450 000 rpm (see Figure 1.1). This is known as the free-running speed, but when the dentist is actually cutting tooth structure it slows down to 250 000–300 000 rpm, and this is known as the cutting speed.

It operates using compressed air, which turns the turbine containing the bur. The first handpiece was designed by John Walsh and first produced commercially by Dr John Borden in the USA in 1950. The handpiece has two main parts:

- The body through which the compressed air and water are channelled
- The turbine that is contained within the head of the handpiece

The turbine is precision made and converts the compressed air into rotational energy. The fins arranged around its periphery are caught by the flow of compressed air and rotate the turbine within the head of the instrument. A bur is held within the central axis of the turbine, and this is then rotated as the turbine turns. The burs inserted into air turbines are known as friction grip burs. Many handpieces now have a fibre optic facility to shine light directly at the tooth being prepared.

Water is also channelled through the handpiece and sprays a mist onto the rotating bur. This has the effect of cooling the bur and the tooth being cut as well as flushing away the cut debris. It is vital that routine maintenance is performed on all handpieces to ensure they are free from abrasive particles that can cause wear in the turbine and allow it to vibrate. Nowadays cleaning and lubrication can be performed in automated machines. The use of a regular maintenance programme will greatly extend the life of these expensive handpieces.

Video 1.1

Contra-Angled Handpiece

These are often referred to as slow-speed handpieces and are used for removing caries or refining the margins of a cavity. These handpieces require a motor to drive them. This can be an air driven

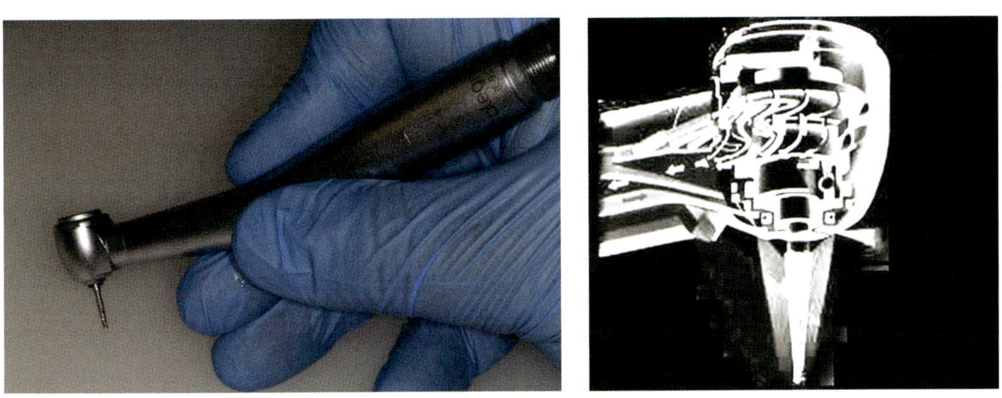

Figure 1.1 The air turbine handpiece is well balanced and operates in excess of 400 000 rpm. It is driven by compressed air that passes over the blades of the turbine and rotates them.

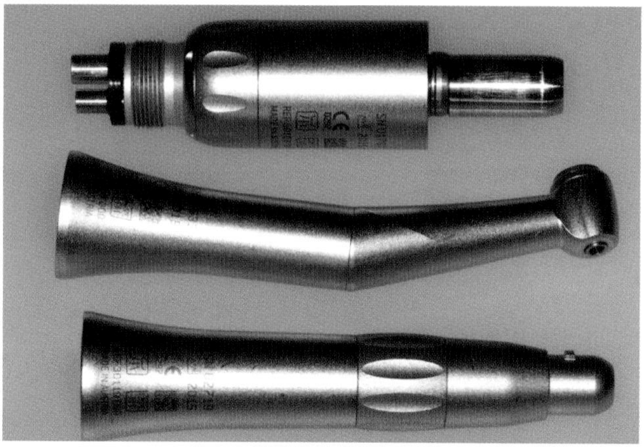

Figure 1.2 An air driven or electric motor can be used to drive the slower-speed handpieces. These can be either straight or contra-angled, and both are designed to be easily held by the operator.

motor or an electric version. The resultant speed of rotation differs between the two with an air motor providing a rotational speed of about 6000 rpm, whereas an electric version can rotate at speeds up to 40 000 rpm. The speed of electric motors can be controlled by rotating a ring at their lower end (see Figure 1.2).

The handpiece connects over the motor shaft and is held in place with a locking device. Both straight and contra-angled handpieces are available. A handpiece with one of more bends in the body allows the bur to lie at an angle to the shaft and is known as a contra-angled handpiece. This allows the bur access to less accessible areas of the mouth. The burs are held within the head of the handpiece by mechanical means and are known as latch grip burs. The body of the handpiece contains a series of gears and is available in a number of versions: speed reducing (4 : 1), speed increasing (1 : 10), and direct (1 : 1).

The torque available with a motor driven handpiece is greater than that of an air turbine, but the speed is lower. In some countries, there is a preference for using a speed increasing handpiece on an electric micromotor because this can produce a speed of nearly 400 000 rpm but with much greater torque than is available with an air turbine. The disadvantage is that there is greater vibration experienced by the patient and a greater potential for rises in pulpal temperature.

Burs

A dental bur is a type of bur or rotary cutter used in a dental handpiece (see Figures 1.3 and 1.4). The burs can be made from steel or tungsten carbide or may be diamond coated. The three parts to a bur are the head, the neck, and the shank.

The heads of steel and tungsten carbide burs contain the cutting blades that remove material. These blades may be positioned at different angles to change the property of the bur. More obtuse angles improve the strength and longevity of the bur, whereas more acute angles produce a sharper blade. Additional cuts across the blades of burs were added to improve their cutting efficiency, but their benefit has been minimised with the advent of high-speed handpieces. These extra cuts are called crosscuts.

The heads of other commonly used burs are covered in a fine diamond grit, which has a similar cutting function to blades but actually abrades the tooth structure and generates more heat.

There are various shapes of burs that include round, inverted cone, straight fissure, tapered fissure, and pear shaped burs.

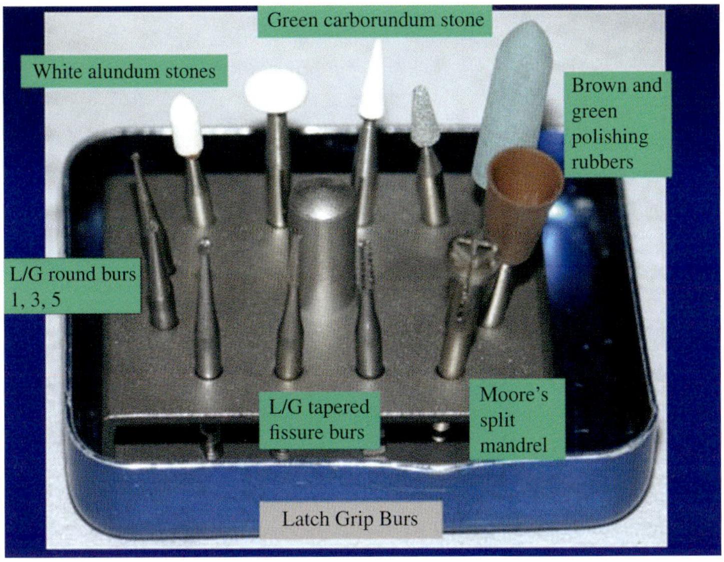

Figure 1.3 A range of steel single use burs for intra-coronal use are shown. In addition, a range of stones and impregnated rubber points are present to smooth and polish restorations.

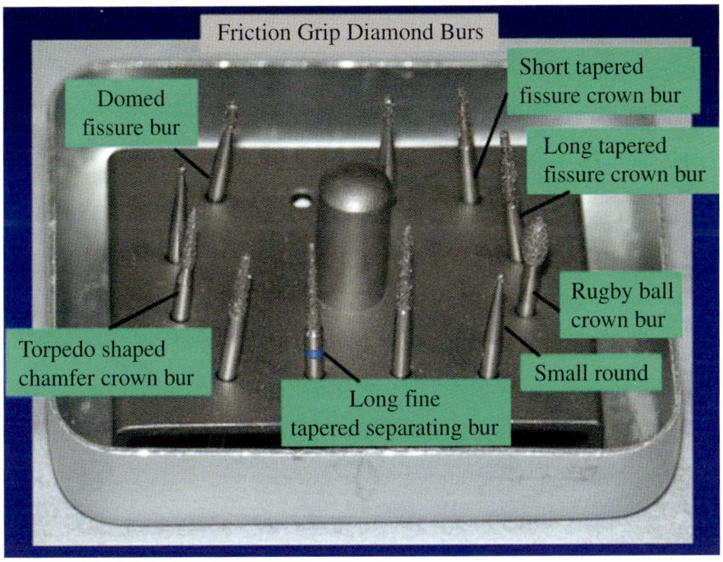

Figure 1.4 A range of friction grip burs for intra-coronal and extra-coronal use. The examples shown are all coated with industrial diamond to make the surface rough and abrade the tooth structure. Similar designs are available made from tungsten carbide that will cut the tooth structure.

Due to the wide array of different burs, numbering systems to categorise them are used and include a US numbering system and a numbering system used by the International Organisation for Standardisation (ISO).

The speed at which these burs operate makes them behave very differently. A bur in an air turbine handpiece will produce a smooth cut with ease, but there will be a high pitched whine while it is operating. A slow-speed bur may be quieter but will produce a courser cut with a lot more

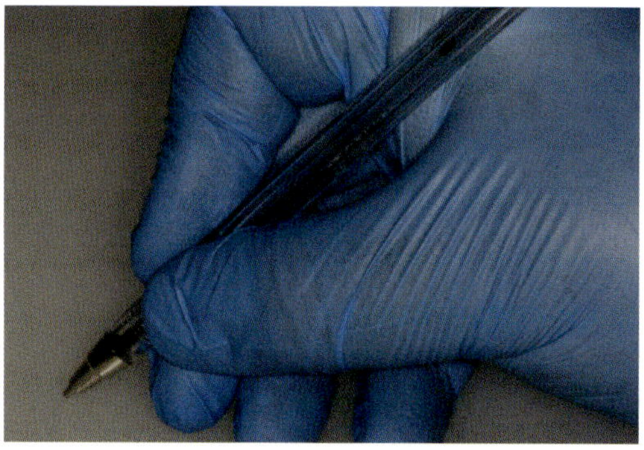

The way in which a person holds a pen gives a great deal of control over the movement of the writing instrument.

Figure 1.5 Handpieces are held using the pen grip to exert maximum control of the instrument.

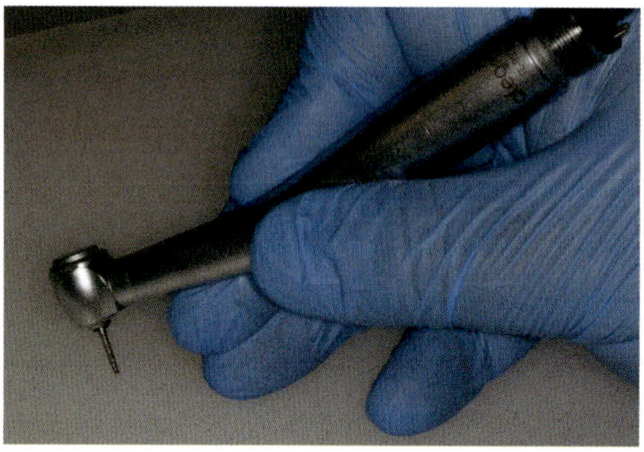

If the pen is replaced with a dental handpiece, a similar level of control can be exerted over the manoeuvrability of the dental instrument. This means that minute movements in a lateral direction can be exerted by small movements of the thumb against the handpiece balanced against the forefinger.

Video 1.2

Figure 1.6 When a handpiece is substituted for the pen, maximum control of the instrument can be used.

vibration experienced by the patient. It is important to check that the bur is running in a clockwise direction, otherwise the flutes will not engage the tooth structure.

It is important that the operator learns to control the handpieces to prevent hard and soft tissue trauma (see Figures 1.5 and 1.6). This can be prevented by mastering

- Grip on the handpiece
- Finger rest positioning on hard non-movable tissues

The fine control of the handpiece using the pen grip requires that a stable finger rest is obtained onto immovable tissue such as adjacent or contralateral teeth or hard tissues. It is really important that a finger rest is never placed on mobile soft tissues (see Figure 1.7).

Matrix Systems

When placing restorative material in a cavity where the proximal wall has been lost due to caries or fracture, the subsequent aim is to restore the contact area and marginal ridge area to prevent food packing. In addition, it is important to have a smooth junction cervically between the restorative material and the tooth surface. However, the cavity does not have walls surrounding it on all sides, and it is necessary to provide one so that the restorative material can be placed. This is done

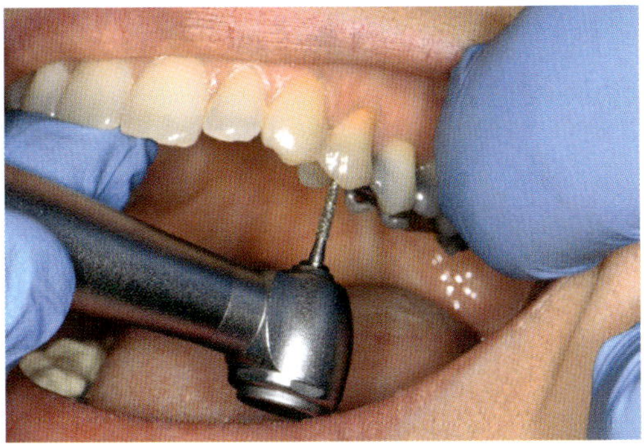

The third or fourth finger is used to rest firmly on adjacent or contralateral teeth to ensure a stable position from which to move the handpiece.

Figure 1.7 It is important that a finger rest is employed when a handpiece is used in the mouth. The finger should be rested on an immovable object, such as adjacent teeth.

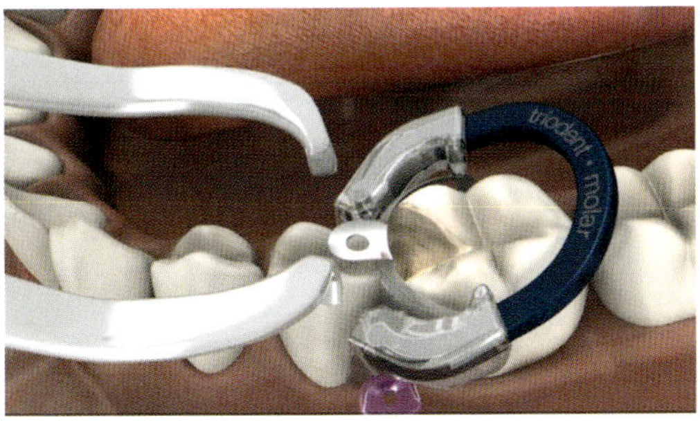

A sectional matrix in place on the mesial aspect of tooth 2.6. The lateral sides of the matrix are adapted to the tooth by the metal ring, and a wedge ensures adaptation to the cervical margin.

Figure 1.8 A modern version of a sectional matrix band that is held in place with a spring ring.

using a matrix band: a clear polyether band anteriorly or a stainless steel band posteriorly. The functions of this matrix band are:

- To retain the filling material in the cavity during placement
- To provide a smooth and close adaptation of the filling material to the surrounding tooth
- To re-establish the contact point and contour of the tooth

There are three types of matrices:

1) Where the band encircles the tooth and is retained by a holder on the buccal or lingual side. The bands held in these holders or retainers can be straight, curved, or contoured. This design allows a firm adaptation to the tooth, e.g. Siqveland or Tofflemire.
2) Where the band encircles only three-quarters of the tooth and the retainer has sharp jaws that impinge into the other tooth embrasure. This type of matrix system is useful when contact points are very tight and resist placement of a matrix bond through the contact, e.g. Ivory or sectional matrix.

   A modern version of this matrix is the newer sectional matrix systems (see Figure 1.8) where a shaped band is inserted and held in place with a metal ring whose sides press against the band and tooth structure to ensure its close adaptation, e.g. Palodent System.
3) In the third type of matrix, there is no retainer. The matrix is held in position using a wedge or may consist of a spring mechanism. The latter has the advantage that no retainer is required and can be used on badly broken down teeth, e.g. AutoMatrix System (see Figures 1.9–1.12).

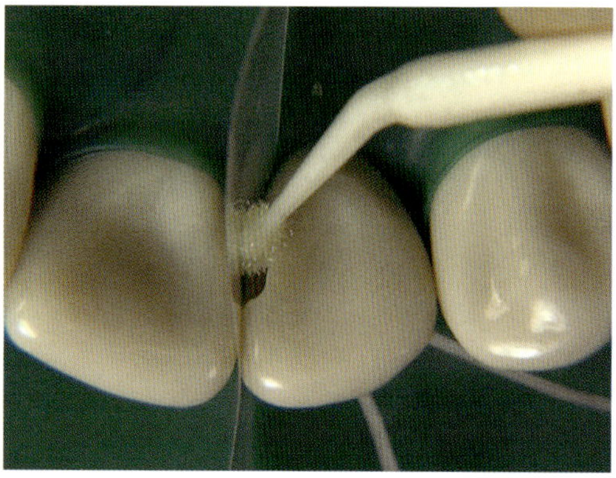

A polyether strip can be placed between anterior teeth to retain composite resin. This is held in place using the operator's fingers.

Figure 1.9 A clear polyether matrix strip can be used when anterior teeth are being restored with composite resin.

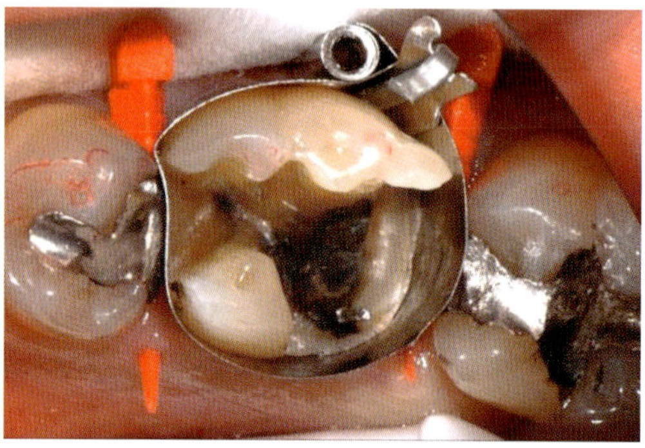

A spring AutoMatrix in place on a heavily broken down tooth. The absence of the matrix holder allows easier access for the restoration of this tooth.

Figure 1.10 A metal AutoMatrix can be useful when restoring very heavily broken down teeth and avoids the presence of a matrix holder in the mouth.

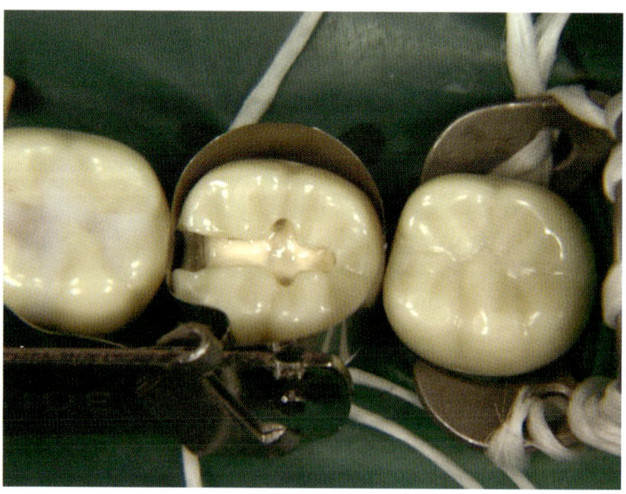

Figure 1.11 A Siqveland matrix band and holder in place on tooth 37. The stages of assembling this matrix are shown in the accompanying video in chapter 6.

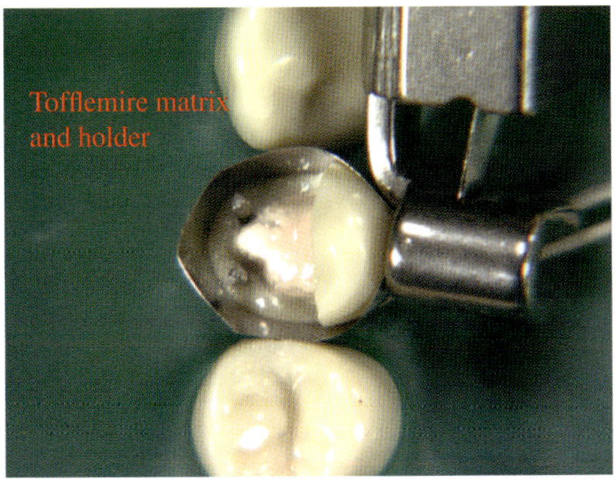

A Tofflemire matrix band and holder applied to a premolar tooth with only a palatal cusp remaining. This system has the advantage that the holder can be removed while still leaving the band in place around the tooth. This allows the band to be removed more carefully.

Figure 1.12 A Tofflemire matrix band and holder in position on tooth 1.4, which has lost its buccal cusp. The holder can be removed from band after the restoration has been placed. This allows removal of the band more easily from around the tooth.

Further Reading

Bartolomucci Boyd, L.R. (2015). *Dental instruments: a pocket guide*. St. Louis, Mo: Elsevier/Saunders.

2

Isolation

It is imperative that the operator keeps control of the operating field during operative procedures. Teeth and cavities must be kept free from moisture during dental examinations and cavity restoration. The moisture can come from saliva, blood, or crevicular fluid. It is important that isolation includes the protection of the soft tissues from potentially caustic materials and the safeguarding of the airway and alimentary canal from instruments and materials. The mucosa of the lips, gingivae, cheeks, palate, and tongue require protection to avoid erosion or traumatic lesions.

Moisture control is required to produce a high quality of restorative care to ensure that lining and filling materials do not become contaminated. Most operative dentistry today involves the use of tooth coloured filling materials and bonding to tooth structure. Salivary contamination cannot be tolerated in adhesive dentistry.

Protection of soft tissues is required during operative procedures. The air turbine handpiece requires a copious water spray to ensure that debris from cavity cutting is washed away and the tooth and bur are kept cool. Isolation should ensure that lips, cheek, and tongue are kept away from the rotary bur. The evacuation of the water spray must be considered carefully to protect these tissues and for patient comfort. During the restoration of the cavity, etchant should be kept away from the surrounding soft tissues so that painful iatrogenic ulceration does not result.

Protection of the airway is vital during all operative procedures as clinicians should 'do no harm' to their patients. The ingestion of cavity debris and water spray can result in reduced patient cooperation, but the inhalation of instruments and debris can be hazardous to health and result in litigation.

Methods of Isolation

High volume aspiration tips can be made of autoclavable metal or disposable plastic. The latter are now the most common in clinical areas. The aspirator tip is useful in retracting lips, cheek, and tongue as well as removing debris and water from the area adjacent to the tooth being treated. Up to 150 ml per second can be removed using this method. This improves vision of the operating field, particularly when indirect mirror visualisation is needed.

A variety of ***saliva ejectors*** are available made from autoclavable metal or disposable plastic. These are placed in the floor of the mouth below the tongue with their tip facing posteriorly. It is important to ensure that the tip is not directly in contact with the mobile soft tissues in this area, otherwise the suction can pull the soft tissues into the lumen of the instrument and result in soft tissue trauma.

A Practical Approach to Operative Dentistry, First Edition. Gordon B. Gray and Alaa H. Daud.

Companion website: www.wiley.com/go/gray/operative-dentistry

Cotton wool rolls and absorbent pads are water absorbent but can also minimally retract soft tissues. Prefabricated rolls and pads provide an acceptable degree of dryness for some procedures, such as examination of teeth, recording an impression, and cementation of crowns and bridges. Absorbent pads are useful in the buccal vestibule because they retract the cheek and absorb saliva from the parotid duct.

Gingival retraction cord can be used to physico-mechanically displace the free gingival margin for the cavity margin in class II and V restorations. This method should only be used where the gingival tissues are healthy and there is an adequate amount of attached gingiva present. A vasoconstrictor or astringent solution of ferric chloride may be added to the cord to improve the efficiency of this method by preventing crevicular fluid exudation by vasoconstriction or haemostasis/astringent. Newer gels are now available that can be syringed into the gingival crevice and would appear to work as effectively without the risk of gingival recession occurring.

Rubber dam provides the ultimate solution to moisture control and soft tissue retraction. Its use was first described by Dr Sandford Barnum in 1864, and much of the original equipment is still used today even if it is in an updated form. Rubber dam provides a dry and clean operating field with good access and visibility from its contrasting background colour (see Figures 2.1–2.3).

The relative merits of using rubber dam must be weighed up by the operator:

Advantages	Disadvantages
Forms a physical barrier to salivary contamination	Gingival damage
Controls movements of the tongue and cheeks	Fracture of porcelain restorations if clamped
Improves access to the operating site	Fracture of heavily restored teeth
Provides gingival retraction	Inhalation or swallowing of clamps
Provides a surgically clean field for endodontics	Contact allergy to rubber dam
Improves vision and contrast at operating site	
Reduces operating time	

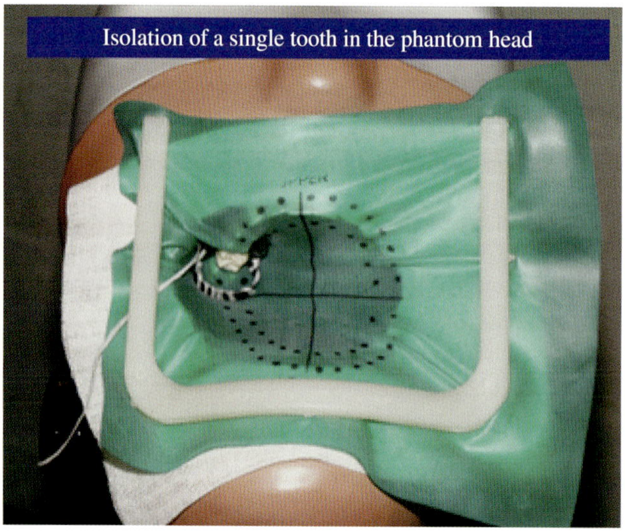

Figure 2.1 Rubber dam can be used to isolate a single tooth for such procedures as endodontics. A radiolucent plastic frame is useful for this procedure.

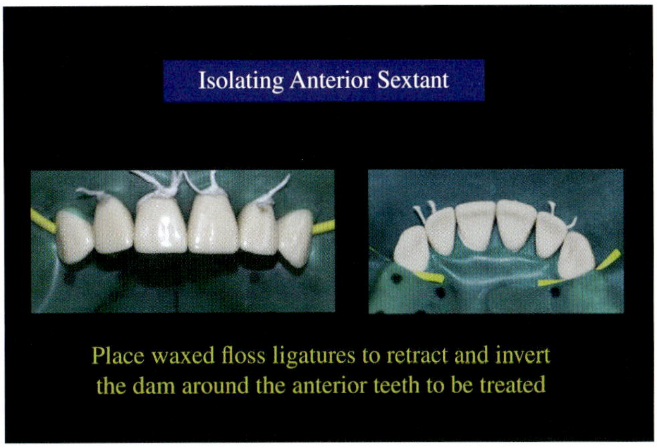

Figure 2.2 Alternatively, rubber dam can be used to isolate a number of teeth. This improves the access to the area and is useful for operative procedures.

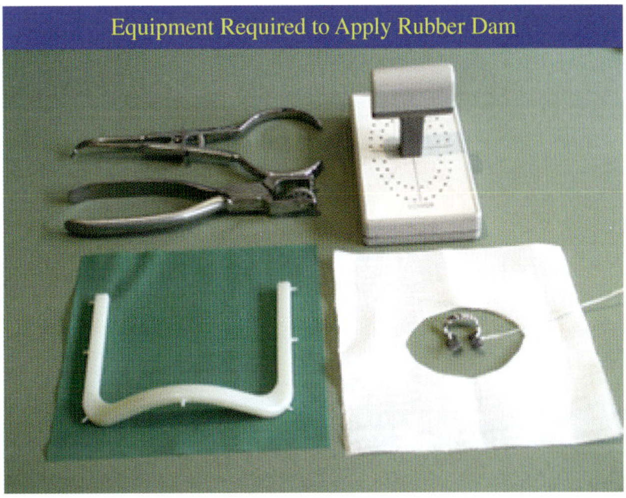

Figure 2.3 An ink stamp is useful to mark the position of the teeth in the dental arches. The holes can be punched in a variety of sizes to accommodate varying tooth sizes. A clamp can be used to anchor the dam, and this is usually placed on the most distal tooth.

The rubber dam is made from natural latex rubber and is available in a variety of colours. It can be purchased in pre-cut squares of 15 cm or on a roll of a similar width that can be cut to length. The thickness of the dam is available from 0.15 to 0.35 mm, with thicker variants offering better soft tissue retraction but being more challenging to pass through the tooth contact points. Generally, a thickness of 0.25 mm is a good compromise. Latex free rubber dam is now widely available and has almost replaced the natural latex version to avoid contact allergy.

Rubber dam clamps may be classified as bland or retentive or, alternatively, as winged or wingless. The jaws of bland clamps approximate each other and are most useful in fully erupted teeth, whereas the retentive clamps have jaws that slope apically and will slide subgingivally on teeth that are partially erupted. The jaws of the clamp are placed at a level below the buccal and lingual bulbosity. It is important that the clamp makes a four point contact with the tooth to prevent it from rotating and causing gingival damage. The clamp is carried to the mouth and placed onto the anchor tooth using rubber dam forceps as shown in Figure 2.4. The bow of the clamp is placed distally to avoid hindering access. Some people favour placing a loop of floss around the bow of the clamp in case of fracture.

The dam can then be supported in front of the face using a rubber dam harness or frame. The latter can be made from stainless steel or plastic and is usually U shaped with retentive tags along the outer surface onto which the dam can be stretched.

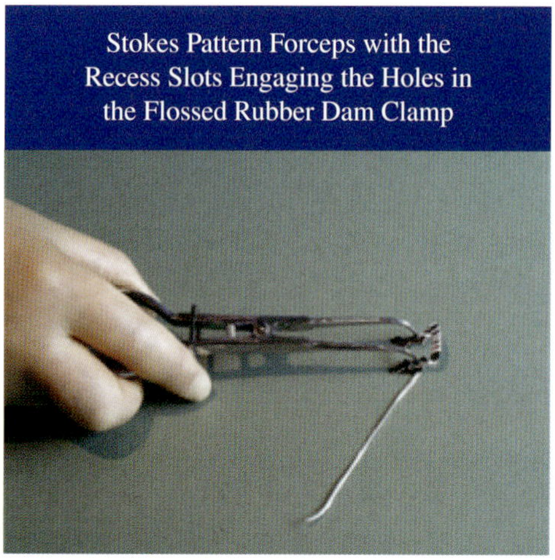

Figure 2.4 The recess slots on the tip of the forceps are placed into the holes on the jaw of the rubber dam clamp. The forceps have a sliding latch that can be pulled back to keep the jaws in an opened position to offer over the anchor tooth.

Further Reading

Al-Amad, S.H., Awad, M.A., Edher, F.M. et al. (2017). The effect of rubber dam on atmospheric bacterial aerosols during restorative dentistry. *Journal of Infection and Public Health* 10: 195–200.

Dahlke, W.O., Cottam, M.R., Herring, M.C. et al. (2012). Evaluation of the spatter-reduction effectiveness of two dry-field isolation techniques. *American Dental Association*: 1199–1204.

Perrine, G.A. (2005). A simplified rubber-dam technique for preparing teeth for indirect restorations. *Journal of American Dental Association* 136 (11): 1560–1561.

3

Dental Charting

Dental charting is an essential part of the preparatory work for patient care. It is a diagrammatic representation of teeth and their surfaces and provides a visual note of the patient's teeth and any treatment he or she has had. Charting shows an immediate representation of the patient's mouth and helps in disease diagnosis and treatment planning. Accurate dental charting can also be used in forensic identification of bodies.

When a patient first attends, a full base chart should be recorded to show all teeth present and any treatment that has been carried out in the past. The charting should be checked each time the patient attends and updated to reflect changes.

There are a number of systems used to chart the dentition and, nowadays, there is even electronic software for this purpose because many practices have gone entirely 'paperless'.

A chart is a diagrammatic representation of the dentition and should show:

- Teeth present
- Teeth missing
- Work to be carried out
- Work completed
- Surfaces with cavities and restorations, etc.

Charting Notations

Zsigmondy-Palmer Notation

R	8 7 6 5 4 3 2 1	1 2 3 4 5 6 7 8	L
	8 7 6 5 4 3 2 1	1 2 3 4 5 6 7 8	

e.g. UR6 or 6┘ has mesio-occlusal caries

LL5 or ┌5 has occlusal restoration

A Practical Approach to Operative Dentistry, First Edition. Gordon B. Gray and Alaa H. Daud.

Companion website: www.wiley.com/go/gray/operative-dentistry

FDI Two-Digit Charting Notation (Fédération Dentaire Internationale)

In this system, the quadrant symbol is replaced by a number. The quadrant number is the first digit while the second number identifies the individual tooth.

In the permanent dentition:

1) for upper right
2) for upper left
3) for lower left
4) for lower right

18 17 16 15 14 13 12 11	21 22 23 24 25 26 27 28
48 47 46 45 44 43 42 41	31 32 33 34 35 36 37 38

e.g. Tooth 16 has mesio-occusal caries
Tooth 35 has an occlusal restoration

Forensic Dental Notation (Box Charting)

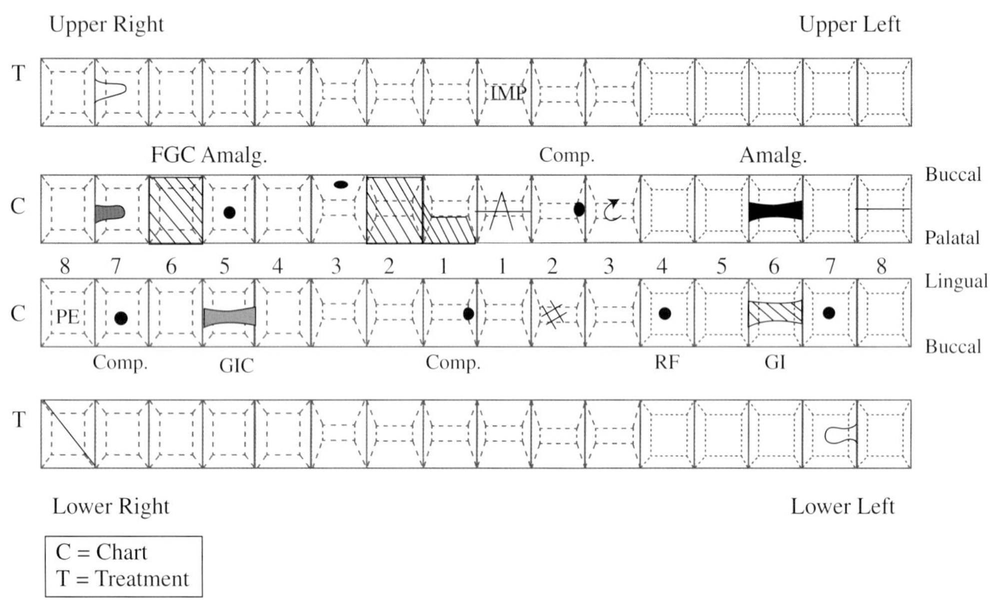

Tooth Surfaces

It is important to be able to identify and note the correct surfaces of teeth. These are defined below:

Occlusal – the biting surfaces of premolars and molars
Mesial – the surface of any tooth nearest to the mid-line of the arch
Distal – the surface of any tooth farthest from the mid-line of the arch
Buccal – the surface facing the cheeks (molars and premolars)
Labial – the surface facing the lips (incisors and canines)
Palatal – the surface facing the palate of all upper teeth
Lingual – the surface facing the tongue of all lower teeth
Cervical – the part of the tooth next to the gingival margin

Abbreviations for Dental Charting

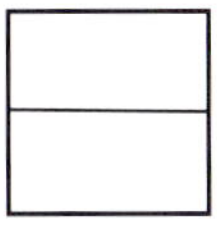

Chart line –tooth absent, draw to → indicate that space has closed between teeth

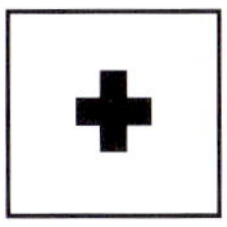

Chart line–a root is present

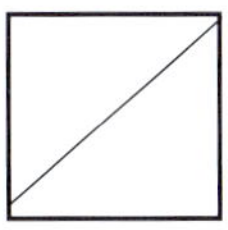

Treatment line – a tooth or roots to be extracted

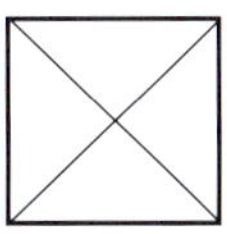

Treatment line –a tooth or roots which have been extracted during this course of treatment

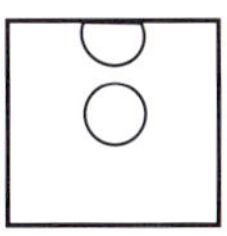

Chart line – primary carious lesion or abrasion cavity present
Treatment line –restoration(s) required during this course of treatment

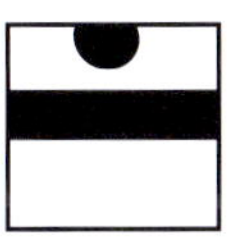

Chart line – restoration(s) present

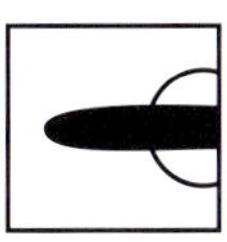

Chart line – secondary carious lesion under part of the restoration
Treatment line – restoration to be partially replaced

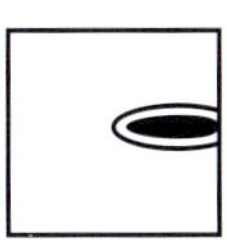

Chart line – secondary carious lesion underlying the whole restoration
Treatment line – restoration to be completely replaced

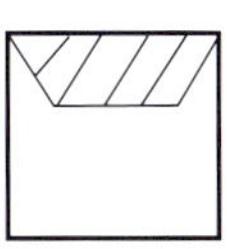

Chart line – labial veneer present

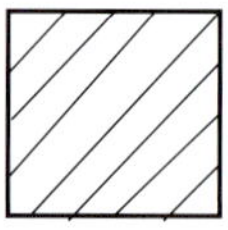

Chart line – crown is present

Treatment line – a tooth that has to be crowned

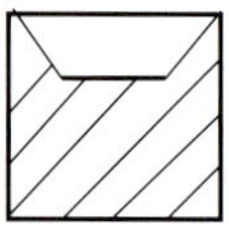

Chart line – ¾ crown is present

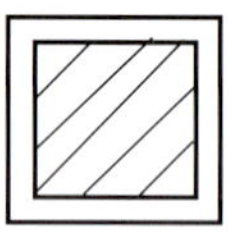

Treatment line – a tooth whose crown is to be replaced

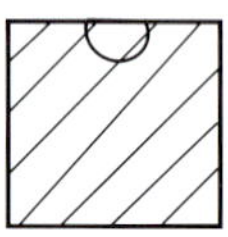

Chart line – crowned tooth with associated marginal caries
Treatment line – restoration to be placed at existing crown margin

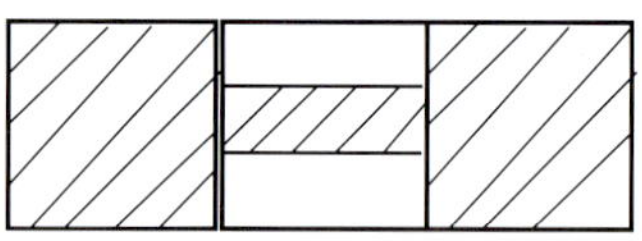

Chart line – conventional three unit bridge
Treatment line – conventional bridge to be replaced (without crosshatching)

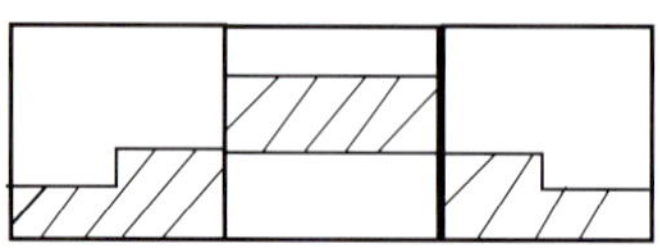

Chart line – resin retained three unit bridge
Treatment line – resin retained bridge to be replaced (without crosshatching)

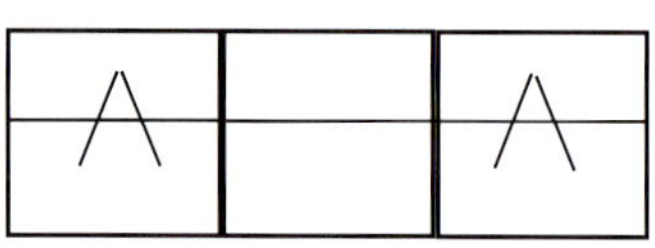

Chart line – denture replacing missing teeth
Treatment line – denture to be replaced

Codes may be written on or beside the chart or treatment boxes. Examples include:

FS	Fissure sealed	v	Veneer
*	Ledge or rough area	GI	Gold inlay
FVG	Full gold crown	GO	Gold onlay
¾ GC	¾ gold crown	CI	Composite inlay
PJC	Porcelain jacket crown	CO	Composite onlay
PFM	Porcelain fused to metal crown	PE	Partially erupted
PC	Post crown	U	Unerupted
RRB	Resin retained bridge	RF	Root filled
CB	Conventional bridge	RCT	Root canal therapy required
AR	Arrest carious lesion	#	Fractured tooth or restoration

Caries status can be inserted adjacent to the box chart:

Ø	No caries detected but operative intervention required, e.g. fracture due to trauma
E1	Caries confined to outer half of enamel
E2	Caries extended to inner half of enamel
A	Caries extended to amelodentinal junction (ADJ)
D1	Caries definitively through the ADJ and into the superficial dentine (less than 0.5 mm when measured on a radiograph)
D2	Caries extended substantially into the dentine (more than 0.5 mm into dentine but more than 0.5 mm away from pulp)
D3	Caries within 0.5 mm from pulp or with pulpal involvement

US Tooth Numbering Notation

There is also an American system of numbering teeth from 1 to 32. This system is not as easy to understand for Europeans as the previously mentioned systems but can often be referred to in American journals and texts. The following diagram describes the system:

UR								UL							
1	2	3	4	5	6	7	8	9	10	11	12	13	14	15	16
32	31	30	29	28	27	26	25	24	23	22	21	20	19	18	17
LR								LL							

Further Reading

Brown, N.L., Jephcote, V.E.L., Morrison, J.N., and Sutton, J.E. (2017). Inaccurate dental charting in an audit of 1128 general dental practice records. *Dental Update* 44 (3): 254.

Shanbhag, V.L. (2016). Significance of dental records in personal identification in forensic sciences. *Journal of Forensic Science and Medicine* 2: 39–43.

4

Minimally Invasive Dentistry

Minimally invasive dentistry (MID) is a philosophy of dental care that is concerned with the early detection of caries and followed by minimally invasive treatment to repair any damage. The concept of MID is based on a better understanding of the carious process and of improved diagnostic techniques. Any damage can then be repaired using adhesive techniques and biomaterials. The main advantages for the patient are to provide a more conservative approach to caries management and to offer a less invasive, health-oriented treatment option.

The philosophy of MID combines all the present knowledge of prevention, remineralisation, ion exchange, healing, and adhesion with the object of reducing carious damage in the simplest and least invasive manner possible. MID is dependent on a number of factors:

1) The demineralisation – remineralisation cycle
2) Adhesion in restorative dentistry
3) Biomimetic restorative materials

Protocol for Using Minimally Invasive Dentistry

- Early caries diagnosis is vital so that preventive measures can be initiated
- Classification of caries depth and progression using radiographs
- Assessment of individual caries risk (high, moderate, low)
- Reduction of cariogenic bacteria
- Arresting active lesions
- Remineralisation and monitoring of non-cavitated lesions
- Placement of restorations in cavitated lesions, using minimal cavity designs
- Repair rather than replacement of defective restorations
- Monitoring

Diagnosis

It is not only important to diagnose carious lesions in teeth early, it is vital to make an assessment of caries activity. The latter is difficult and challenging. It begins with the presence of dental plaque on the teeth, but an assessment of demineralisation must be done over a period of time. Often such adjuncts as radiographs and electronic caries detectors or laser fluorescence are used. Some are

A Practical Approach to Operative Dentistry, First Edition. Gordon B. Gray and Alaa H. Daud.

Companion website: www.wiley.com/go/gray/operative-dentistry

better on occlusal rather than interproximal surfaces. Diagnostic and therapeutic protocols are being developed to aid treatment decisions. These are based on clinical indicators of caries activity and caries risk, e.g. the International Caries Detection and Assessment System (ICDAS) scores.

Alternative Cavity Classification System

A system based on the site and size of carious lesions was suggested by Mount and Hume in 1998 and is shown in the following table:

	Cavity Size				
	Non-cavitated	Minimal Size 1	Moderate Size 2	Large Size 3	Extensive Size 4
Site 1 Pit and fissure	1.0	1.1	1.2	1.3	1.4
Site 2 Interproximal	2.0	2.1	2.2	2.3	2.4
Site 3 Cervical	3.0	3.1	3.2	3.3	3.4

Pit and fissure caries are difficult to diagnose because the white spot lesion (WSL) arises bilaterally on the side walls of the fissure where it cannot be seen. Preventive fissure sealing before caries arise is a sound practice, particularly in patients who have more than two other carious lesions in their dentition. Fissure sealing is a particularly good practice if the fissure can be obliterated by resin before it becomes occluded by pellicle and plaque or any WSL progresses into the underlying dentine. An alternative to a resin fissure sealant is the use of a polyalkenoate cement (glass ionomer). The technique using this material is known as a fissure protection and has the added benefit of fluoride release.

As fissure lesions progress into the dentine, they are still difficult to diagnose because dentine cones on a bitewing radiograph may mask a radiolucency near the enamel dentine junction, and the lesion will only become visible when it has progressed well into the dentine. Electronic and laser fluorescence methods of fissure caries diagnosis have limitations. Often an 'enamel biopsy' may be carried out in the suspect area of a fissure using a small round bur. This has the advantage that only a discrete area of the fissure will be involved, and the remaining sound area of fissure can be left intact. In these circumstances, a sealant restoration can be provided in which the cavity is restored with either glass ionomer cement or composite resin and the adjacent fissures obliterated with a fissure sealant.

Assessment of Caries Risk

Caries activity is the process that begins with the presence of dental plaque that leads to demineralisation. Caries activity cannot be determined at only a single point in time but by monitoring the lesion over time and using such adjuncts as radiographs and electronic means of determining the presence and extent of caries.

Reduction in Cariogenic Bacteria

The first step is to improve the patient's plaque control by demonstrating toothbrush technique and interproximal plaque control. Agents such as chlorhexidine and topical fluorides can be applied to encourage remineralisation. Chlorhexidine acts by reducing the number of cariogenic bacteria. Topical fluorides increase the availability of fluoride ions for remineralisation and the formation of fluoroapatite.

Arresting Active Lesions

It is possible to arrest and even reverse early carious lesions before cavitation takes place. If the lesion is allowed to progress, it will advance towards the underlying dentine and spread along the enamel dentine junction. This can eventually result in the enamel becoming undermined, and the lesion may then cavitate. It is not easy to control plaque once this has happened, and the availability of the ions required for remineralisation is also compromised. It is for this reason that operative intervention becomes necessary at this stage.

Remineralisation of Carious Lesions and Monitoring

The cycles of the carious process demineralise the enamel surface when the oral pH falls below 5.5, and this results in the subsurface carious lesion known as the WSL. However, in between the cycles of demineralisation, the tooth can be remineralised by replacing the lost calcium and phosphate ions, providing that the local environment is conducive. Fluoride is important in enhancing the uptake of these ions and produces fluoroapatite, which is less soluble in the acidic conditions found in a demineralisation cycle. In this way, a lesion can be arrested, provided that plaque control is improved, the frequency of refined carbohydrates is reduced, the clinician checks that there is adequate salivary flow, and the patient is educated on the need for these regimes.

Restoration of Cavities Using Minimal Cavity Designs

Not all dentists can agree when surgical treatment is indicated, but when it is, it should be minimally invasive. Such minimally invasive techniques as air abrasion are used to prepare cavities for restoration with adhesive materials. Such restorations are discussed below. In contemporary dental practice, operative intervention of lesions confined to the inner half of enamel and even slightly into dentine is not indicated. This approach is justified on the basis that caries progression through the enamel is very slow. This is especially true in patients exposed to fluoride. In fact, in some populations, it takes six to eight years for a lesion to progress through enamel. It is estimated that a 50% reduction in restoration placement could result from focusing on infection control rather than surgical intervention.

Cavitation makes plaque control difficult or impossible. Therefore, we may rely on a surgical approach when there is cavitation. Infected tissue is removed and replaced with a suitable restorative material, keeping in mind that nothing can equal natural tooth structure. Adhesive dental materials make it possible to conserve tooth structure using minimally invasive cavity preparations, because adhesive materials do not require the incorporation of mechanical retention features. There are several materials that can be used: glass ionomer cements, resin-based composite with bonding agents, and a laminated restoration using these materials.

The advantage of using ***glass ionomer cement*** (GIC) is that this material adheres to tooth structure and releases fluoride. It performs well in low stress areas. Mature GIC is 'rechargeable' and forms a reservoir for fluoride ions, meaning it can take up fluoride from the environment exposure to fluoride treatments and toothpaste. Theoretically, this fluoride uptake and slow release can have an anticariogenic effect. On the other hand, GICs are technique sensitive. The handling properties and brittleness of the material can be partially overcome by adding resin to the material. The resulting resin-modified glass ionomer cements (RMGICs) are easier to place, have command curing, and have improved aesthetics. However, the introduction of the resin component introduces polymerisation shrinkage to the material. GICs and RMGICs are satisfactory in cervical restorations, fissure sealants, proximal lesions in anterior permanent teeth, and proximal lesions in anterior and posterior primary teeth.

Composite resin when combined with enamel and ***bonding resins*** allows strong bonding to tooth structure and virtually eliminates microleakage around enamel margins. Cavity preparations for this material are designed to conserve enamel and can eliminate the need for macro-mechanical retention.

Simultaneous etching of dentine and enamel and the formation of a hybrid layer has improved the quality of the bond. The technology is constantly improving, but polymerisation shrinkage and marginal leakage at dentine margins are still considered to be problematic. Newer flowable materials have low viscosity and often are used in smaller preparations as well as in cervical cavities.

Repairing Defective Restorations

It is currently thought that dentists working in general dental practice spend between 50% and 70% of their time replacing restorations. Each time a restoration is replaced, the cavity increases in size and the tooth becomes weaker. This, in turn, leads to larger restorations with a potentially shorter life span. The reason dentists replace rather than locally repair 'failing' restorations is a fear of inadequate bond strength to the remaining restorative material and a fear of leaving residual caries in the tooth.

However, caries under well sealed restorations fail to progress, so repairing a defective margin rather than replacing the restoration is a valid and conservative treatment option. The treatment decision must balance the patient risk of developing further caries versus the risks and conservative management.

Monitoring

A MID approach can work well, but, because this is a treatment modality for established carious lesions, it is important that a regular monitoring regime is embarked upon to ensure that lesions do not progress. Remineralised lesions are more resistant to further acid attack. WSLs initially have a matt surface, but following remineralisation, they can arrest and then have a smoother shiny surface. The colour of these lesions may also change, and they may take on a darker or brown appearance.

It is important to monitor the patient to ensure good plaque control is being maintained because, without this, the lesions may not arrest. Therapeutic fissure sealants also need to be checked to ensure they remain intact because they form a barrier that cuts off the nutrient supply to any incarcerated bacteria within the fissure system.

Cavity Preparation

A cavity is only prepared where it is not possible to arrest the carious lesions using any other means. The smallest size of bur possible should be used, and the process often requires the help of magnification. As an alternative to the traditional use of handpieces, air abrasion and lasers may be used to localise the cavity preparation.

Air abrasion uses a fast but narrow stream of aluminium oxide particles in air. These interact with the tooth structure and abrade it. It is particularly useful in diagnosing and preparing cavities in pit and fissure lesions. There is no vibration and minimal noise when using this technique, and therefore it is good for patient cooperation. However, the powerful stream of particles is not effective at removing soft carious material. Soft dentine caries can be removed conventionally using a hand excavator or a round bur in a dental handpiece. Alternatively, chemo-mechanical methods can be used to dissolve the soft dentine caries. This method is atraumatic and bactericidal. It uses a gel composed of sodium hypochlorite and three amino acids: lysine, leucine, and glutamic acids. This technique uses specially designed hand instruments and is particularly useful with phobic patients.

Lasers may be used to prepare cavities. Erbium: yttrium aluminium garnet lasers and erbium, chromium: yttrium-scandium-gallium-garnet lasers are the most common types. These lasers can remove soft caries as well as hard tissue. Lasers reportedly can allow the dentist to remove caries selectively while maintaining healthy dentine and enamel. They may be used without a local analgesic, but some researchers have suggested that there may be a rise in pulpal temperature when this technique is employed.

MID for Pits and Fissures

Molar teeth with deep fissures are one of the most susceptible areas to become carious. The early application of a ***preventive fissure sealant*** will obliterate these stagnant areas and does not require any tooth cutting (see Figure 4.1).

Where areas of the fissure are decalcified and there is some surrounding opacity in a localised area, a sealant restoration may be provided. This requires the local investigation of the suspect area of fissure and its restoration using a composite resin filling before a fissure sealant is applied to all pits and fissures in the tooth (see Figure 4.2).

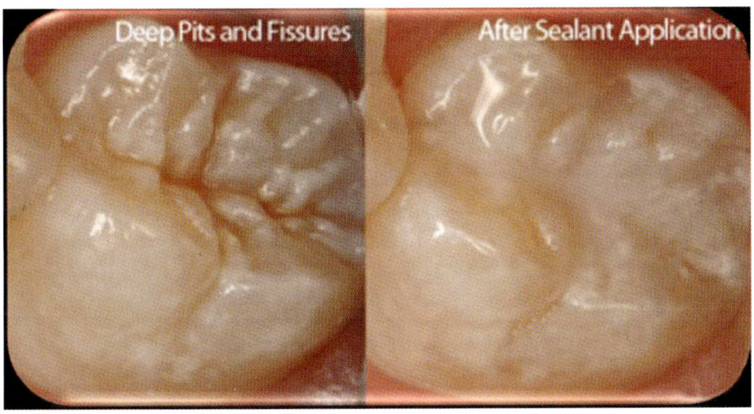

Figure 4.1 Note the steep cuspal inclines and the deep fissures. These can be obliterated by using a resin of low viscosity.

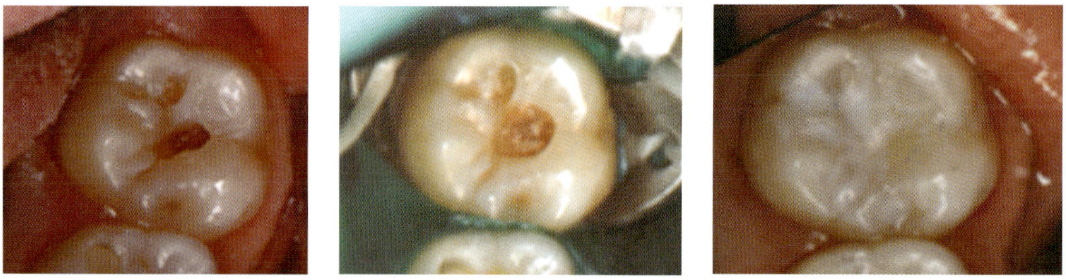

Figure 4.2 The last standing molar tooth in the above pictures had two separate localised areas of staining and decalcification. The more mesial of the two lesions also had some localised breakdown of the enamel. The two cavities were prepared with no 'extension for prevention' and restored with composite resin, and a fissure sealant was applied to all adjacent sound fissures.

MID for Interproximal Lesions

Tunnel Restorations

A tunnel restoration is an alternative to an interproximal box preparation but is more conservative of tooth structure. This type of restoration is more complex to perform well but is more conservative and maintains the tooth integrity and strength. The use of magnification and handpieces containing LED lights has facilitated the readying of tunnel preparations. There are some disadvantages associated with the tunnel restoration in that the marginal ridge may fracture if less than 2.5 mm of tooth structure remains from the occlusal cavity access to the marginal ridge. In addition, damage to the interproximal surface of the adjacent tooth can result in caries. A tunnel preparation can be situated within a millimetre of the pulp, whereas a conventional box preparation can leave a greater thickness of dentine for protection (see Figure 4.3).

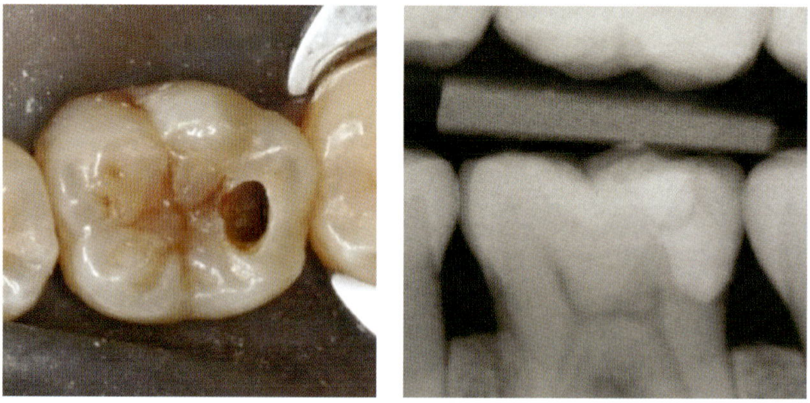

Figure 4.3 A tunnel preparation on the distal surface of the lower left first molar tooth. Note the distance from the occlusal access cavity to the marginal ridge. The bitewing radiograph shows the extent of the glass ionomer cement and surface layer of composite resin.

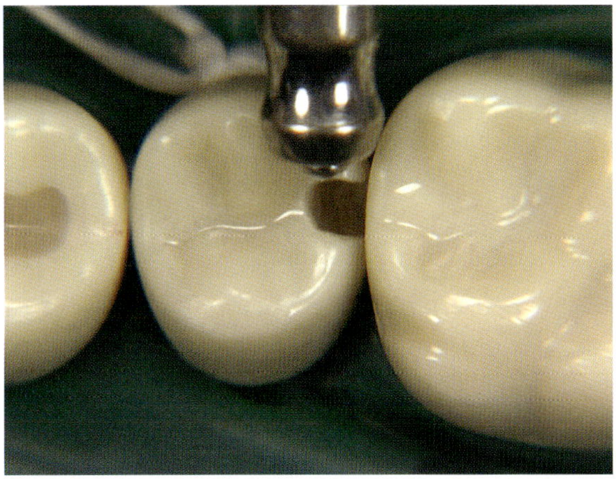

Figure 4.4 A proximal slot has been prepared in the distal of upper left second premolar tooth. This can be restored using composite resin.

Box Preparation

Almqvist described the first slot preparation for amalgam in 1973. In 1978, Simonsen described a modified cavity without mechanical retention for restoration with composite resin. The slot technique is superior to tunnel restorations (see Figure 4.4). This is likely due to improved operator visibility but also possibly due to removal of all demineralised enamel.

Icon

When an interproximal lesion is diagnosed on a bitewing radiograph, it is important to be able to determine if the lesion has cavitated. This can be done by separating the teeth with an orthodontic separator and recording an impression with a light bodied silicone impression material (see Figure 4.5). A non-cavitated lesion can be sealed in much the same way as a therapeutic fissure sealant can be used to seal an incipient lesion in a fissure. Icon from DMG America is a system that can deliver an etchant to penetrate the pseudo-intact surface zone of the WSL and then deliver a resin that can be taken up into the porosity of the lesion. This effectively obliterates the porosity within it and prevents the ingress of cariogenic acids and the loss of further calcium and phosphate ions. In addition, because the WSL can have up to 30% porosity, the enamel structure can be supported by the resin.

Other Examples of a More Minimal Approach to Treatment

Micro-Abrasion

Enamel micro-abrasion can eliminate enamel irregularities and areas of discoloration. This can improve the appearance of teeth with minimal destruction of tooth structure. It has been shown that teeth that have been treated with micro-abrasion can appear yellowish because the enamel has been made thinner, allowing the colour of the underlying dentine to influence the final appearance. This technique was developed in the mid-1980s as a method of improving the appearance of teeth – particularly those affected by fluorosis, where the discolouration is located in the outer layer of enamel. Fluorosis is a hypomineralisation of enamel resulting

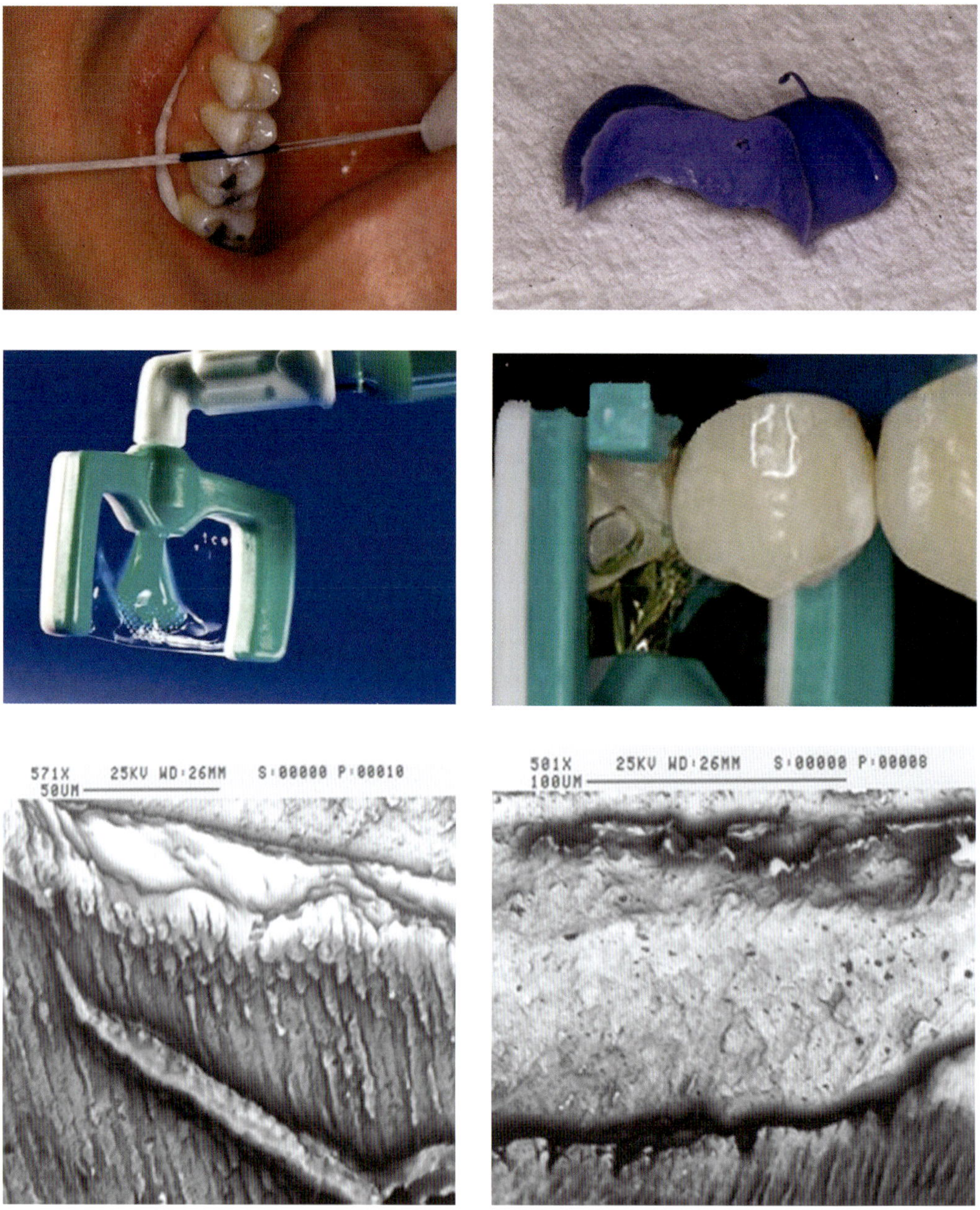

Figure 4.5 The interproximal space is opened using an orthodontic separator to allow an impression using a silicone material. The Icon can then be employed to deliver a flowable resin that will be taken up by capillary action. The SEM pictures show the resin has infiltrated into the white spot lesion.

from excessive intake of fluoride during tooth development. Patients can benefit from enamel micro-abrasion to yield impressive cosmetic results. Micro-abrasion uses 18% hydrochloric acid and pumice made into a slurry and applied using a slowly rotating rubber cup. Sometimes this technique may be combined with bleaching or the addition of composite resin to achieve an aesthetic result. These techniques may be used in isolation or combination and are minimally invasive compared to older techniques, such as crown preparation.

Veneers

Teeth that are discoloured, chipped, mal-aligned, or of an unpleasing shape can be corrected by using veneers. An alternative to providing veneers for discoloured teeth could include the use of bleaching or tooth whitening techniques. Veneers can be made from a thin layer of composite resin or porcelain and are under a millimetre thick. These restorations are more conservative of tooth structure than crowns because the latter require radical tooth reduction. The most natural looking and durable veneers are made from porcelain, but the use of composite resin is more economical and can be readily repaired. No-prep veneers are available or, alternatively, a small amount of tooth enamel can be removed to prepare the surface of the tooth and allow enough space for the dental veneer to be bonded.

Adhesive Bridges

A dental bridge consists of an artificial tooth or pontic that is bonded to one or both of the adjacent natural teeth. This is an example of an adhesive bridge that is not removable by the patient. The bridge can be made from porcelain bonded to nickel chromium alloy or, alternatively, can be made from metal free zirconia. The bridge has either a single wing or retainer projecting from one side of the pontic (a cantilever design; see Figure 4.6) or two retainers (a fixed design; see Figure 4.7) that attaches to the adjacent teeth. It is held in place using an acid etch technique and a specialised bonding resin. The tooth supporting the bridge is known as the abutment tooth, and this must be unrestored or minimally filled.

The adjacent teeth do not require to be reduced to receive full coverage retainers as would be required in a traditional style dental bridge. The adhesive bridge is a good example of MID because little or no enamel reduction is required.

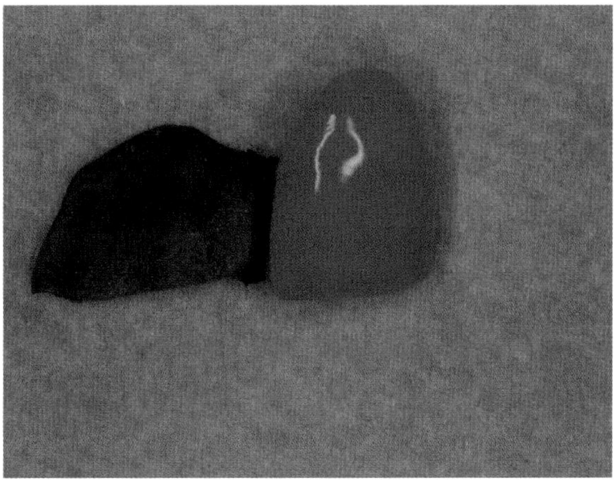

Figure 4.6 This is an example of a cantilever adhesive bridge. The fit surface of the metal retainer has been sandblasted to roughen it and create micromechanical retention for the adhesive cement lute.

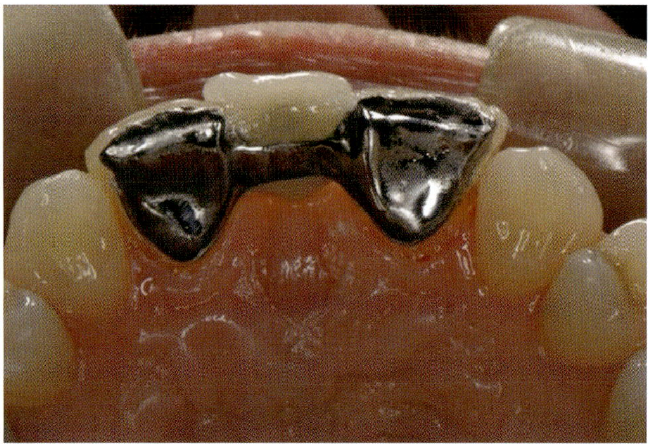

Figure 4.7 This is a fixed design of adhesive bridge that utilises two unrestored adjacent abutment teeth. The disadvantage of metal retainer wings is that they can impart a grey colour to the abutment teeth.

Adhesive Onlays

An adhesive onlay can be made from gold alloy or tooth coloured ceramic or composite resin. An onlay by definition is a restoration that covers the cusps of premolar or molar teeth. It is usually made indirectly by the technician but can also be made using computer aided design/computer aided manufacturing (CAD/CAM) so that the restoration can be fitted at the same appointment rather than the patient having to return for a second visit.

An adhesive onlay is a minimal restoration compared to the alternative of building the tooth up in restorative material and preparing it for a crown (see Figures 4.8 and 4.9).

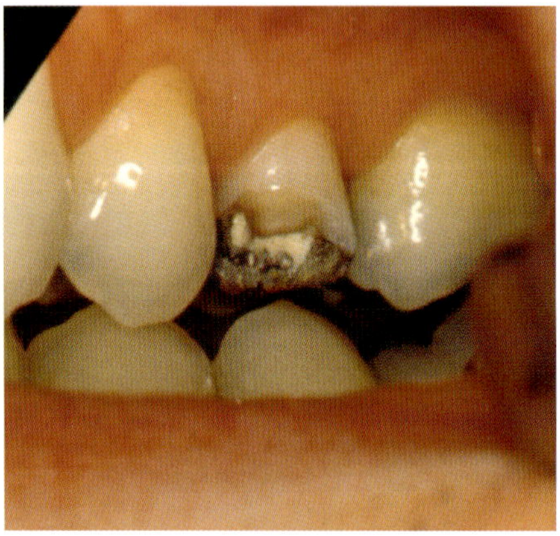

Figure 4.8 The buccal cusp of this maxillary left premolar tooth fractured as it had been left thin following the placement of a widen amalgam filling. It would have been prudent to have considered an onlay at this time.

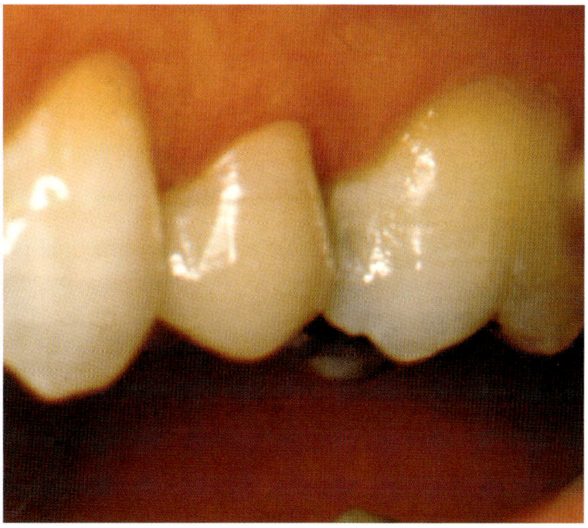

Figure 4.9 The amalgam restoration was removed and a chamfer finishing line prepared buccally at the level of the edge of the fracture. The palatal cusp was reduced and a similar finishing line prepared. This indirect ceramic restoration was made.

Further Reading

ICDAS

Gugnani, N., Pandit, I.K., Srivastava, N. et al. (2011). International Caries Detection and Assessment System (ICDAS): A New concept. *International Journal of Clinical Pediatric Dentistry* 4 (2): 93–100.

Research Behind Icon

Gray, G.B. and Shellis, P. (2002). Infiltration of resin into white spot caries-like lesions of enamel: an *in vitro* study. *European Journal of Prosthodontics and Restorative Dentistry* 10: 27–32.

Review Paper on Minimally Invasive Dentistry

Walsh, L.J. and Brostek, A.M. (2013). Minimum intervention dentistry principles and objectives. *Australian Dental Journal* 58: 3–16.

Pickard's Guide to Minimally Invasive Operative Dentistry

Avijit Banerjee, Timothy F. Watson, H. M. Pickard, Oxford, UK: Oxford University Press, 2015

Minimally Invasive Dentistry: The Management of Caries

Nairn H. F. Wilson, Batavia, IL: Quintessence, 2007

Section II

Intra-Coronal Restorations

5

Pit and Fissure Caries

During the past three decades, the prevalence of dental caries in schoolchildren has fallen in Western Europe and in the USA. Despite this overall reduction in caries prevalence, there has been a reported increase in the proportion of pit and fissure lesions (see Figure 5.1). This is thought to reflect the protection afforded to smooth tooth surfaces by fluoride. Even in areas with a low concentration of fluoride in the water supply, the level of caries has fallen due to the increased use of fluoridated toothpastes. Occlusal caries have been shown to account for 83% of the total caries experience of children between the ages of 5 and 17 years, with the first permanent molar being the most frequent site of fissure caries. An appreciable number of pit and fissure caries have been found in the late teens and early twenties. This shows that fissure caries continue to develop throughout the teens and early twenties and are no longer restricted to the first few years following eruption. New lesions can develop at any age.

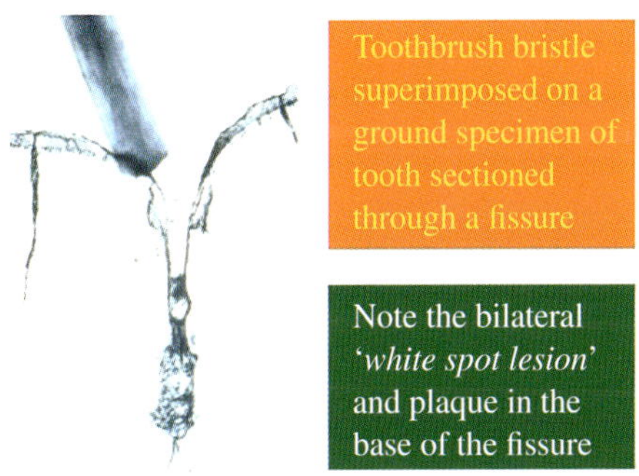

Figure 5.1 A section through a fissure with a toothbrush bristle superimposed.

Fissure morphology is a variable entity. Some fissures are little more than shallow grooves, whereas others can be deep invaginations that can almost reach the enamel dentine junction. There is no established method of determining the depth of fissures *in vivo* without preparing a cavity. Caries commence bilaterally on the side walls of the fissure, which cannot be inspected directly. Like all caries lesions, one commences as a white chalky decalcified area with sub-surface porosity. Fissure caries are no different from those occurring on smooth surfaces in that the dental plaque utilises carbohydrates from the diet to produce a range of organic acids that demineralise the enamel. This is not a gradually progressive process but one in which there are periods of demineralisation followed by phases of remineralisation when the circumstances are

A Practical Approach to Operative Dentistry, First Edition. Gordon B. Gray and Alaa H. Daud.

Companion website: www.wiley.com/go/gray/operative-dentistry

favourable. It is possible to arrest lesions by changes in the local environment where plaque control is improved and the number of cariogenic challenges is reduced. This is particularly the case when fluoride becomes incorporated into the remineralised lesions. The process of arresting lesions is often termed cariogenic priming. Fissure caries are more prevalent due to the sheltered environment in the fissure system, where the flow of saliva is reduced. This means the buffering capacity is lowered and the rate of carbohydrate clearance is reduced. If the lesion progresses and reaches the scalloped enamel dentine junction, it may then spread laterally as well as progressing towards the pulp at a faster rate than that through the enamel. It is in this way that a dark shadow can been seen surrounding a fissure.

Once a carious lesion has established in the dentine, it contains bacteria and there is a pulpal response where secondary dentine is laid down at the pulpal end of the dentinal tubules to help protect the pulp. It has been shown that the body of the dentine lesion is softened and infected while at the advancing front the lesion the dentine is slightly demineralised but still contains histologically recognisable features with no bacterial invasion. This area can be remineralised following placement of a restoration and provision of a good peripheral seal.

The occlusal surfaces of permanent teeth account for only 12.5% of the total tooth surface area, although it has been reported that 60% of all new restorations are placed in this surface. The diagnostic aids that may be employed for fissure caries diagnosis can be divided into two groups: invasive and non-invasive methods:

Non-invasive	**Invasive**
Probe	Diagnostic cavity or
Visual inspection	'Enamel biopsy'
Magnification	
Radiographs	
Transillumination	
Electronic methods	

One of the greatest challenges facing clinicians today is the correct diagnosis of fissure caries. Dental health educators and most of the general public believe that a regular dental examination plays an important role in preventing dental disease. Accurate diagnosis is essential in providing patients with the best possible care, but some studies using extracted teeth have shown that operators have great difficulty with the accurate diagnosis of carious fissures and, in addition, have problems in correctly identifying fissures that are sound. The detection of small occlusal lesions is difficult. It is appropriate to consider the relative merits of all methods of diagnosis to allow the clinician to select the method of diagnosis with the greatest accuracy (sensitivity) and the fewest disadvantages (specificity).

Dental Probe

Traditional teaching advocated the use of the dental probe to search out 'sticky fissures' where the probe would resist withdrawal. It is recognised, nowadays, that the probe may resist withdrawal when the tip is inserted into sound fissures that are sufficiently wide and deep to grip the tip of the instrument. This practice results in a false diagnosis with the placement of an

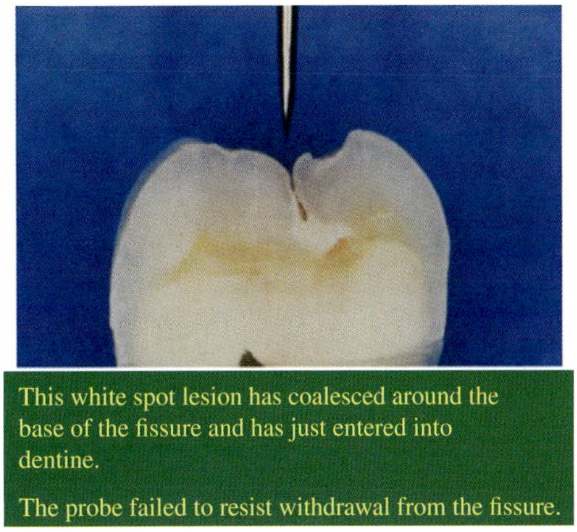

Figure 5.2 A dental probe superimposed on a section of tooth that shows decalcification along the walls and base of the fissure. The carious lesion has just reached the enamel dentine junction.

unnecessary filling. The relationship between 'stickiness' on probing and the shape and size of the probe tip and the fissure being examined was realised more than 65 years ago. It was observed that narrow fissures would fail to grip the probe tip and that, in some instances, the probe would only stick once caries were well established in dentine. As all restorations have a finite life, repeated replacements will produce a cavity form that is wider than the original. The surrounding cusps will also be weakened and may be at risk of fracture. In a survey of a group of general dental practitioners, up to 50% were still using the probe as their main method of fissure caries diagnosis (see Figure 5.2).

The practice of probing fissures also carries with it some other disadvantages. Irreversible traumatic defects may be produced if early fissure caries lesions are probed. Probing of carious fissures renders them more susceptible to the progress of caries. In addition, cariogenic bacteria may be transferred into non-infected fissures by probing. The results of laboratory studies using extracted teeth have shown no difference in diagnosis between operators using a probe and those using a visual only technique. In the light of the disadvantages of using a probe, it can be concluded that the use of this method of diagnosis should be abandoned.

Visual Method

Good lighting and clean teeth are essential for accurate fissure caries diagnosis using a visual inspection technique. The signs that the operator should look for include (see Figure 5.3):

- Staining
- Decalcification
- Cavitation

As the initial white spot lesion (WSL) cannot be inspected directly, many operators rely on staining in the fissures as a diagnostic sign. This is inaccurate because brown or black staining may arise from extrinsic sources in the diet. The clinician must look for signs of decalcification, and this can only be achieved when the surface of the tooth is clean and dry.

When the tooth surface is dried for 5 seconds using compressed air from the triple dental syringe, water is removed from the WSL, making it contrast with the surrounding tooth, which has more translucent enamel. It does this by changing the refractive index. Spread of the initial WSL brings

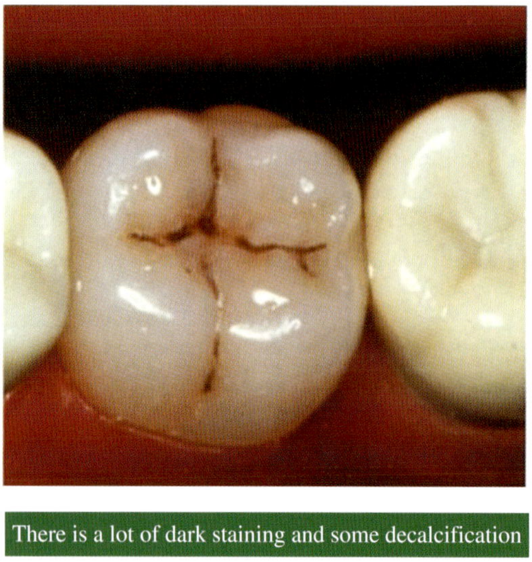

Figure 5.3 The fissures in this mandibular molar tooth are stained and show some areas of decalcification.

the margins to a position at the fissure orifice, where it can be seen. Drying the teeth is critical to good diagnosis, with more lesions being diagnosed compared to teeth that had been left wet.

Visual Method with Magnification

When the clean and dry tooth is inspected under a ×2.5 – ×4 magnification, the validity of the diagnostic decision is improved. Figure 5.4 shows the same tooth viewed at different magnifications. The decalcified areas are easier to see at the higher magnification, but it should be noted that the staining in the fissure pattern is of no relevance unless accompanied by decalcification.

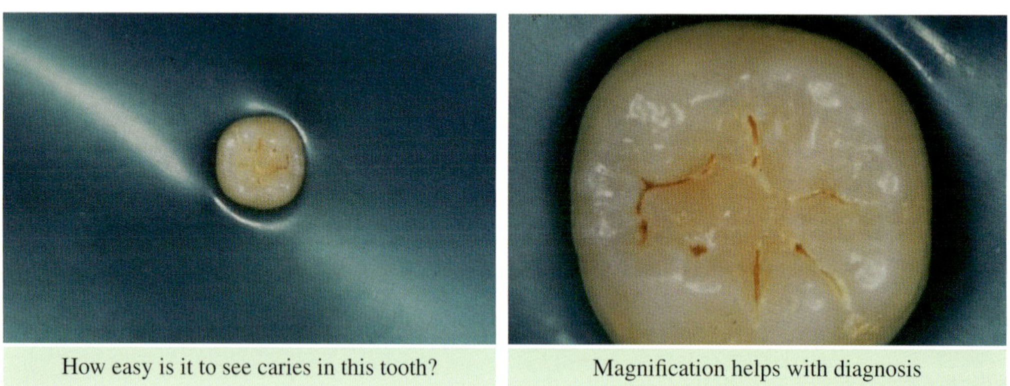

Figure 5.4 The use of magnification in visual diagnosis is of considerable help.

Transillumination

The use of transillumination of the teeth is not a new technique for caries diagnosis but never gained widespread popularity. The recent improvements in fibre optics has led to renewed interest. Fibre optics allows the light source to be used in all areas of the mouth. Studies have reported on the use of this technique in comparison with radiographs in the detection of interproximal caries. This technique also has the advantage of being free from possible health hazards of ionising radiation associated with conventional radiography.

Figure 5.5 shows the use of fibre optic transillumination (FOTI) on a molar tooth. The teeth should be illuminated from both the buccal and the lingual surfaces. When FOTI is being used, the operating light should be switched off to maximise the contrast between the normal and carious tooth structures. The presence of a carious lesion in dentine is depicted as a dark shadow where the passage of the light is impeded.

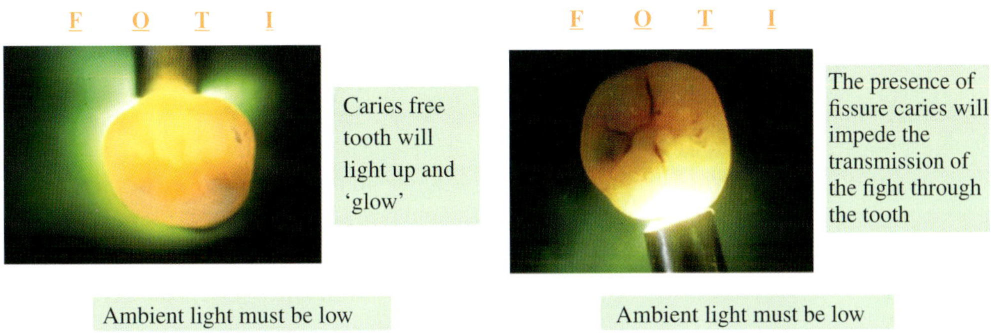

Figure 5.5 The use of FOTI can be a useful adjunct in diagnosis.

There are two problems associated with transillumination as a diagnostic aid. Very small carious lesions do not show up clearly, and the technique is of limited value if restorations are present in the tooth.

Bitewing Radiograph

Bitewing radiographs have been used for many years in the detection of interproximal carious lesions. The use of intraoral radiographs as a diagnostic tool to determine the presence of pit and fissure caries has been the subject of much debate. The tide of opinion about the use of this diagnostic aid is now turning. It has a key role to play in the detection of hidden progressive dentinal caries. Such lesions are called 'occult caries': spreading dentinal caries lying below an apparently intact occlusal surface (see Figure 5.6).

Figure 5.6 It is not always easy to see a radiolucency just below the enamel dentine junction.

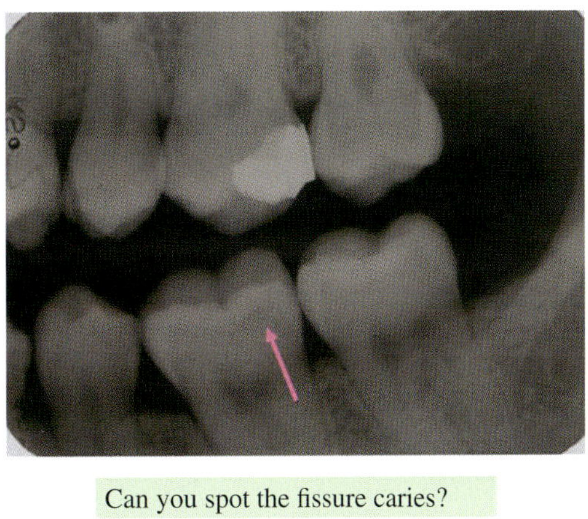

When a clinician fails to detect radiographic signs of occlusal caries, the only firm conclusion that can be reached is that a large dentine lesion is absent. This diagnostic technique cannot show early enamel caries related to pits and fissures. Conversely, when a dentine caries is visible on the film, the lesion should be investigated and restored. In a study, the radiographs of 2623 teenage patients were scrutinised. The authors found that 12.1% of lower molar teeth and 3.1% of maxillary molars that were judged to be clinically sound showed radiographic evidence of caries. FOTI has been said to be almost as reliable as bitewing radiographs once the caries has progressed into dentine.

When bitewing radiographs are being taken, it is important that clinicians remember that it is a technique sensitive examination. Setting the exposure factors and processing the films correctly are critical to the overall diagnostic value of the films. Small changes to the angulation of the tube head can make smaller dentine lesions disappear. The use of routine radiographs should vary according to the needs of individual patients. The age, caries status, and perceived caries risk of each patient should be assessed. Although x-ray dosage should be kept to a minimum, it is reasonable to expose a bitewing film in response to a specific clinical problem, such as the suspected presence of an occlusal caries lesion. In the radiograph shown in Figure 5.6, the dentine lesion was not seen on careful clinical examination of the cleaned and dried tooth surface but was evident on the radiograph.

Electronic Methods of Fissure Caries Diagnosis

Electronic methods of detecting demineralised fissures is not a new technique. It was first described in 1951, and the technique has been developed subsequently. The increased conductivity of the porous carious lesion reduces the impedance between a blunt probe applied to a suspect fissure and an additional electrode placed on the patient's lip.

Recent improvements to electronic methods of fissure caries diagnosis have been reported, and a clinical trial has shown a high degree of accuracy in the detection of carious and sound teeth. This diagnostic method can be used to monitor the progress of an individual lesion. The VistaProof from Dürr Dental uses a high energy violet light with a wavelength of 405 nm (see Figure 5.7). This fluoresces the porphyrin metabolites in caries that show up as red on the computer image. Sound tooth structure will appear green in such images.

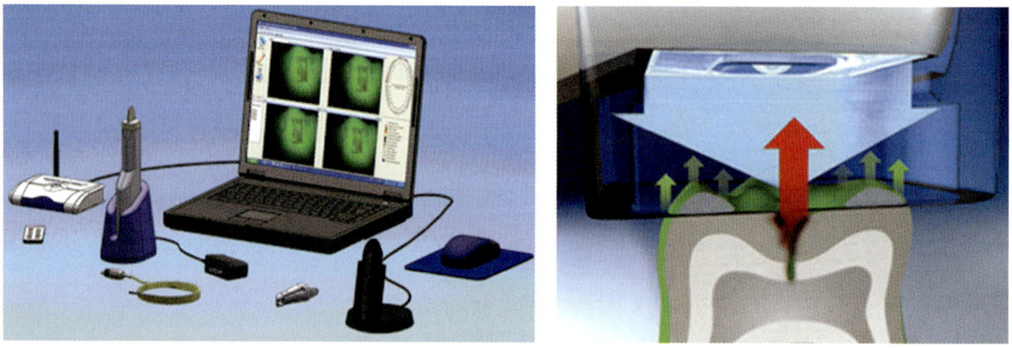

Figure 5.7 Dürr Dental have developed a method of fluorescing the tooth with a violet light and picking up the resulting image electronically. Because this can be shown on a laptop screen, it can be used to demonstrate to the patient. *Source:* Printed by Kind Permission of Durr Dental.

Enamel Biopsy

Even after a careful clinical inspection of an occlusal surface, there may be doubt about the presence of caries in a fissure. If this lesion is investigated with a small round bur (ISO 008) in an air turbine handpiece, the extent of the caries will be determined (see Figure 5.8).

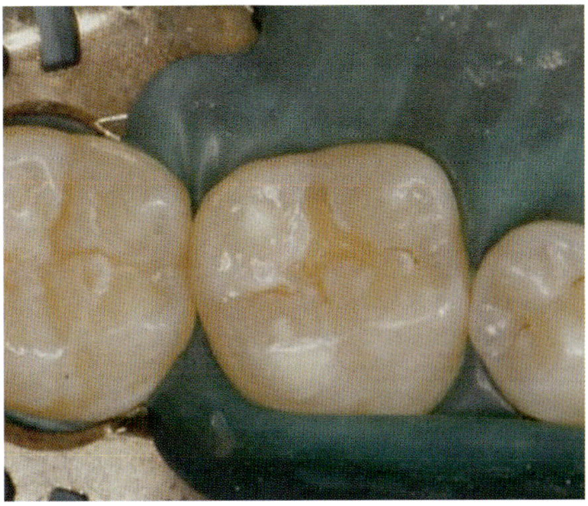

Figure 5.8 A small enamel biopsy has been performed on this mandibular molar, but the lesion has been found to burn out in the enamel.

This technique is known as the 'enamel biopsy'. A light stroking action is employed to open the fissure and to allow inspection of the floor and side walls of the small cavity. The outcome of the enamel biopsy is not predictable. Sometimes, it will be found that the lesion 'burns out' in the enamel, while in other instances the clinician will be surprised at the extent of the underlying dentine lesion that is present. While the enamel biopsy is the most accurate method of determining the presence and extent of fissure caries, it has the disadvantage of possibly committing a tooth to a restoration when no lesion is present. Restoration of such a tooth has been made easier by the use of the sealant restoration technique.

'Occult caries' has been described, where a large dentine lesion is present below what appeared to be a clinically intact occlusal surface. The occult lesion is thought to be the result of the use of topical fluoride that enriches the enamel surface so that breakdown will only occur when an underlying dentine lesion is very large. Many clinicians are no longer prepared to adopt a 'wait and watch' approach once they have observed a decalcified fissure.

However, they do face a dilemma in which they have to balance between carrying out treatment that may be unnecessary and missing a carious lesion that could be in dentine. The use of new diagnostic procedures using soft laser fluorescence may remove some of this diagnostic uncertainty (see Figure 5.9).

The management of suspect or problematic fissures was simplified by the introduction of the 'preventive resin restoration' that was first described in 1988. In this technique, only the local carious tooth structure was removed and the cavity restored using either composite or diluted composite in combination with fissure sealant. Subsequent modifications to this technique have been considerable as adhesive materials, and dentine bonding resins have become available. Today, a range of techniques have been described, and these are collectively known as 'sealant restorations'. Sealant restorations now provide the dentist with a wider range of management options for fissure

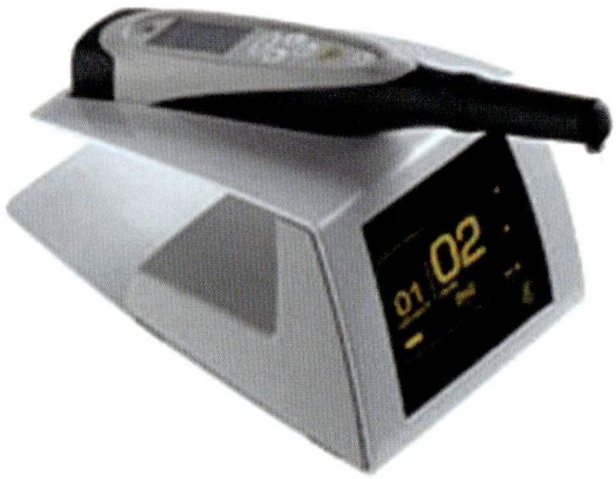

Figure 5.9 The DIAGNOdent from KaVo uses natural fluorescence of the tooth to a red light and compares it to sound area of the same tooth. *Source:* Printed by kind permission from KaVo.

caries. These techniques are more conservative of tooth structure and give more pleasing and cosmetic restorations, where previously only amalgam was available for this purpose. Successful management of fissure lesions can only be achieved when two specific areas are addressed: caries risk assessment and early diagnosis before extensive dentine involvement.

Caries Risk Assessment

It is not possible to make a diagnosis by examining one tooth only. It is vitally important that a wider examination of the patient is undertaken to make an assessment of the overall caries risk for that individual. The factors that should be considered include:

Time since tooth eruption: It is generally thought that the first few years following tooth eruption is the peak time for new caries to develop. In this age group more rapid progression of the lesion has also been noted. It should be remembered, however, that in a survey of new recruits to the armed forces, many were found to be presenting as late as their early twenties with new fissure caries. This may imply that fluoride is having a delaying effect on the onset of fissure lesions.

General condition of the mouth: When examining a patient the dentist should not only look at the level of plaque control that the patient is able to maintain but should also ask about dietary habits. A record should be made of all new carious lesions in teeth that previously have not been restored, and all existing restorations should be charted. This provides the most reliable guide to the caries risk for an individual patient. An 18-year-old patient may be assigned to a high caries risk group if he or she has a decalcified fissure and has other restorations and cavities as well as unfavourable dietary findings. On the other hand, a middle aged or elderly patient with a similar decalcified fissure in a well maintained mouth with few fillings would be placed in a low risk category.

The age of the patient: Unlike patients in their teens, those in the twenties and above are not so prone to caries but are most at risk to periodontal disease. The high risk group of patients, therefore, is those under 20 years old.

Attendance record of the patient: The decision to intervene operatively with a decalcified fissure may be postponed if the patient is a regular attender and there are no other carious lesions present.

Medical conditions: In a medically compromised patient where the sequelae of dental disease are likely to place the patient's general health at risk, early intervention is required. This may take the form of fissure sealing a decalcified fissure lesion at an early stage.

Categorising Fissure Lesions and Selecting a Management Option

The best method of diagnosing fissure caries is by visual inspection of the cleaned and dried tooth surface using magnification and radiographs where indicated. In some instances when the risk assessment is also taken into account, it may be decided that an 'enamel biopsy' should be performed using a small round bur (ISO 008) to be able to categorise finally the extent of the lesion. The status of the fissure can be categorised.

The progress of caries through the enamel is slow with its periods of demineralisation and remineralisation. It can take up to a few years for the lesion to reach dentine, but thereafter, progress is much faster.

Next, a management option must be selected for the restoration of the tooth. This may range from the provision of minimally invasive and conservative sealant restorations to an amalgam or posterior composite restoration.

Available Management Options for Fissure Lesions:

- No active treatment required
- Observation and prevention
- Preventive fissure sealant
- Therapeutic fissure sealant
- Enamel biopsy
- Sealant restoration
- Conventional composite restoration

The only time that observation should be used as a management option for a fissure is when that fissure is diagnosed as sound. In a medically compromised patient, even a sound fissure should receive a fissure sealant. A ***preventive*** fissure sealant would be the most appropriate treatment because future caries could jeopardise the health of the patient. Similarly, active intervention may require the administration of a regional block analgesia that may result in bleeding and trismus in a patient with a bleeding disorder. Not all fissure lesions are suitable for restoration using the sealant restoration technique. Where there has been extensive spread of caries at the EDJ below a seemingly intact enamel surface, it is unlikely that the cavity will be suitable for restoration using a minimally invasive procedure. Such a tooth will require restoration using either amalgam, an indirectly placed inlay of gold or tooth coloured material, or a directly placed posterior composite restoration. The other categories of fissure caries are suitable for restoration using a range of more conservative and cosmetic restorations that involve the application of fissure sealant as an added preventive element.

Sealant Restorations

Four types of sealant restoration have been described, and each has its own specific indications according to the individual clinical situation.

Type 1 (***therapeutic*** fissure sealant): These are indicated where the patient is in a low risk group with two or fewer other carious lesions in a well maintained mouth. Bitewing radiographs should be taken where clinically necessary to exclude the presence of occult caries. There is evidence to suggest that a carefully applied sealant may arrest caries because it cuts off the nutrient supply to the organisms in the fissures. Fissure sealants are available as opaque or translucent materials that can be filled or unfilled. The use of opaque sealant may mask leakage and prevent detection of underlying caries, but they are easier to detect at clinical review than translucent materials.

Type ll: Where a decalcified fissure has been noted but the patient is in a high caries risk group, a fissure biopsy would be advocated. Many investigations reveal caries that are much greater than anticipated from the clinical picture. Where the lesion is found to burn out in enamel, the operator may stop at this stage and restore the cavity with an acid etch composite restoration covered with fissure sealant extended into the adjacent fissures.

Type lll: If the cavity resulting from the enamel biopsy investigation extends just into dentine but with no lateral spread, the cavity and the adjacent fissures could be etched and restored using composite resin or compomer and fissure sealant. Alternatively, a glass ionomer cement could be inserted to restore the cavity before the occlusal surface is fissure sealed. It is important to remember that a radio-opaque cement should be used to avoid confusion at later radiographic investigations. Studies have shown minimal microleakage with these restorations.

Type lV: Where investigation of a suspect fissure shows the cavity to have established well into dentine in a localised area of the occlusal surface, the margins of the cavity are likely to be in occlusion. In this situation the operator would be advised to restore the tooth using a hybrid composite resin designed for use in posterior teeth. The lost dentine may be replaced using a radio-opaque glass ionomer cement that will adhere the dentine, release fluoride, and have a similar thermal expansion coefficient to the lost tooth structure. The remaining cavity can then be restored using an acid-etch composite resin. Recent practice advocates the restoration of the cavity without the need for a lining or base. The dentine and enamel are etched and a layer of bonding resin applied before the cavity is restored with an obliquely layered restoration of hybrid composite resin. The disadvantage of this technique is that at any future removal of the restoration, there is no visual layer of cement to warn the clinician he or she is approaching dentine. Adjacent fissures are protected from further caries exposure by fissure sealing.

Evidence Based Dentistry

The astute dentist should question the value of various procedures both in terms of life expectancy of the restorations and their ease of clinical use. It is not unreasonable to expect newer types of restorations to last at least as long as the more tried and tested alternatives.

Although sealant restorations may lose some fissure sealant from areas of the fissure pattern, it is a simple procedure to add further fissure sealant to allow them to continue to function satisfactorily. The presence of small composite restoration does not appear to adversely affect the retention of the fissure sealant.

Summary

Management of fissure caries can only be undertaken once the results of all appropriate diagnostic test have been confirmed. The probe is not a reliable method, and it may damage the tooth.

Accurate diagnosis of fissure caries challenges clinicians.

The best methods of diagnosis are:

- Visual inspection with magnification of clean and dried teeth
- Transillumination
- Enamel biopsy in patients with high risk factors
- Bitewing radiographs, a useful screen to detect hidden occult dentine caries
- Use of electronic means can be a helpful adjunct

Caries in pits and fissures can be restored using a variety of techniques ranging from sealant restorations using adhesive tooth coloured filling materials to more conventional direct and indirect restorations where the cavity is large and has left few if any remaining areas of fissure.

International Caries Classification and Management System

A system was developed in 2002 by academics from a number of international centres to assess the evidence around caries detection and assessment and to create the International Caries Detection and Assessment System (ICDAS). The group merged some existing caries classification systems, some of which involved both visual assessment and histological validation, to produce an integrated caries classification system known as the International Caries Classification and Management System (ICCMS). There are seven codes to this classification, as follows:

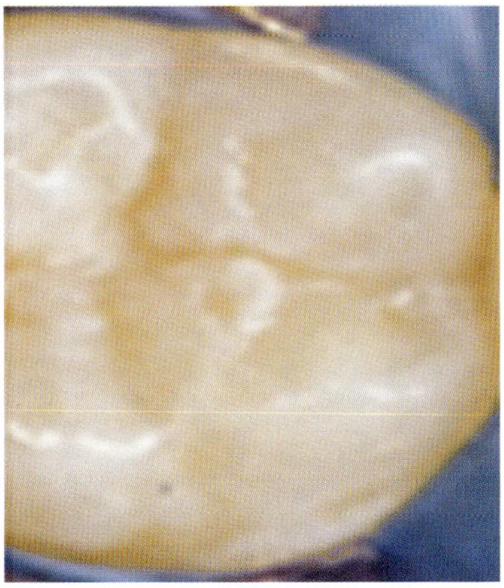

Code 0 refers to sound tooth surfaces that show no evidence of visible caries when viewed following prophylaxis and air-drying for 5 seconds.

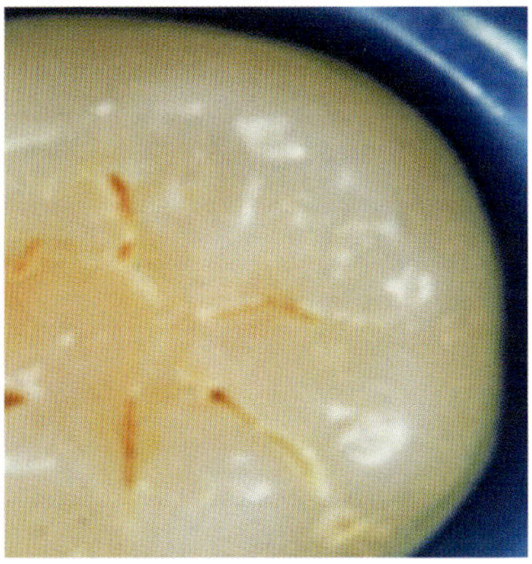

Code 1 refers to the first visual change in enamel. This can be an opacity or discolouration that is visible at a stagnation area, such, as an interproximal space, cervical margin, or, fissure entrance. The discolouration can be white or brown and should be visible after prolonged air-drying

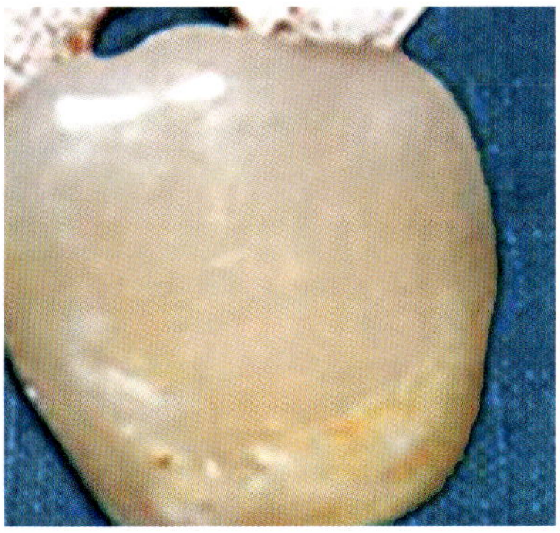

Code 2 refers to a distinct visual change in the enamel that can be seen even when the tooth is wet.

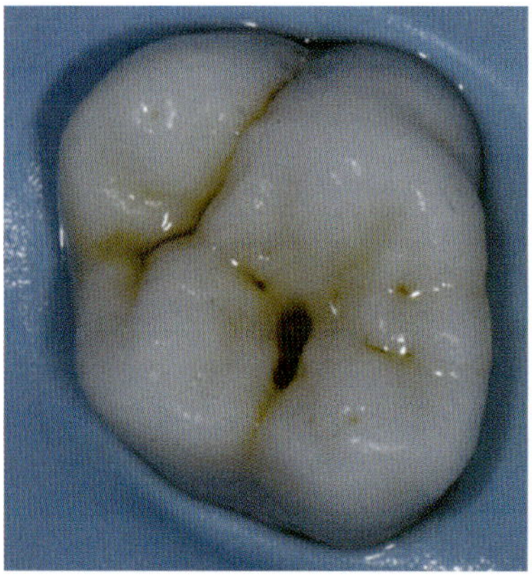

Code 3 refers to localised enamel breakdown that can be seen even when the tooth is wet. There should be no visual signs of underlying dentine involvement. The ball end of a WHO probe will confirm the defect in the surface.

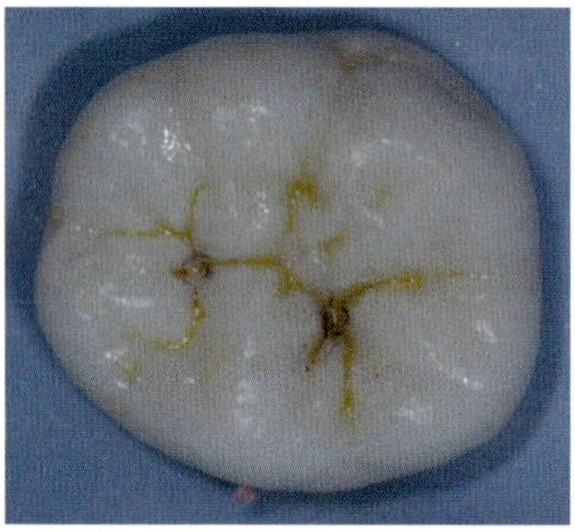

Code 4 refers to surface appearance where there is a dark shadow in the dentine underlying the surface enamel. The ball end of a WHO probe will confirm the defect in the surface.

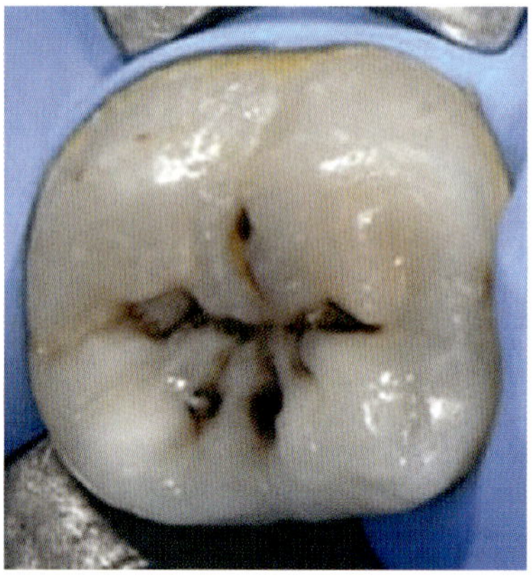

Code 5 refers to a distinct open cavity in the dentine. A WHO probe should be able to confirm dentine involvement.

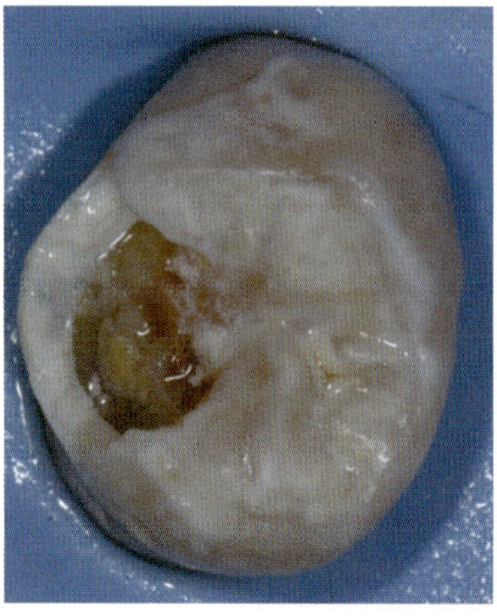

Code 6 refers to an extensive distinct open cavity with dentine visible. It should involve more than half of the tooth surface. A WHO probeshould be able to confirm dentine involvement.

Clinical Guide to Restoring a Tooth Using a Sealant Restoration Technique

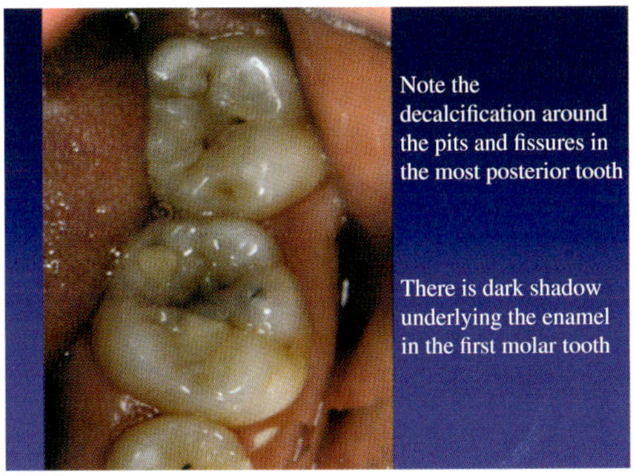

This clinical case shows two mandibular molars with fissure caries.
Note the staining and decalcification visible in the last molar tooth, whereas in the other molar, a dark shadow below the surface enamel can be seen.

Fissure caries are difficult to diagnose accurately.

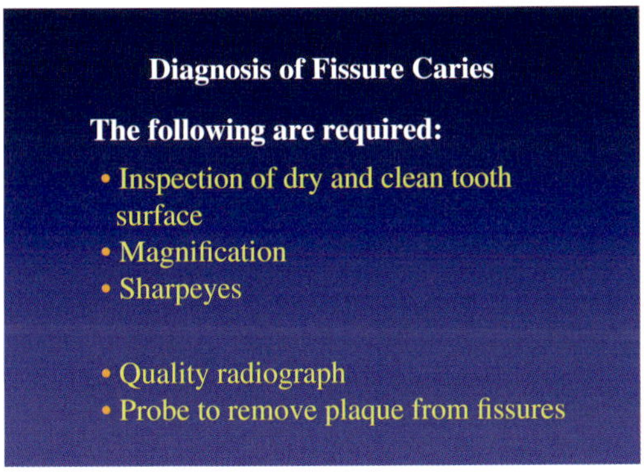

Before a diagnosis can be made, the tooth should be cleaned thoroughly to allow visual inspection.
Use of probes is not encouraged unless it is to remove plaque from the fissure orifice.
Magnification will improve diagnostic ability of operator.
A radiograph is useful only to exclude occult caries, i.e. large dentine lesions underlying seemingly intact enamel.

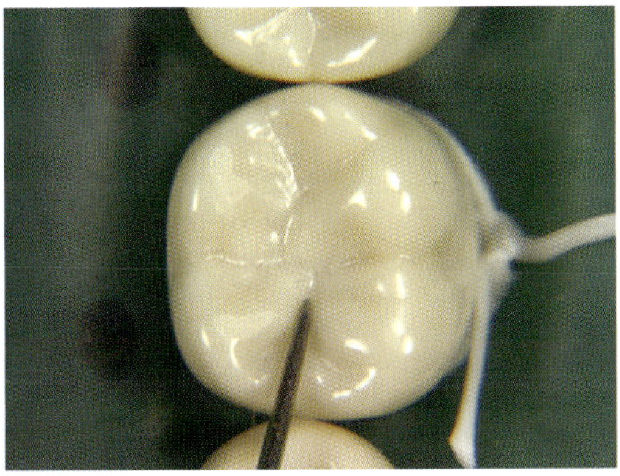

In this casein tooth it should be imagined that there is decalcification in the distal fissure and another area of staining and decalcification in the mesial fissure.
The latter area has not only decalcification but also a surrounding area of discolouration underlying the enamel.
A radiograph of this tooth ***may*** show a small radiolucency just under the enamel in this area.

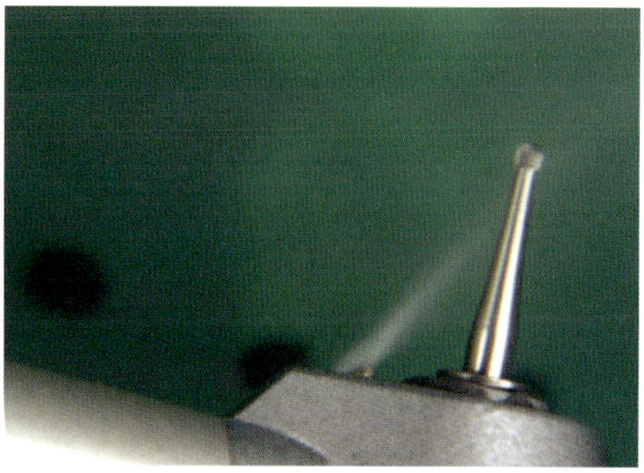

An enamel biopsy is performed using a small round bur.
The bur in the accompanying slide is a round F/G diamond bur that is 0.8 mm in diameter.
It is used in the air turbine handpiece operating at a free-running speed of 450,000–500,000 rpm.
Water spray is needed to cool bur and tooth and keep the investigation site clear of debris.

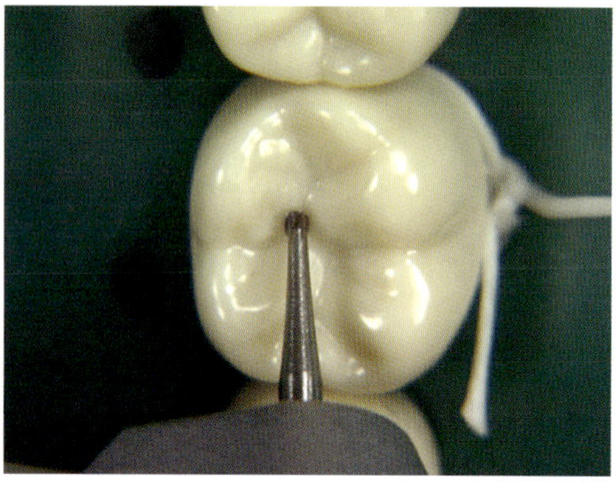

Using a L/G round steel bur in the slow contra-angled handpiece, the caries can be removed from around the enamel dentinal junction (EDJ) of the more mesial cavity.

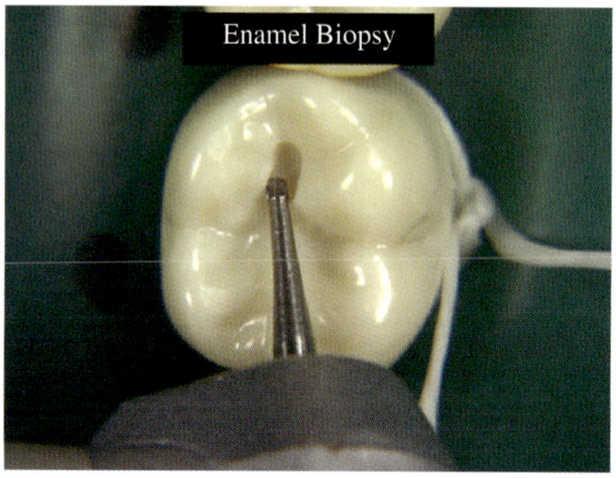

In this example imagine that there is a decalcified lesion in the fissure and it has 'burnt out' within the enamel.
This can usually be detected when the lesion gets smaller as the investigative cavity progresses towards the enamel dentine junction.
With a sealant restoration there is no need to cut further into the dentine as would be required for an amalgam cavity.
This small cavity in enamel is all that would be required to manage this carious lesion using an adhesive filling material.

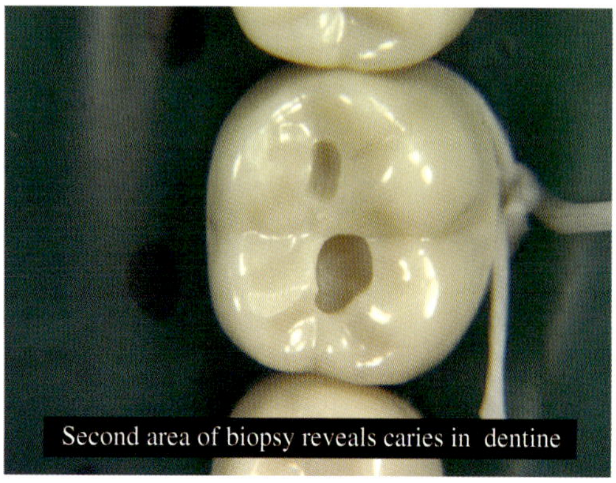

Investigation of the other suspect area of fissure reveals that the decalcification in the fissure has progressed through into the dentine.
Once established in the dentine, the lesion spreads along the dentine at the EDJ. This has undermined the enamel surface.

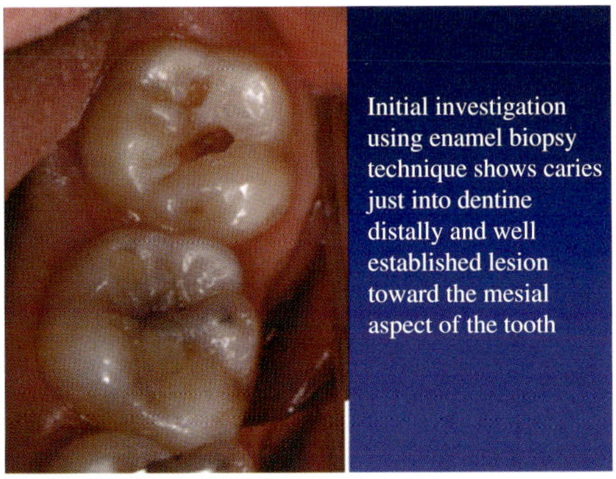

In this clinical case, the same situation is present as in the casein tooth.
Note the stained dentine in the mesial of the two cavities in the last molar tooth.

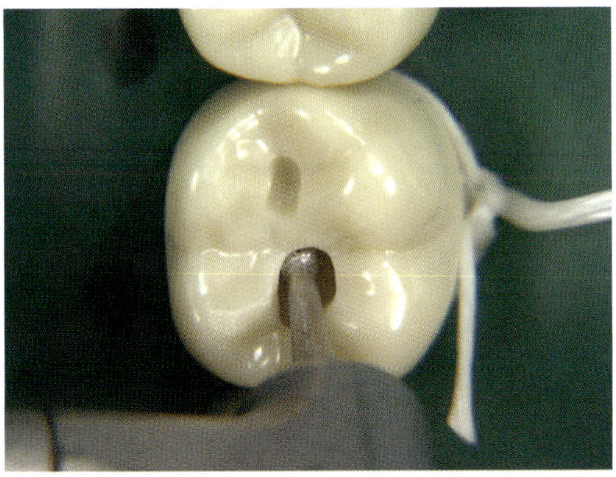

Using a L/G round steel bur in the slow contra-angled handpiece, the caries can be removed from around the EDJ of the more mesial cavity.

This bur is worked in a systematic manner around the EDJ to remove all staining and decalcification.

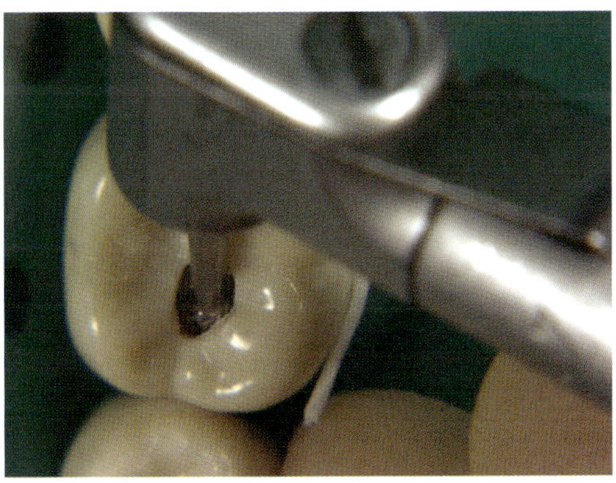

Frequent breaks in cutting may be required to inspect the EDJ for the presence of staining.
Use of compressed air from the triple dental syringe will aid in this inspection.
It may also be necessary to wash the cavity periodically.

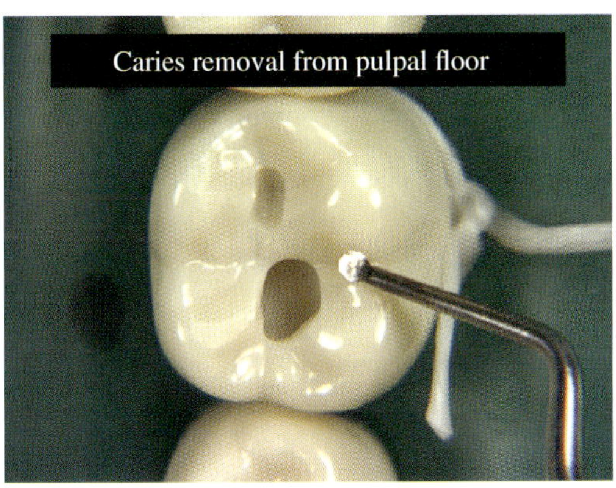

Following the principles of cavity preparation, the caries is then removed from over the more central area of pulp.
Hand instruments such as this discoid excavator are useful for this purpose.
Remember that slow-speed burs will remove even sound dentine.

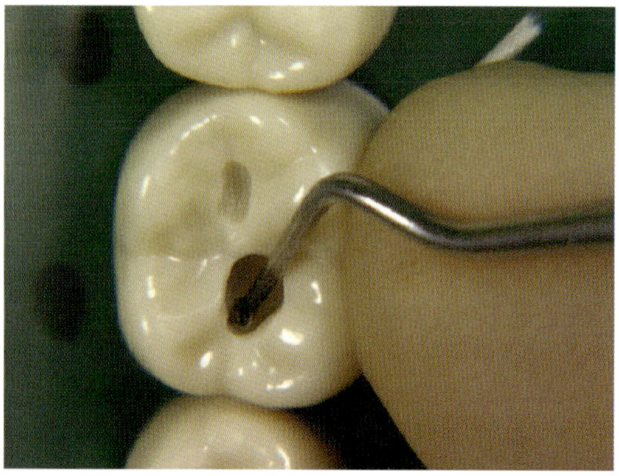

The sharp cutting edge is placed centrally on the carious lesion and worked with a scraping action towards the periphery of the cavity.

This is effective at cutting through the denatured dentine matrix.

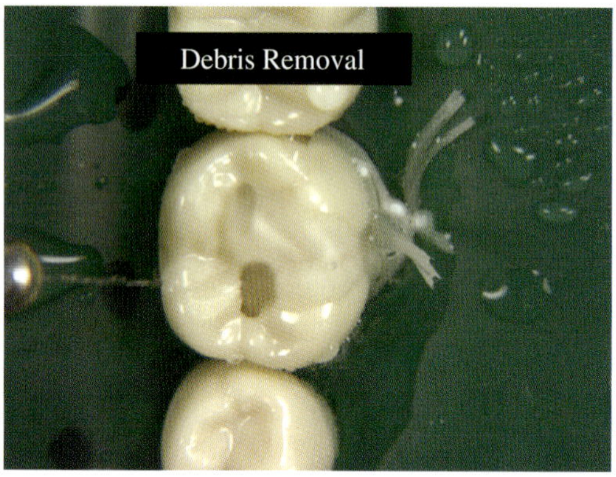

At the end of the cavity preparation stage, the cavity is washed to remove debris.

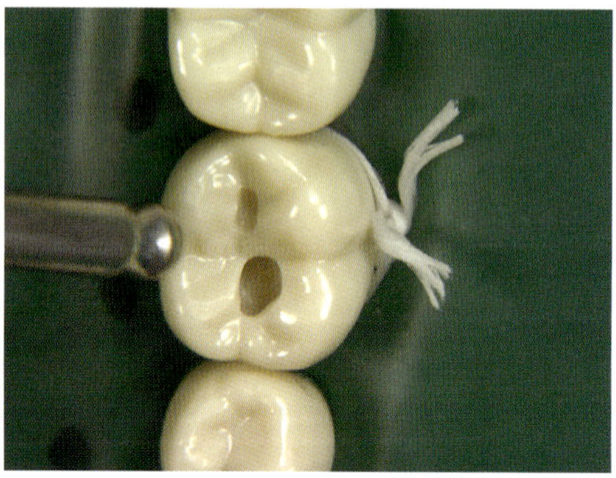

... and carefully dried without desiccating the dentine. Therefore, the drying stage should not exceed three seconds.
The cavity can then be inspected.

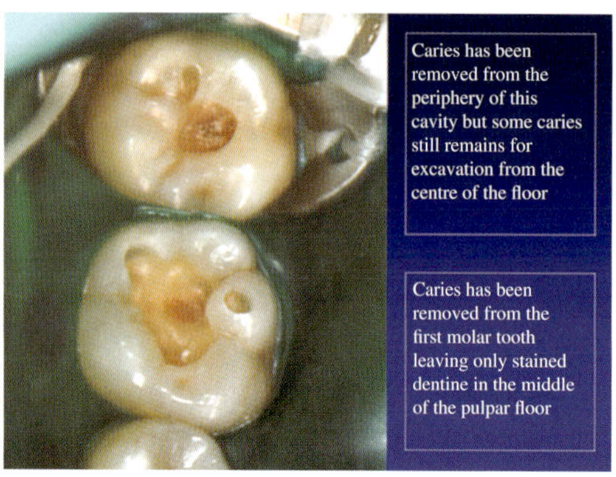

In the clinical case, the active caries has been removed from the cavity periphery and floor.
The periphery is now free from caries both to a visual inspection and to exploration with a probe.
The pulpal floor has some stained dentine but this is firm to probing.

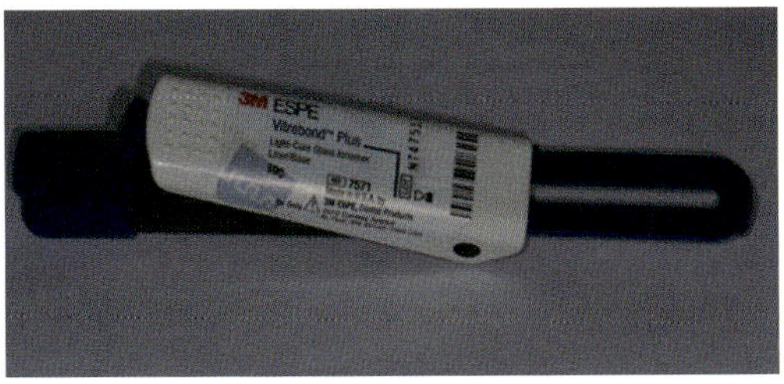

In this slide sequence a L/C glass ionomer lining will be placed in the deeper cavity.
It has the advantage of :
* adhering to the dentine floor
* releasing fluoride
* allowing a bond to the overlying composite resin

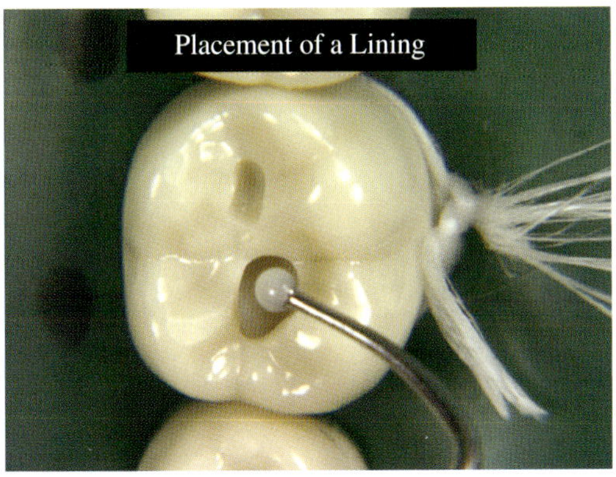

A creamy mix can be achieved by mixing equal amounts of the two pastes from the syringe.
From the paper pad the material can be transferred to the cavity on the ball end of a PF10 instrument.
Only the deeper more mesial cavity requires a lining.
In some contemporary practices no lining would be placed and the composite resin would be etched and bonded to the dentine.

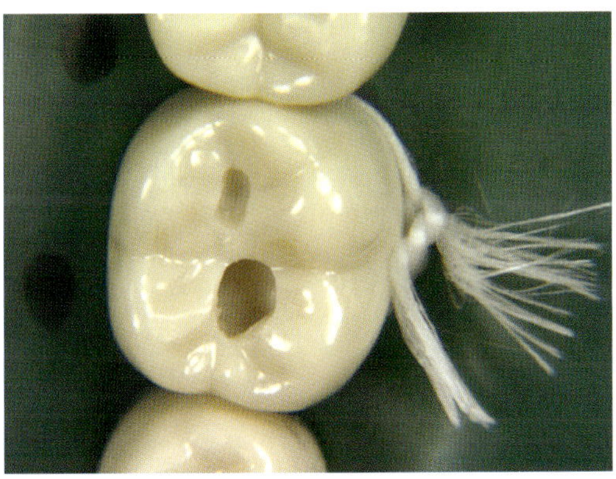

The instrument is used to spread the material over the dentine on the pulpal floor of the mesial cavity.
It is difficult to see in this slide as the colour is similar to that of the casein tooth structure.
Care should be exercised to ensure that the material is kept away from the enamel and the cavity margins.
If material is left on the cavity margins it could gradually dissolve and lead to microleakage around the restoration.

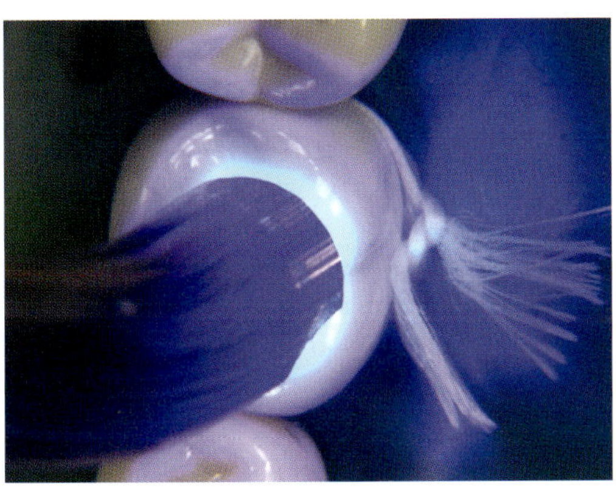

The material will set by a free-radical polymerisation reaction when exposed to visible blue light of 470 nm. A 20 second exposure from the occlusal surface should ensure an adequate cure. The manufacturer's instructions should always be followed.

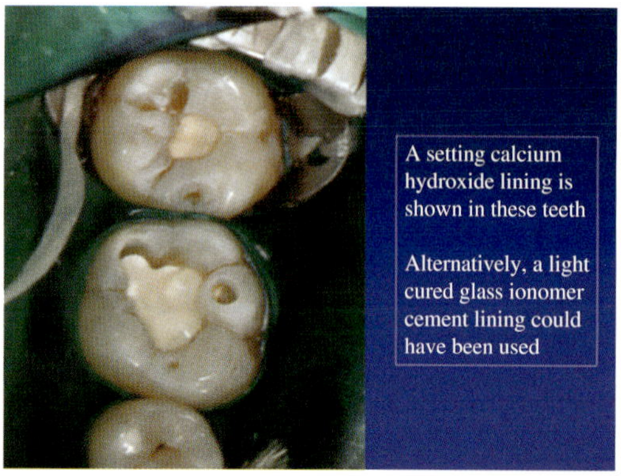

As an alternative, a setting calcium hydroxide cement may be used.

This clinical case shows this material in place- note how its colour contrasts against that of the dentine.

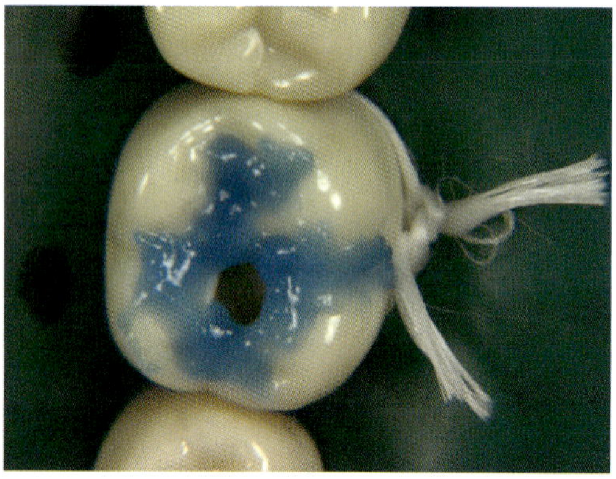

The two cavities in the tooth are now ready to be filled using composite resin. An acid etch procedure is needed for micromechanical retention of the filling material.
Stage 1 involves placing the etching gel onto the enamel for a ***minimum*** of 15 seconds -but not exceeding 30 seconds. This gel contains 36% buffered ortho phosphoric acid.
As fissure sealant will be applied into all adjacent fissures in this procedure, the entire fissure pattern and the enamel walls of the cavity are covered in contrasting coloured gel.

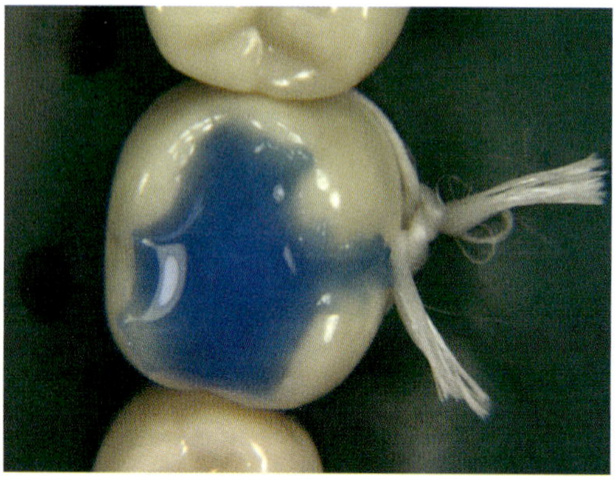

The gel is then allowed to cover the dentine and lining of the mesial cavity for a ***maximum*** of 15 seconds in the second stage of the etching procedure.

The gel can be seen to fill the deeper mesial cavity.

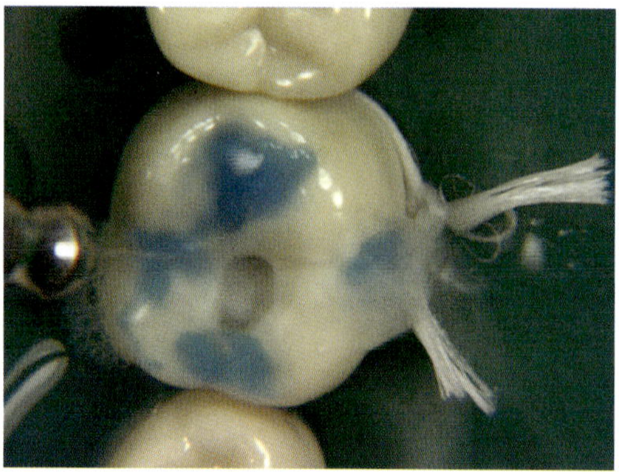

The next stage is to remove the gel using the triple dental syringe.

Water is used initially to remove the etchant gently and avoid it spattering onto the surrounding tissues

An air and water spray can be used once the bulk of the gel has been removed.

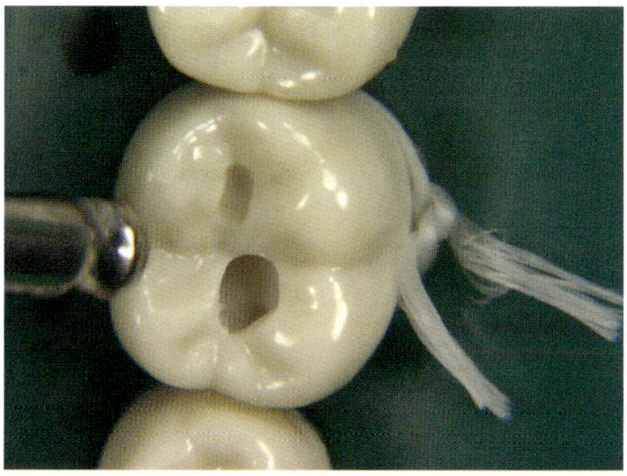

After carefully drying the cavity but ensuring it does not become dessicated, the cavity can be inspected to ensure that enamel frosting is visible.

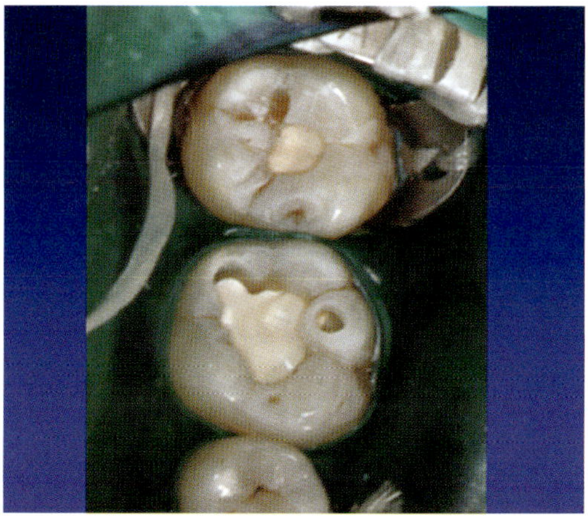

Chalky or frosted appearance like this must be visible after etching. If it is not present on natural enamel, the procedure should be repeated.

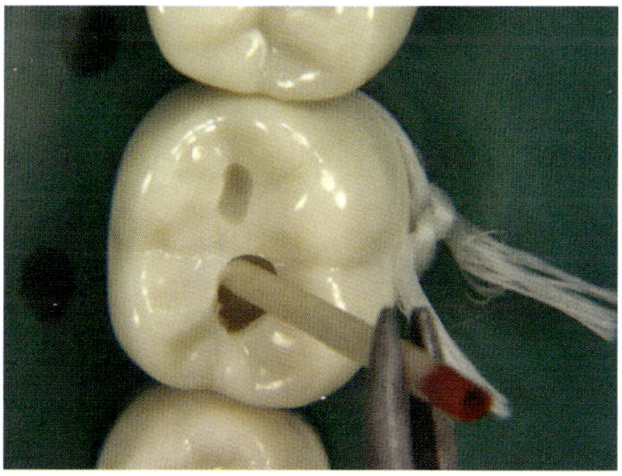

Bonding resin is applied and left undisturbed for 30 seconds to penetrate into the tubules of the dentine and into the small pores created in the enamel.

A microbrushor short section of endodontic point may be used to apply the bonding agent onto the cavity walls and floor.

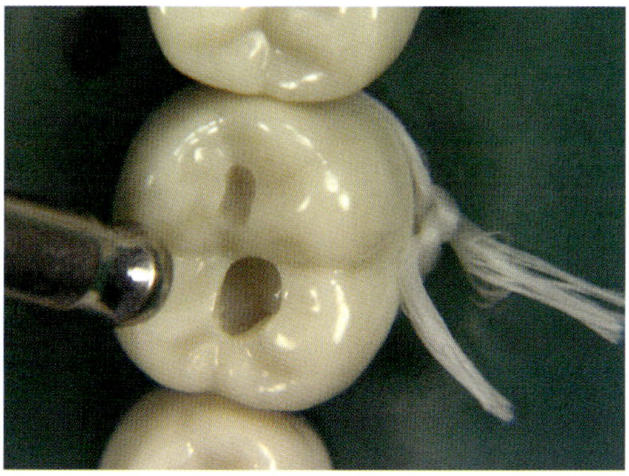

After the 30 seconds, the resin is gently air-dried with the triple dental syringe.
This removes the butanol solvent for the resin

Only a gentle air jet is required for this stage of the procedure.

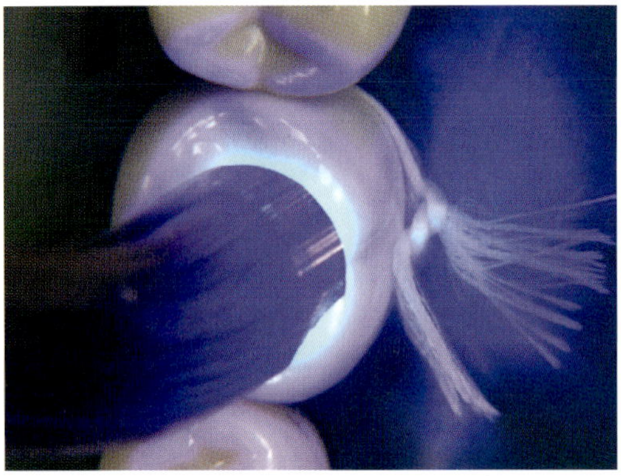

The resin is light cured for 10 seconds.

It is important not to look directly at this high intensity light source as damage may be caused to the retina of the eye.

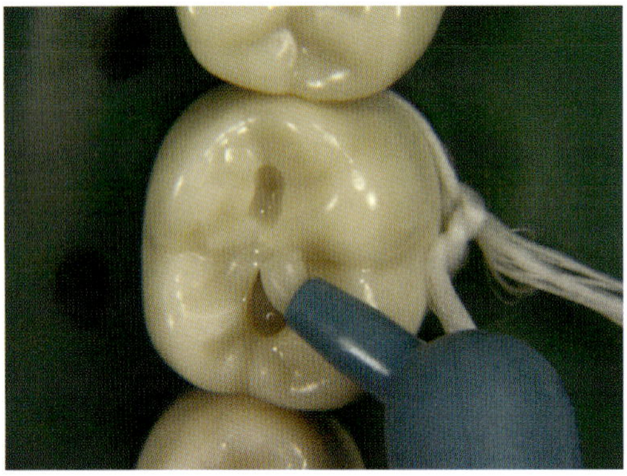

Only small increments of composite should be placed and cured at each stage.

Most manufacturers recommend that a layer of material not exceeding 3 mm should be placed.

The first increment of shade-matched composite is expressed from the small compuledirectly into the larger of the two cavities…

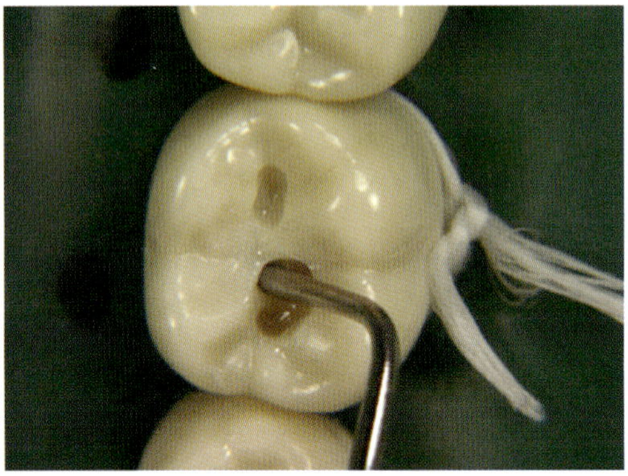

... and adapted to the floor and walls of the cavity using a ball ended instrument.

Preferably, a Teflon coated instrument should be used to prevent the material adhering to the instrument and being pulled away from the cavity floor.

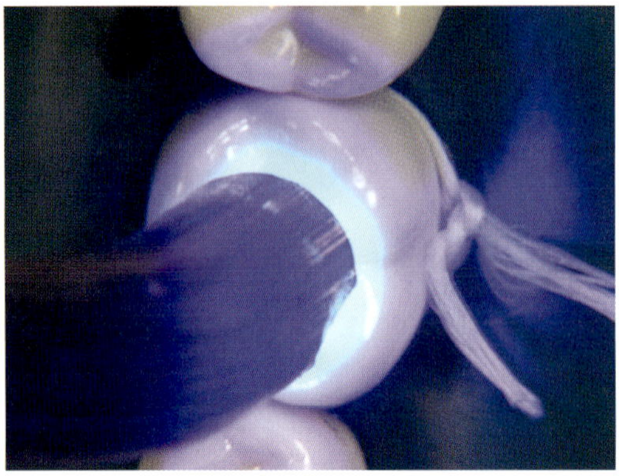

On polymerisation, the composite shrinks towards the surface that offers the greatest bond strength. In this case, the composite resin would shrink towards the enamel.

The composite should be cured from multiple surfaces.

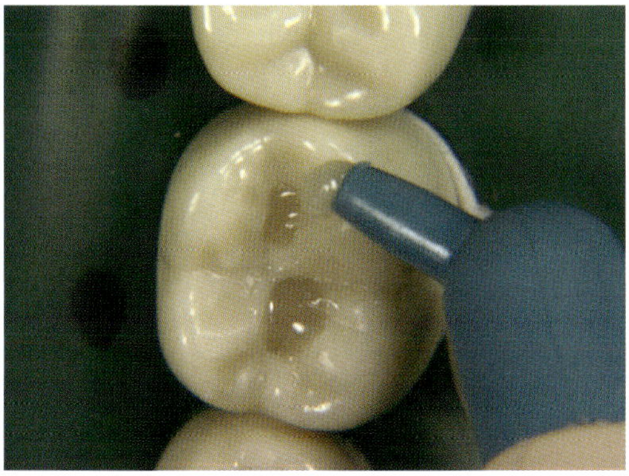

Another increment of composite is added and shaped. Simultaneously, the smaller intra-enamel cavity can be restored in one stage.
The oblique incremental packing procedure seen with the occlusal composite restoration is difficult to achieve with these small cavities.

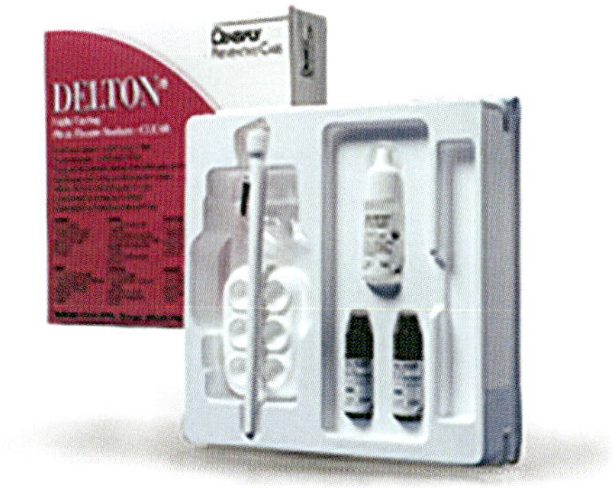

A fissure sealant is applied over the composite resin restorations and into all of the adjacent pits and fissures. In this way, it will act to prevent further caries developing in these areas.

The resin isolates the bacteria remaining in the sealed fissures, preventing them from using carbohydrates in the diet to produce organic acids.
Source: Dentsply Sirona

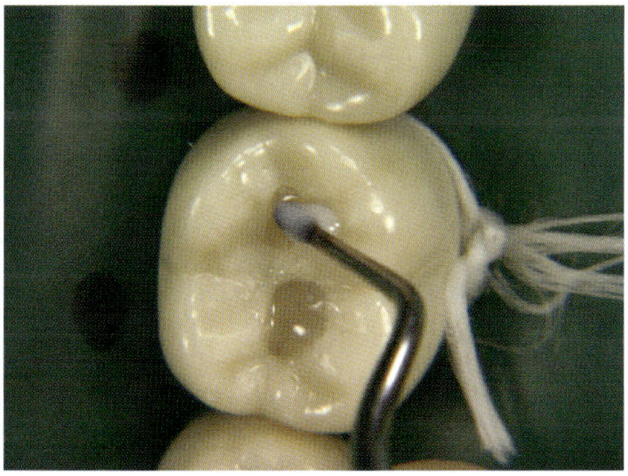

This fissure sealant is classified as an unfilled material – the white colour comes from inclusion of only 0.5% TiO_2.
It can be transferred to the fissures on a small excavator.
By moving the leading edge of the instrument along the fissures, the material is spread without introducing air blows.

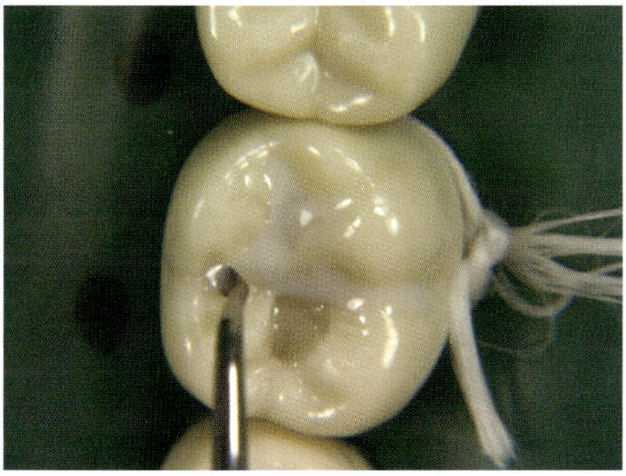

Further increments can be applied to cover all fissure areas up to about halfway up the surrounding cusp slopes.
Remember that the buccal fissure in mandibular teeth is a site frequently affected by caries. This surface should also be covered.
The palatal fissure in maxillary molar teeth should be treated similarly.

Video 5.1

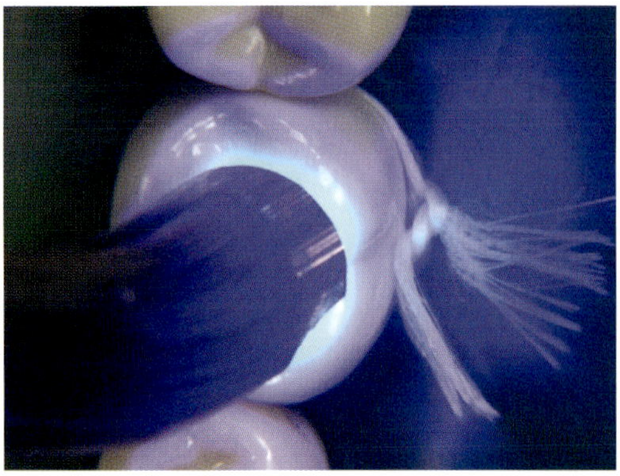

The material is polymerised with the same curing light used as for the composite resin.

It is impossible to over-cure resin materials, but under-curing is a real risk.

A 40 second exposure should be satisfactory.

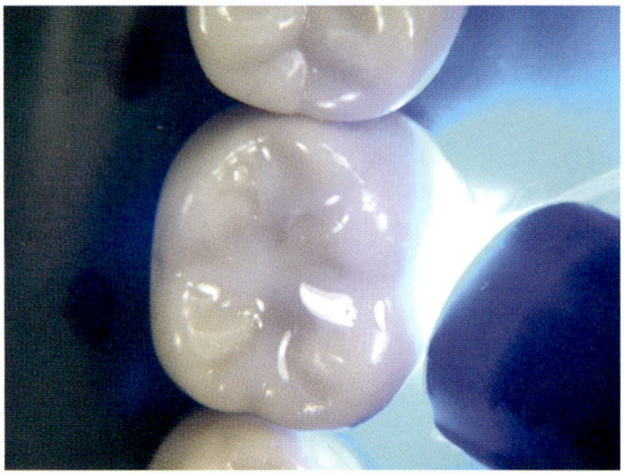

Where buccal or palatal fissures have been sealed, they should be polymerised with a separate 40 second exposure.

The tip of the light guide should be placed as close as possible to the surface without touching it.

The intensity of the light reduces inversely by the square of the distance from the surface.

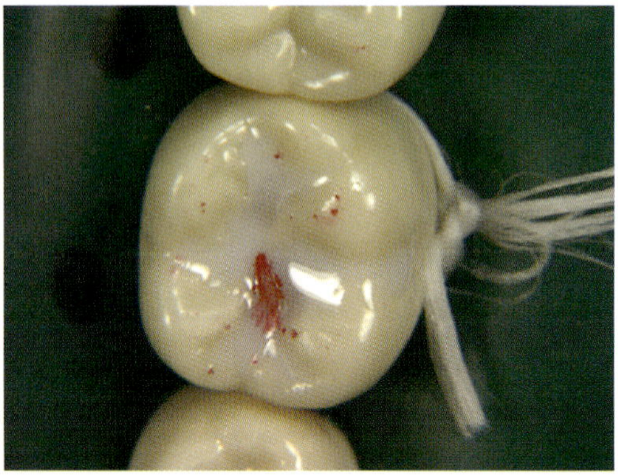

In a clinical case, the rubber dam would be removed and the occlusion checked using articulating paper. High spots should be adjusted as required to allow the patient to bring the upper and lower teeth into occlusion without interference.

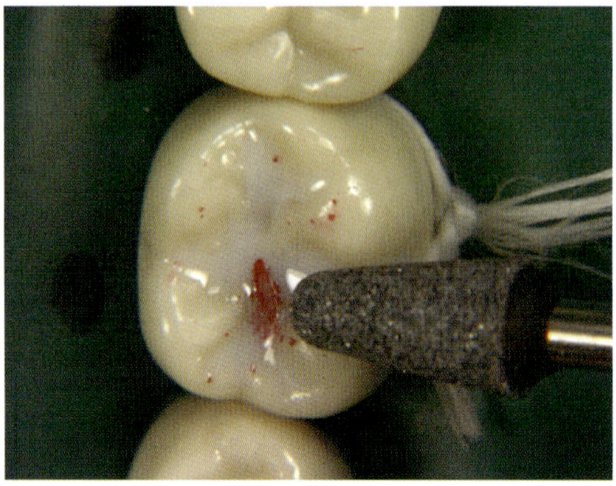

Adjustment can be made with stones or fine diamond burs.

Where only fissure sealant is causing an interference, adjustments can be made using a brown rubber point containing abrasive silica particles.

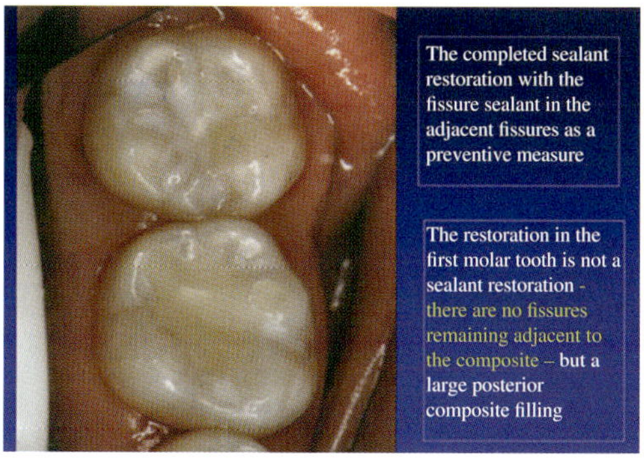

In the clinical case, the tooth has been restored and the rubber dam removed.

The minimal nature of these aesthetic restorations can be contrasted with that of large directly placed restorations.

Clinical Guide to Restoring a Posterior Tooth with a Composite Resin

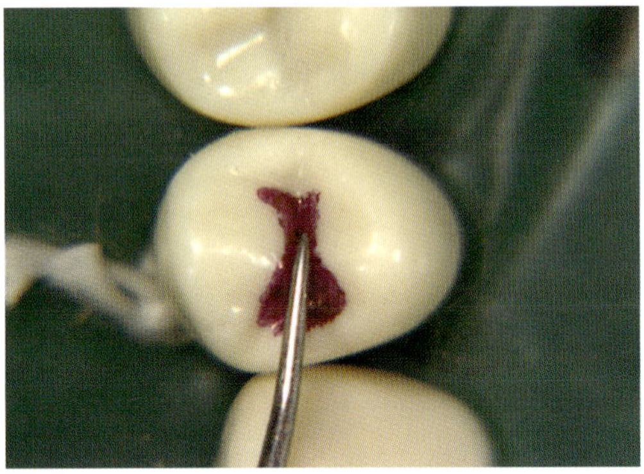

In this sequence, the coloured area indicates the extension of the caries at the EDJ underlying the tooth surface. A dental probe indicates the fissure pattern.
The coloured area represents a carious lesion 2 mm wide at the EDJ in the mesial part of the fissure. The lesion narrows in the central and distal portions of the fissure pattern.
The lesion extends 2 mm deep into the dentine underlying the mesial half of the fissure. Under the remaining fissures, the lesion just reaches into the dentine.

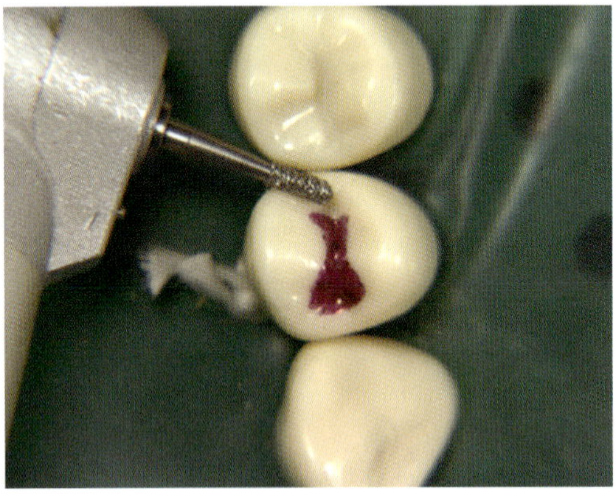

A dome ended cylindrical fissure bur is used in the air turbine (operating at a free running speed of 450,00–500,000 rpm).

As this bur cuts into tooth structure, the abrasion causes heat generation, and it is therefore imperative that the bur is cooled with a water spray. The spray should be directed at the tip of the bur.

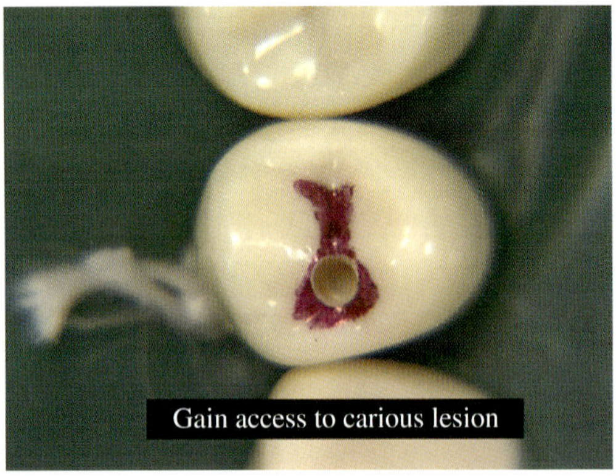

Video 5.2

The initial cut into the dentine should be made above the most extensive aspect of the carious lesion. In this case this is in the mesial half of the occlusal fissure.

The bur should be held in the long axis of the tooth and at right angles to a line drawn across the cusp tips.

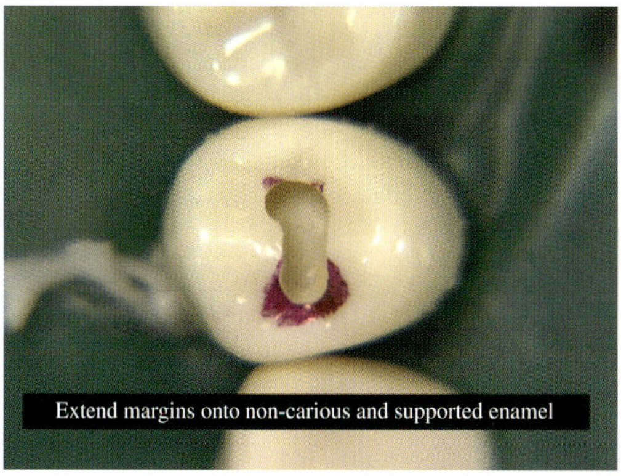

The cavity should be extended minimally throughout the length of the carious part of the fissure pattern to expose the full extent of the caries.

At this stage the extension should be limited to the width of the bur.

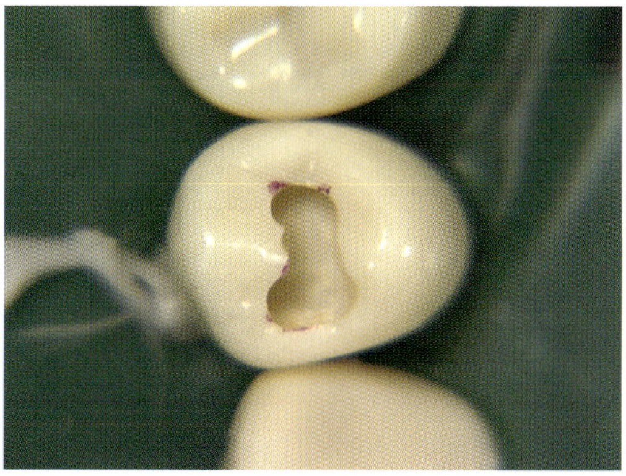

The caries is most widely spread mesially and, within the dentine, will extend well beyond the cavity margins, causing the dimensions of the cavity to be greater below the EDJ.

Unlike a cavity for restoration with amalgam, cavo-surface angles in a cavity suitable for restoration with composite resin are not so critical, and the cavity does not need to be prepared to be mechanically retentive.

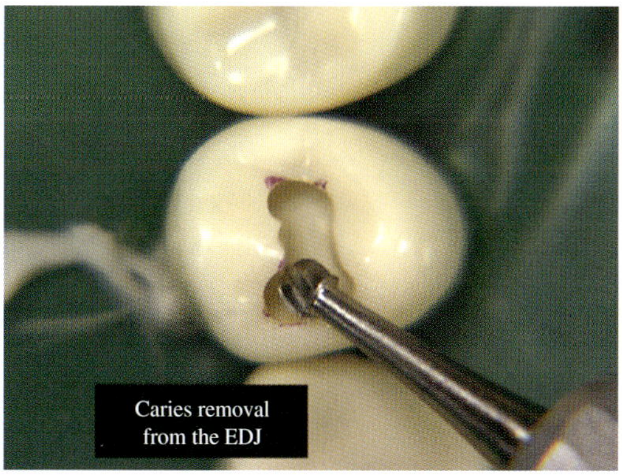

The remaining caries is removed using a large steel latch grip round bur in the slow-speed contra-angled handpiece. This is run at a slow-speed of less than 1000 rpm and does not require a water coolant.

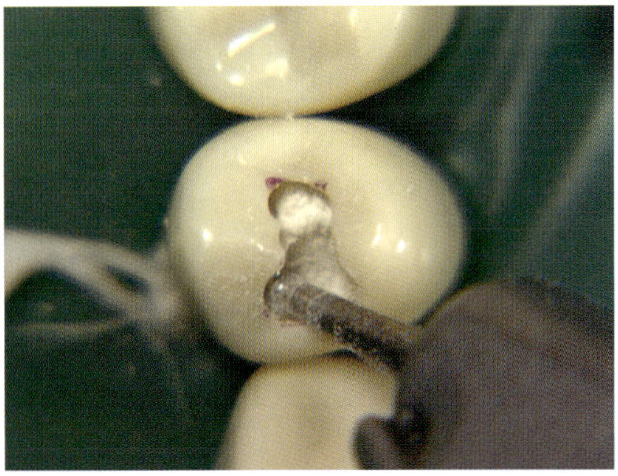

The bur should be used initially around the EDJ of the cavity. The largest bur that will fit into the cavity should be used at this stage.

In this slide the dentine debris is readily visible. This needs to be washed away frequently using the triple dental syringe.

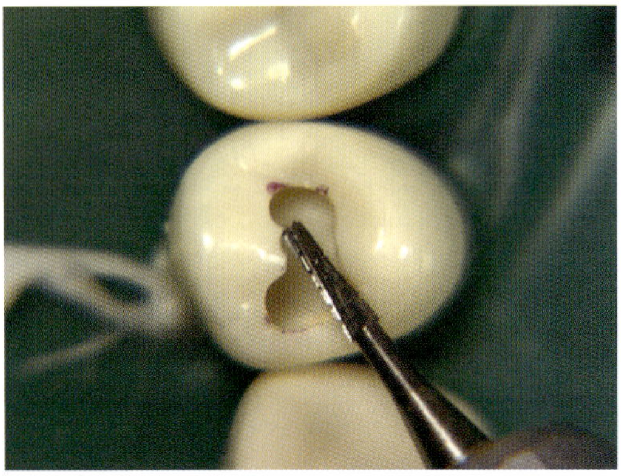

The cavity has been washed and gently dried such that it can be examined clearly for residual caries. A careful check should be made for sound but unsupported tooth substance on the cavity margins.

A fissure bur should be used in the contra-angled handpiece to refine the cavity margins. Plain-cut and cross-cut fissure burs are available.
The cross-cut bur is a more aggressive cutting instrument than the plain-cut version but has the disadvantage of leaving the surface rougher.

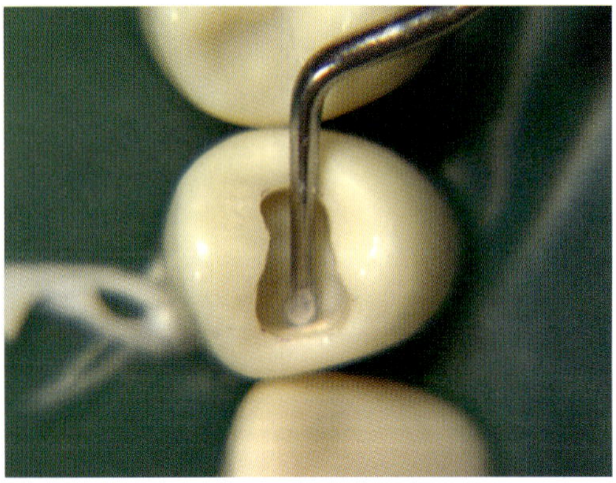

Remaining caries in the depth of the cavity can be removed using an excavator. The instrument should be used with firm stroking action, working from the central area of the cavity towards the periphery, which has already been rendered caries free by using the round bur.

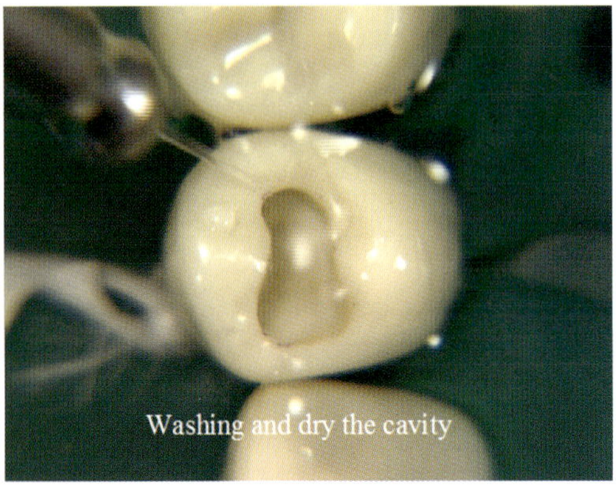

The cavity should now be washed as the last stage of cavity preparation.

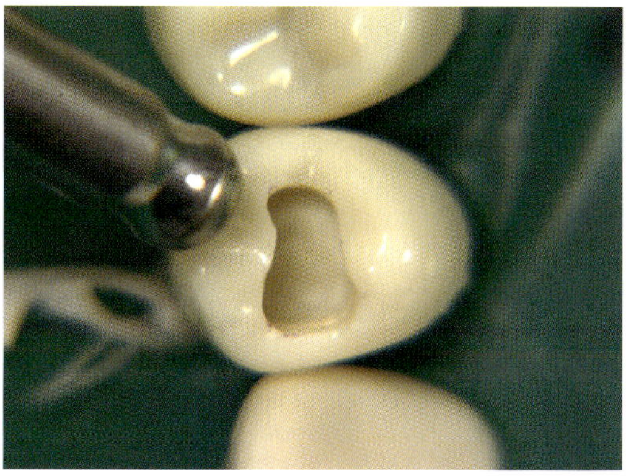

...and dried without desiccation of the dentine.

This cavity is quite large and is what the clinician could expect in a patient who has not been under regular professional supervision.

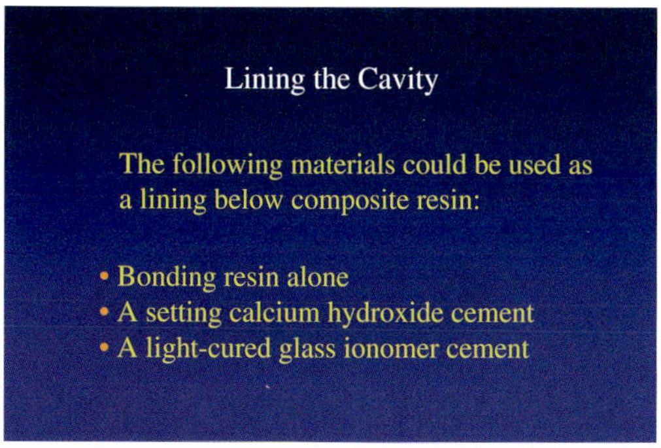

In contemporary dental practice many operators do not place a dental cement as a lining but allow the infiltration of the bonding resin to seal the dentinal tubules.

Others prefer to use either a glass ionomer cement or a setting calcium hydroxide cement below composite restoration. This will also act as a visual barrier if or when this restoration requires replacement.

A eugenol containing material should never be used because it will plasticise the resin base.

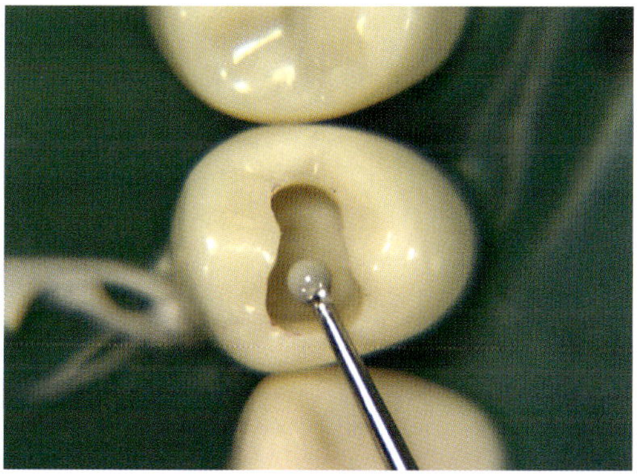

Video 5.3

In this simulated clinical case a light-cured glass ionomer cement lining is being used as an alternative to calcium hydroxide cement. This glass ionomer cement has the advantage of command curing, fluoride leach, and bonding to dentine. It also has a similar coefficient of thermal expansion to dentine.

A PF10 instrument is used to place the lining material. A globule of the material can be seen on the instrument in the slide.

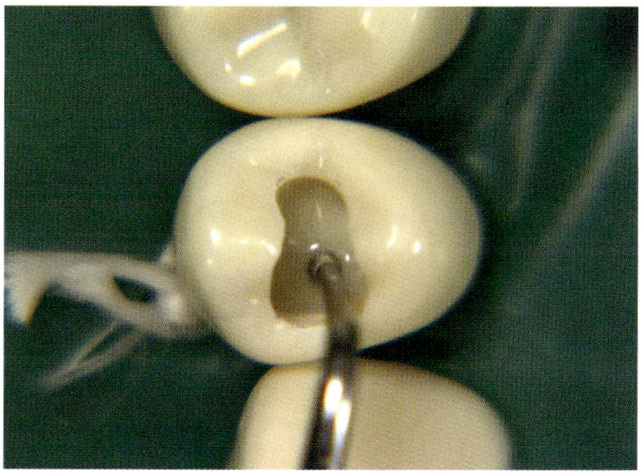

The material is applied along the pulpal floor of the cavity without lifting the instrument. In this way the material is uniformly placed over the entire floor of dentine.

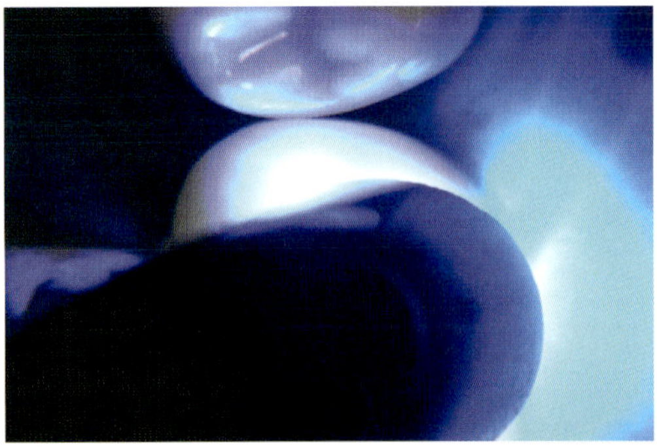

The lining material is polymerized using a visible blue light of 470 nm wavelength. A 30 second curing time is recommended.

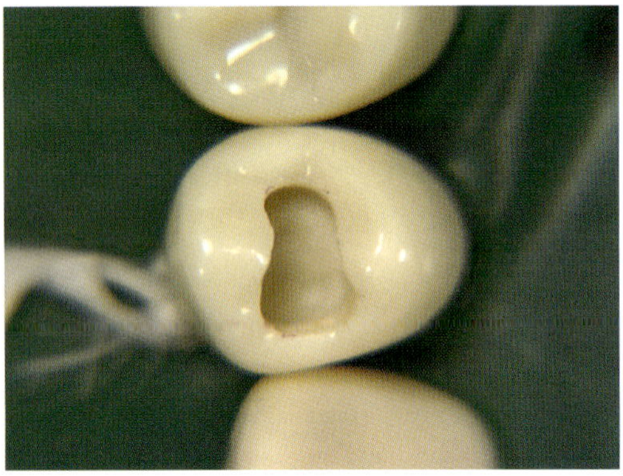

The polymerized lining material is difficult to see because it is colouredsimilar to the structure of these casein teeth. A setting calcium hydroxide is easier to inspect because it has a contrasting opaque shade to that of the dentine.

The placed and cured cement can be seen in the slide covering the pulpal floor of the cavity.

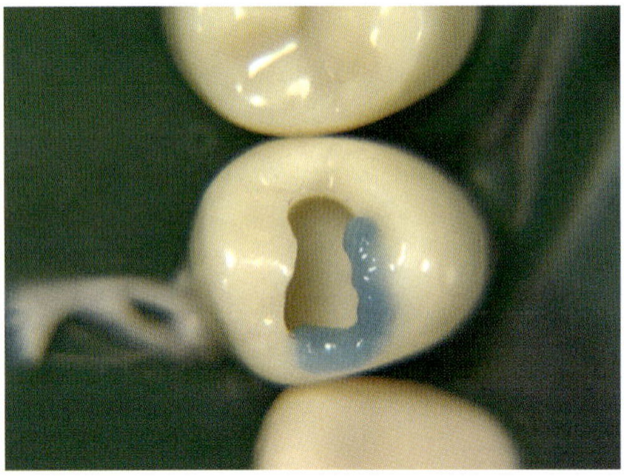

Etching

Acid etching (36% phosphoric acid) allows composite resin to be bonded to both enamel and dentine

- Start by etching the enamel
- Minimum of 15 seconds
- The etchant is dispensed from a syringe using a small blunt tipped needle and is continued around all enamel margins

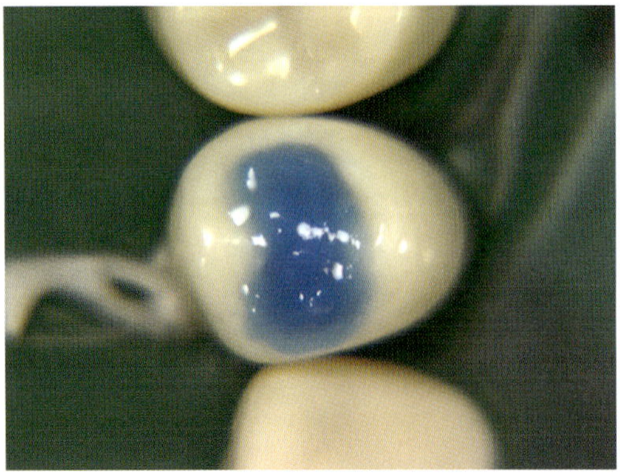

This slide demonstrates the extension of the etchant to contact all areas of the cavity including the dentine.

The etchant should only be left covering all surfaces in this manner for a maximum of 15 seconds.

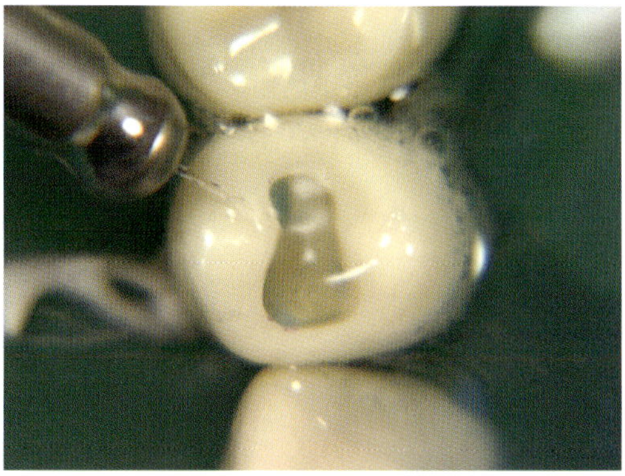

The cavity should be washed for at least as long as the etching procedure has taken.

Start with only water from the triple dental syringe to avoid spatter of the gel onto the operator and patient.

Later introduce air into the water jet for more efficient elimination of the gel.

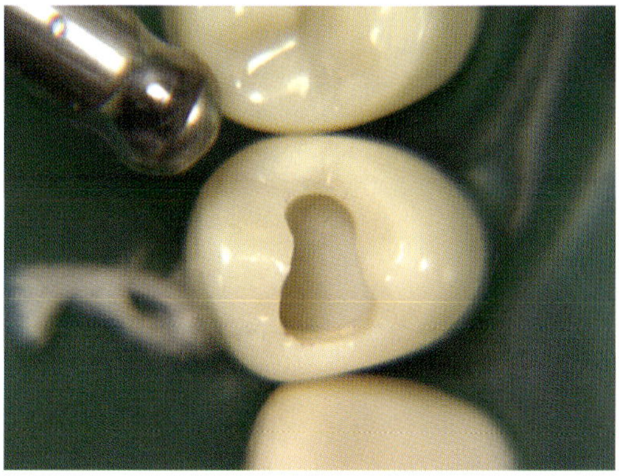

The cavity should be dried, but once again, care should be taken not to desiccate the dentine.

Limit the drying procedure with the triple dental syringe to a maximum of 5 seconds.

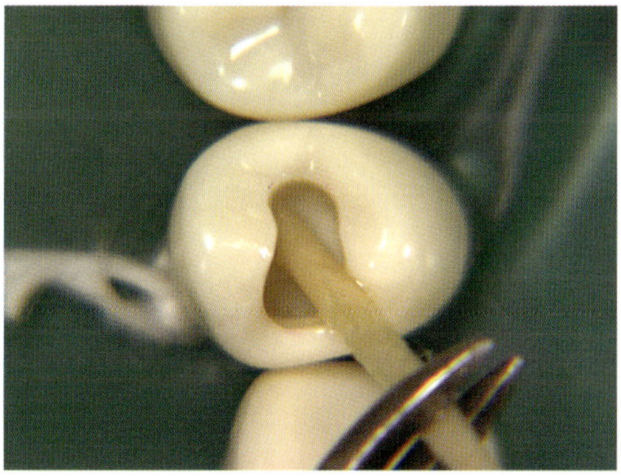

The dental bonding resin can be applied readily using a micro-brush or a section of endodontic paper point.

The bonding resin can be applied to the glass ionomer cement lining and the enamel and dentine cavity walls.

It should be left for 30 seconds to penetrate the pores and tubules so that micro-mechanical retention is achieved.

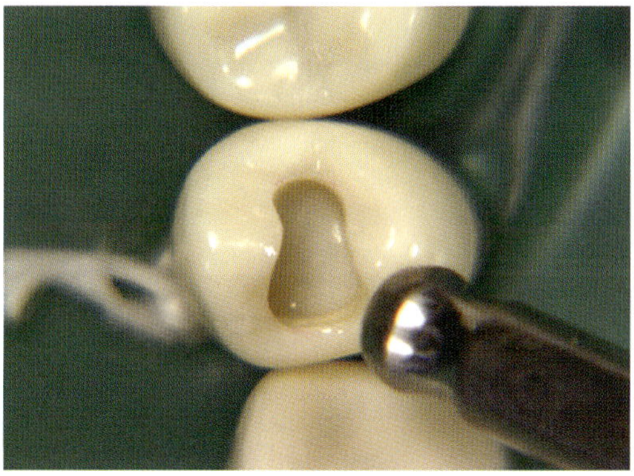

Gentle blowing with air removes the solvent of acetone or alcohol but leaves the active organic resins on the tooth.

Many bonding resins also contain nano-fillers to improve the physical properties.

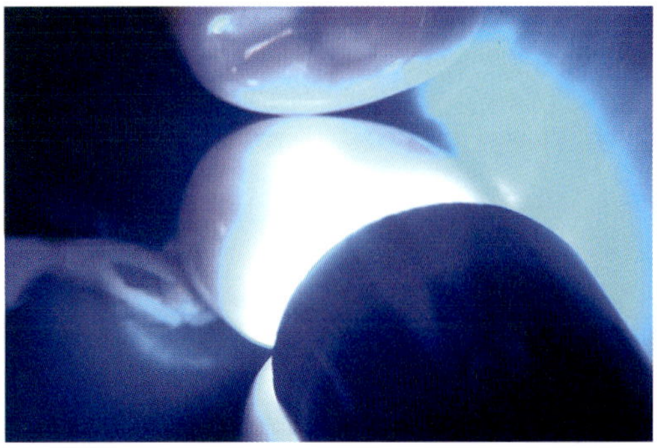

A 470 nm visible blue light source is used to cure the bonding resin. A 10 second exposure is required to optimize the bond with the tooth structures.

Do not look directly into this light because it may cause retinal damage.

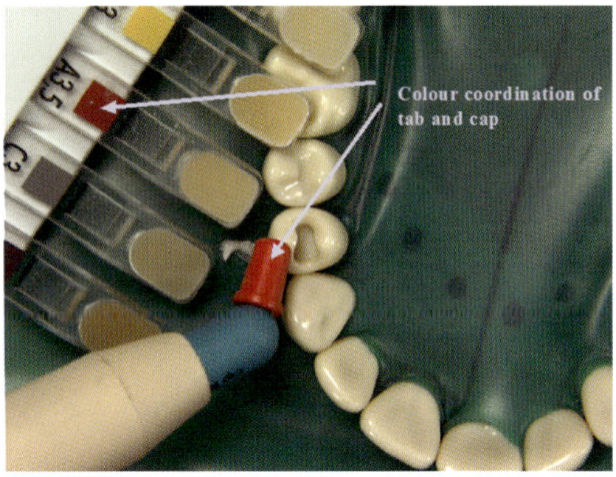

A hybrid composite is used for the restoration of a posterior tooth. It is supplied in either a small capsule for single use or in a large syringe that is expressed onto a paper pad.

There is a wide variety of shades; the colour coding on this guide tab matches the cap on the capsule.

A3.5 is the shade selected here and has a red tab.

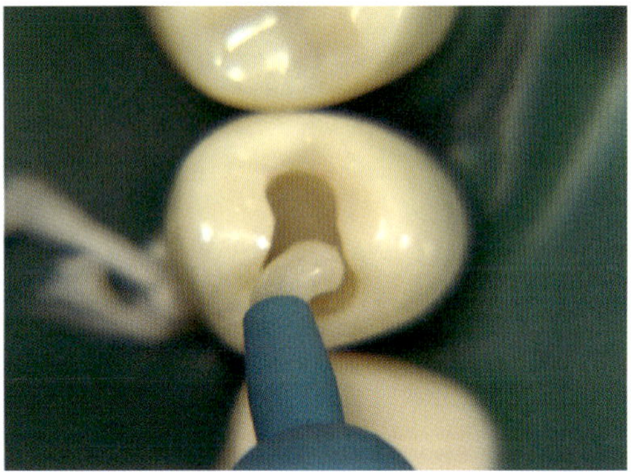

The composite resin should be placed in increments with a 3 mm layer being the most common thickness.

The initial increment of composite is used to cover the floor of the cavity and adapt well to the tooth structure.

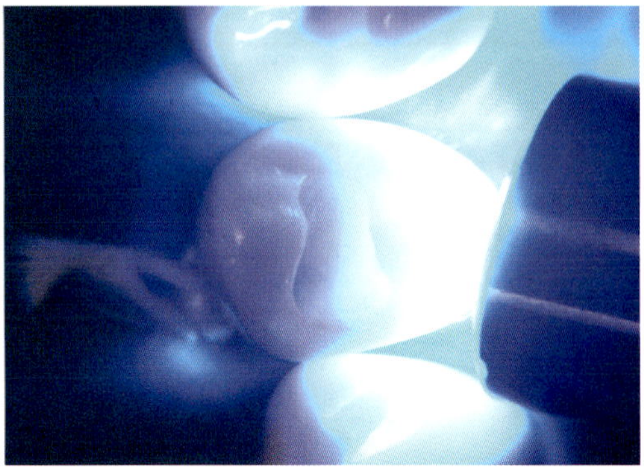

Once adapted, the material is light cured and each increment is cured for 40 seconds.

During polymerization, the composite resin will shrink towards the surface to which it has the greatest bond strength.

Typically 20–25 MPa to dentine and > 30 MPa to enamel.

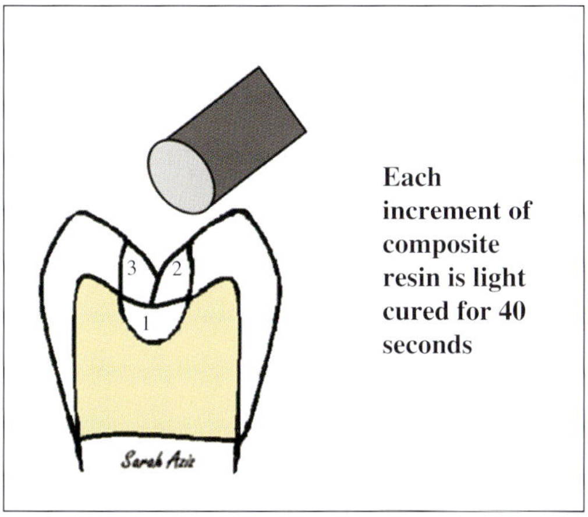

This diagram shows how the increments of composite resin are placed to avoid shrinkage. Shrinkage can create small gaps at the margin of the cavity and result in microleakage.

Increments 2 and 3 are added obliquely so that they only touch one wall and the initial increment.

The polymerising shrinkage vector will be towards the cavity walls.

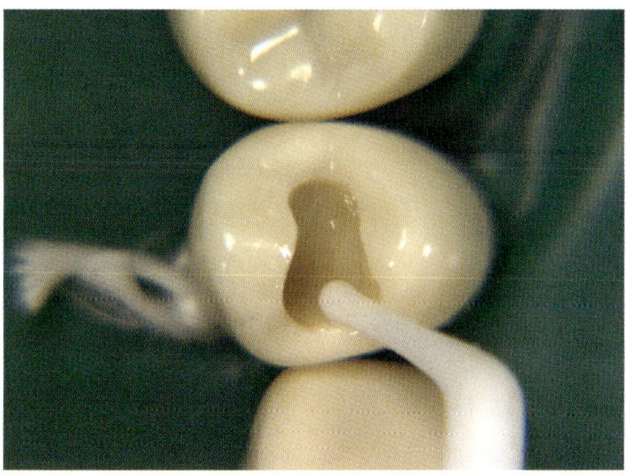

The second increment of composite resin has been placed – in this the material has been placed against the palatal margin of the cavity.

At this stage care should be exercised to ensure that material is not placed against the buccal wall to avoid the risk of material creating a marginal gap during polymerisation.

Video 5.4

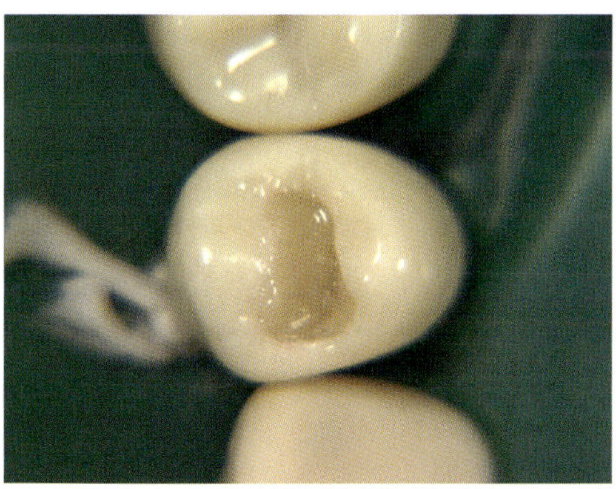

A third increment is added to the buccal side of the cavity.

The procedure of placement and polymerisation is identical to that described above.

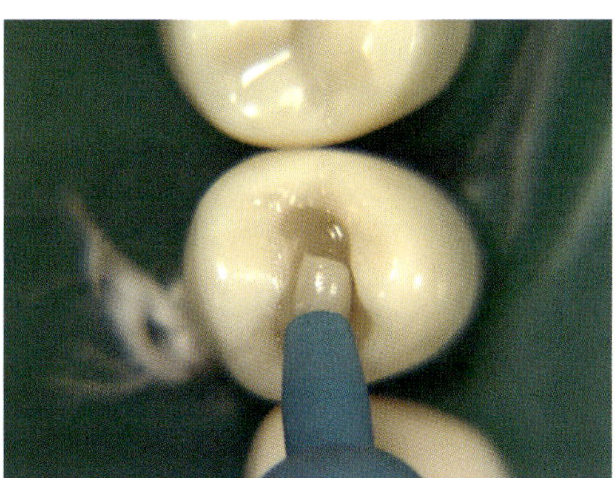

A final small increment of material may be placed to achieve good occlusal contour of the restoration. There are a variety of instruments for working with composite resin that facilitate shaping due to their shape and how they resist the material adhering to their surface.

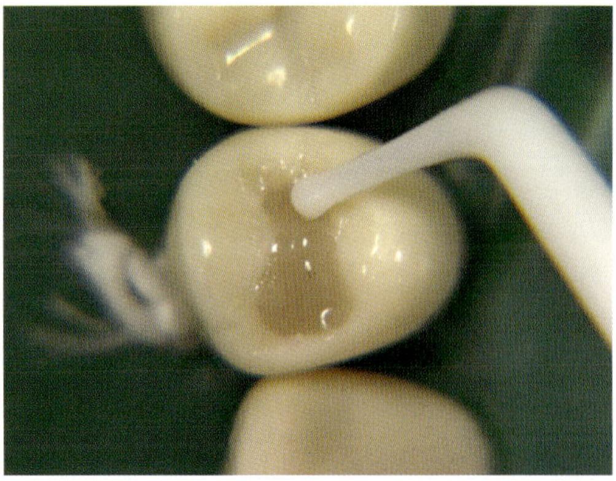

This Teflon coated instrument reduces the adherence of the composite resin to its surface.

Note that a small excess of material has extended onto the occlusal enamel surface. This will make it more difficult to finish and polish.

The ideal goal is to have no excess over the cavo-surface margin of the cavity.

Video 5.5

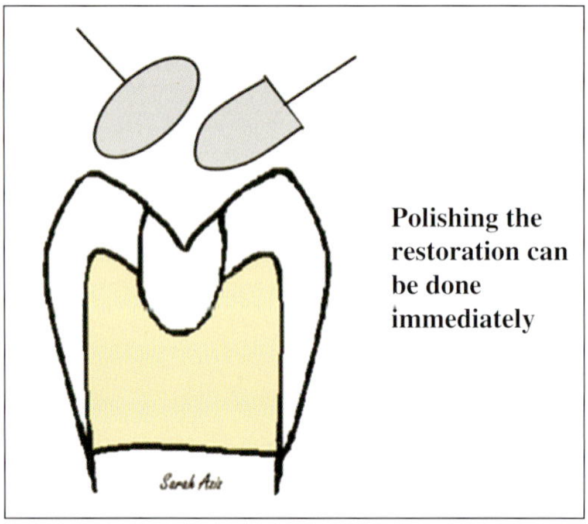

Composite Finishing

Finishing and polishing can be done immediately.

- Contouring stones can be used initially, or fine diamond or tungsten carbide burs
- The final gloss finish is achieved using polishing impregnated silicone cups, discs, or points

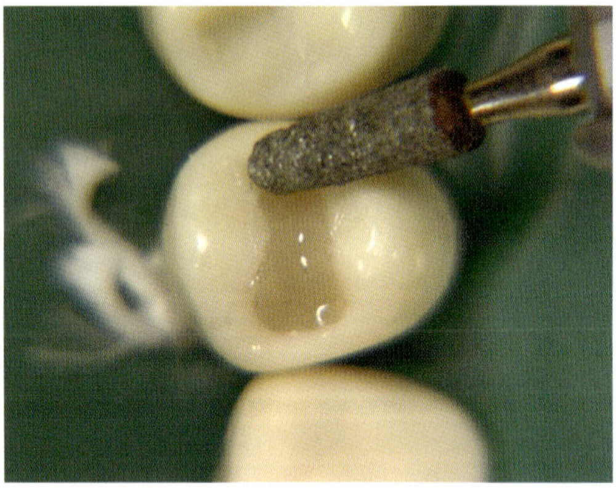

Initially, a selection of stones can be used in the contra-angled handpiece using conventional speeds to remove excess material covering the enamel surface around the cavity margins. This process will roughen the composite and the enamel surfaces. This process, if required, will recreate the anatomical features of the restored area.

Alternatively, fine diamond or multi-fluted tungsten carbide burs may be used at high speed, but fine control of the cutting is not so readily achieved.

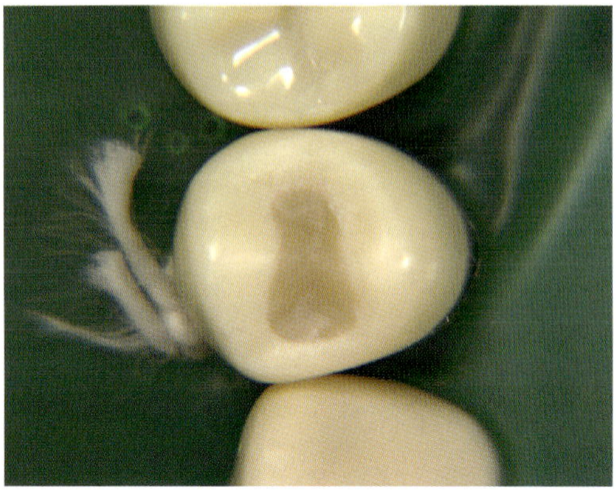

Following completion of contouring with the rotary instruments, the surface of the restoration appears matt.

At this stage, the fissure pattern and, in particular, the Y shaped marginal spillways can be seen clearly now that the anatomical detail has been re-introduced.

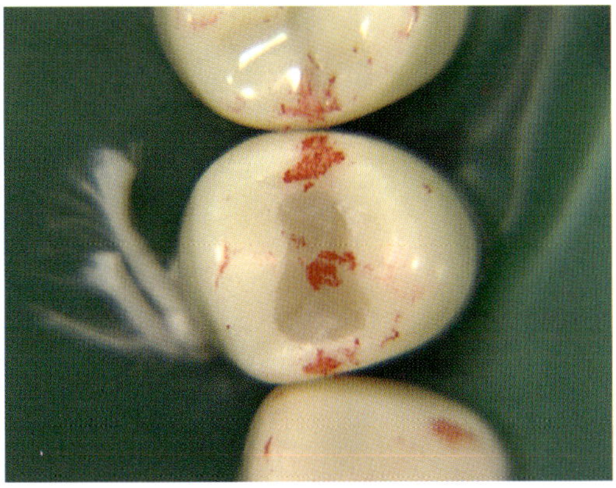

In the clinical situation the rubber dam would be removed and the occlusion checked using articulating paper. Adjustment with rotary instruments may be necessary to ensure that are no premature contacts on the new restoration.

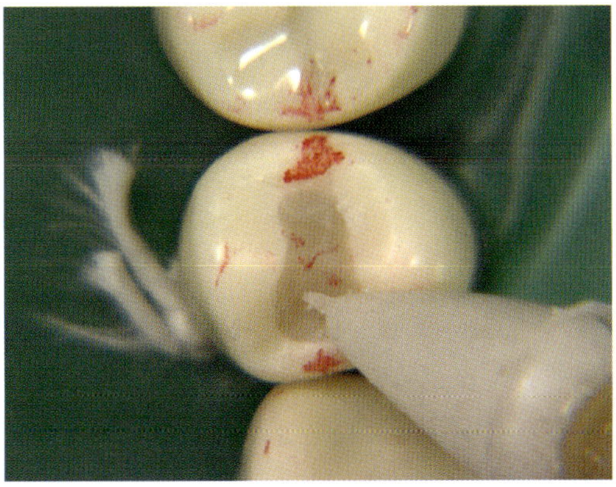

The surface of the restoration is then polished using impregnated silicone points, discs, and cups in the contra-angled handpiece using conventional speeds.

It is important not to apply too great a pressure because overheating of the pulp may ensue and result in postoperative pain.

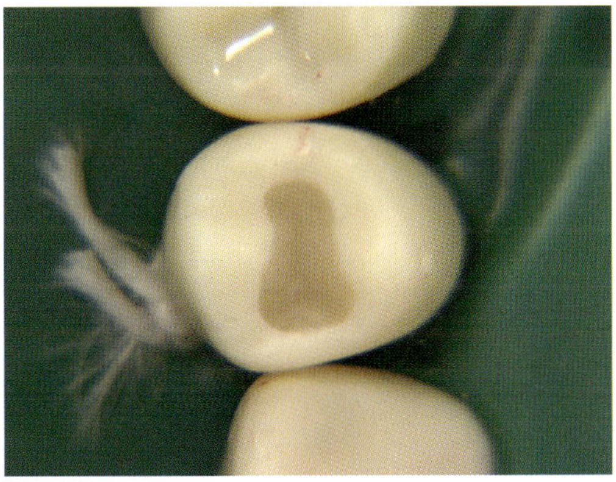

A much smoother surface can now be seen

It should not be possible to feel the margins when a dental probe is moved across the restoration margin from enamel to composite resin and back again to the enamel surface.

If any catch is heard or felt, that area should be re-finished using rotary instruments.

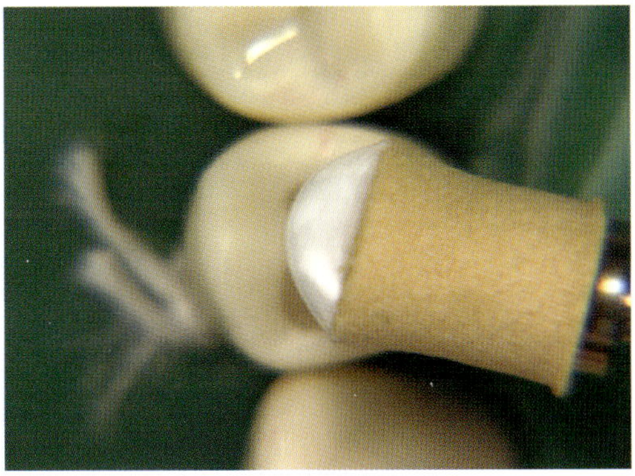

Some polishing systems for composite resin contain finishing pastes – fine and extra-fine. The surface can be polished to a high lustre using these materials. A designated felt cup is supplied with these materials.

The polish is worked onto the surface of the restoration at conventional speed using the contra-angled handpiece.

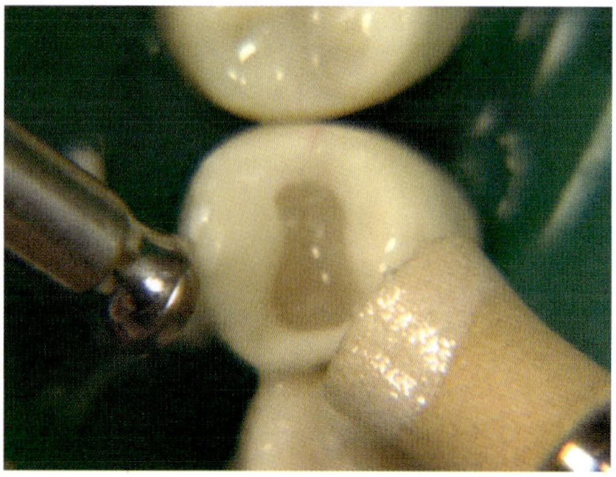

The tooth, restoration and felt cup are washed thoroughly and rinsed before the final application of the extra-fine.

This is used in the same manner as before using a light pressure but moderately high speed.

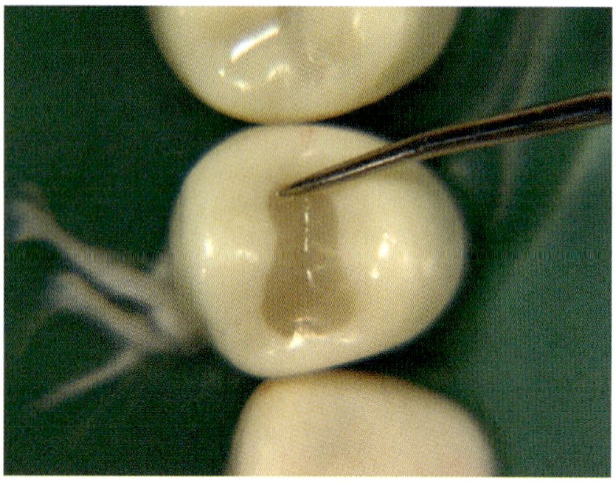

The restoration margins are explored again using a dental probe on completion of the polishing. The probe should be used to explore from filling onto tooth and back again onto the restoration surface.

If any restoration margins can be detected with the probe, they should be eliminated to prevent the development of marginal stain.

The finished restoration can be seen to have a good anatomical contour and a lustrous surface finish.

A Clinical Case

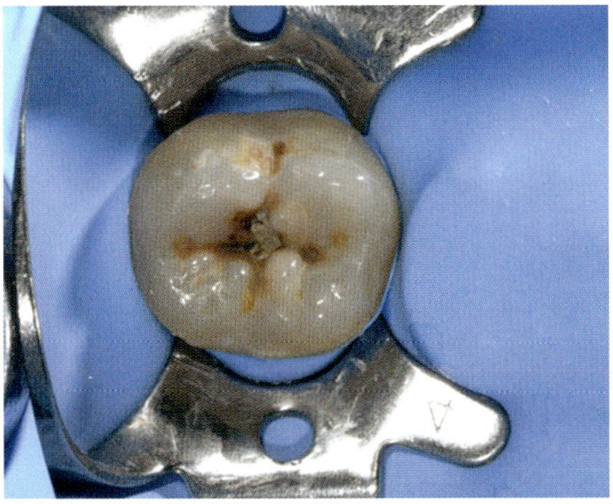

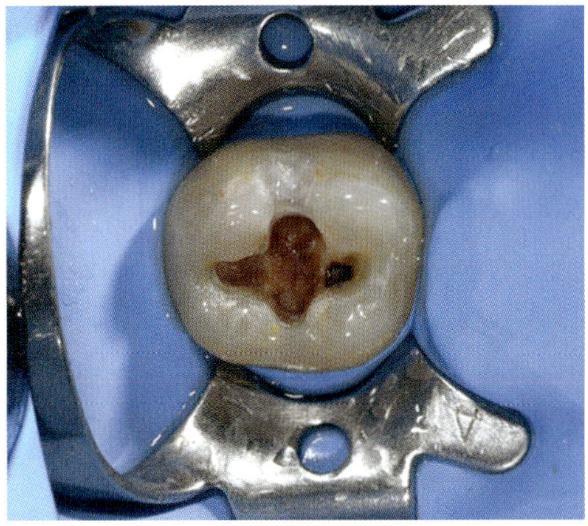

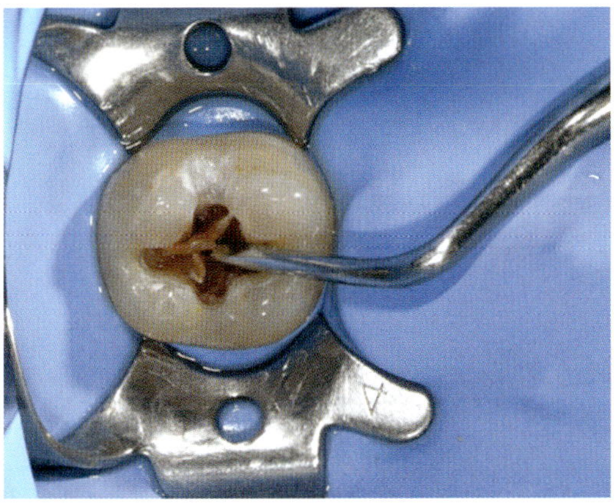

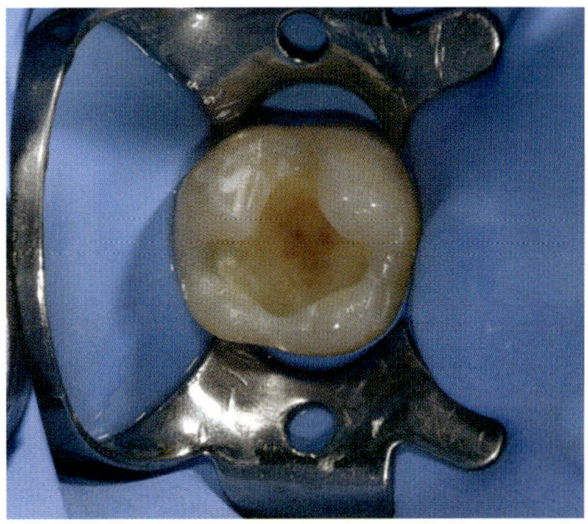

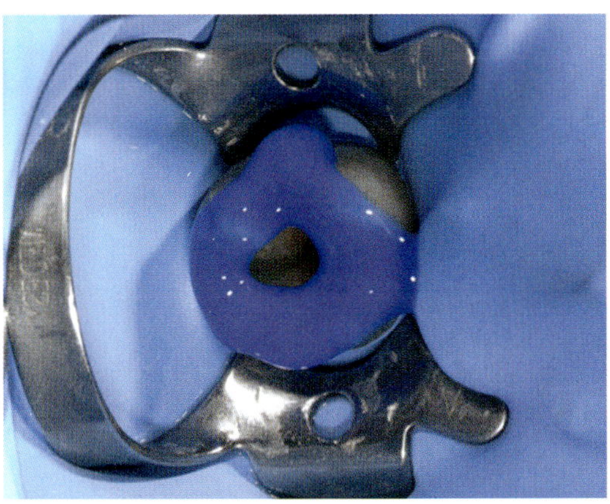

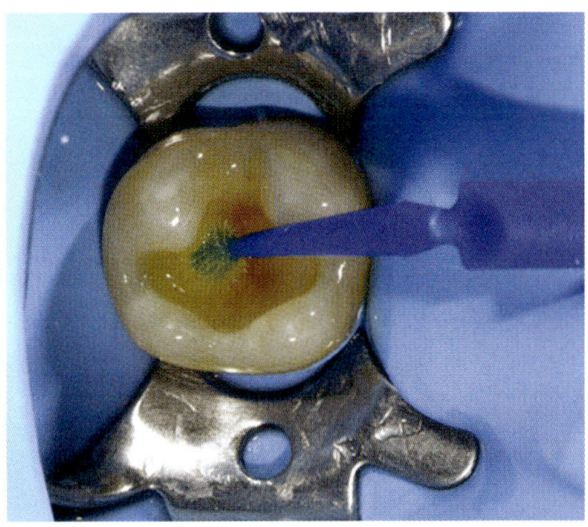

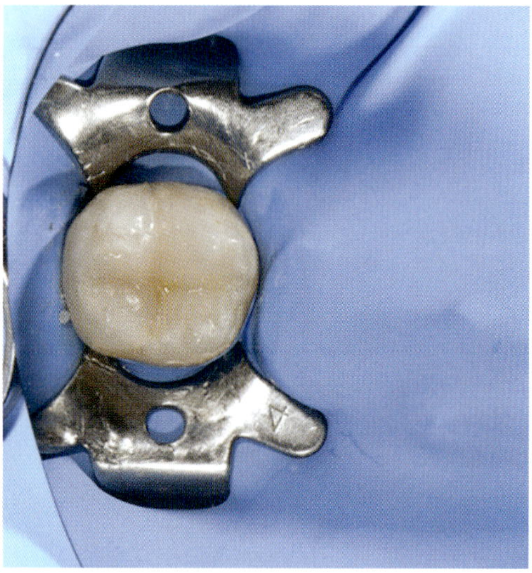

This clinical case shows the investigation and restoration of a mandibular second molar tooth

Source: Printed by permission of Dr Osama Alkhatib.

Further Reading

Chu, C.H., Lo, E.C.M., and You, D.S.H. (2010). Clinical diagnosis of fissure caries with conventional and laser-induced fluorescence techniques. *Lasers in Medical Science* 25: 355–362.

Gomez, J., Zakian, C., Salsone, S. et al. (2013). *In vitro* performance of different methods in detecting occlusal caries lesions. *Journal of Dentistry* 41: 180–186.

Ismail, A.I., Sohn, W., Tellez, M. et al. (2007). The International Caries Detection and Assessment System (ICDAS): an integrated system for measuring dental caries. *Community Dentistry and Oral Epidemiology* 35: 170–178.

Lussi, A. (1993). Comparison of different methods for the diagnosis of fissure caries without cavitation. *Caries Research* 27: 409–416.

Opdam, N.J.M. and Bronkhorst, E.M. (2010). Loomans BAC12-year survival of composite vs. amalgam restorations. *Journal of Dental Research* 89 (10): 1063–1067.

Pit and fissure sealants evidence-based guidance on the use of sealants for the prevention and management of pit and fissure caries. University College Cork, funded by the Health Research Board 2010. https://www.ucc.ie/en/media/research/ohsrc/PitandFissureSealantsFull.pdf

Pretty, I.A. (2006). Caries detection and diagnosis: novel technologies. *Journal of Dentistry* 34: 727–739.

Schwendicke, F., Frencken, J.E., Bjørndal, L. et al. (2016). Managing carious lesions: consensus recommendations on carious tissue removal. *Advances in Dental Research* 28 (2): 58–67.

Selwitz, R.H., Ismail, A.I., and NB, P. (2007). Seminar Dental caries. *Lancet* 369: 51–59.

Zandoná, A. and Zero, D.T. (2006). Diagnostic tools for early caries detection. *Journal of the American Dental Association (Chicago, IL)* 137 (12): 1675–1684.

6

Posterior Approximal Restorations

A class II carious lesion may develop cervical to the contact points of premolar and molar teeth. These areas form natural stagnation points on teeth where plaque may develop and mature. Toothbrushing alone will not remove the plaque from these areas as interproximal cleaning tools are needed. The most common of these include dental floss and interproximal cleaning brushes, e.g. TePe brushes. The plaque uses thc rcfincd carbohydratcs in the diet to produce a range of organic acids that gradually demineralise the enamel to result in a cavity. Unfortunately, the early carious lesion cannot be seen directly but only on good quality bitewing radiographs (see Figure 6.1).

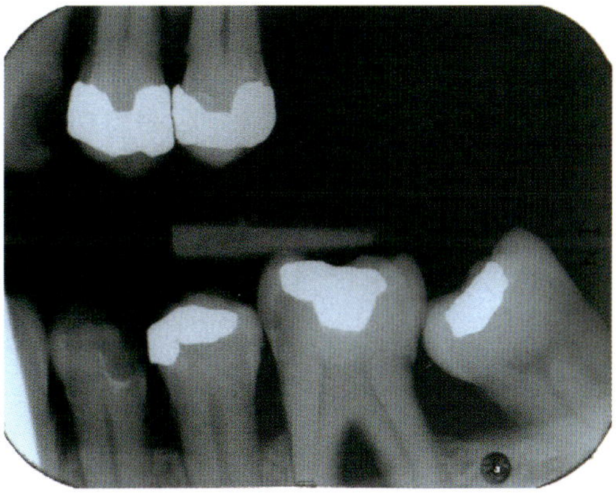

Figure 6.1 This bitewing radiograph shows a large carious lesion on the mesial aspect of the first lower molar tooth that has been previously restored. There is also an early carious lesion confined to enamel on the distal aspect of tooth 35.

The manner in which the class II is managed depends on the stage of disease process. Where lesions are confined to enamel, a preventive approach should be adopted to encourage the lesion to arrest. This would include not only good toothbrushing technique but the use of interproximal brushes or floss. In addition, reducing the number of cariogenic challenges and the application of fluoride in the form of toothpaste, mouthrinses, and professionally applied fluoride varnish should be encouraged. It is imperative that any early lesion is professionally reviewed at regular intervals. Once the lesion has entered dentine and the interproximal surface has cavitated, operative intervention is indicated as well as reinforcing the patient's preventive home care regime (see Figure 6.2).

A Practical Approach to Operative Dentistry, First Edition. Gordon B. Gray and Alaa H. Daud.

Companion website: www.wiley.com/go/gray/operative-dentistry

Classification of Class II Lesions

➢ E_1	Caries confined to outer ½ of enamel
➢ E_2	Caries confined to inner ½ of enamel
➢ D_1	Caries 0.5 mm into dentine
➢ D_2	Caries >0.5 mm into dentine but <0.5 mm from the pulp
➢ D_3	Caries within 0.5 mm of the pulp

Foster LV, 1998

Figure 6.2 The classification by Foster is based on research showing that 92% of D2 carious lesions progressed over the following 3 years compared to shallower dentine lesions.

It is a challenge for the clinician to accurately diagnose when an interproximal lesion has cavitated in posterior teeth, yet this is the main indicator for operative intervention. One way in which an accurate diagnosis can be achieved is to separate the teeth temporarily with an orthodontic elastic separator and record an impression using a light bodied silicone impression (see Figure 6.3).

If it is found that the interproximal surface has not cavitated, the white spot lesion seen on a radiograph can be infiltrated using an organic resin. This is a minimal technique but is very demanding to carry out. The surface must be etched initially, and the lesion can then be dehydrated using absolute alcohol before the resin is applied and polymerised. This technique will work in a similar manner to fissure sealing occlusal surfaces, and in addition, the resin will support the porosity within the lesion.

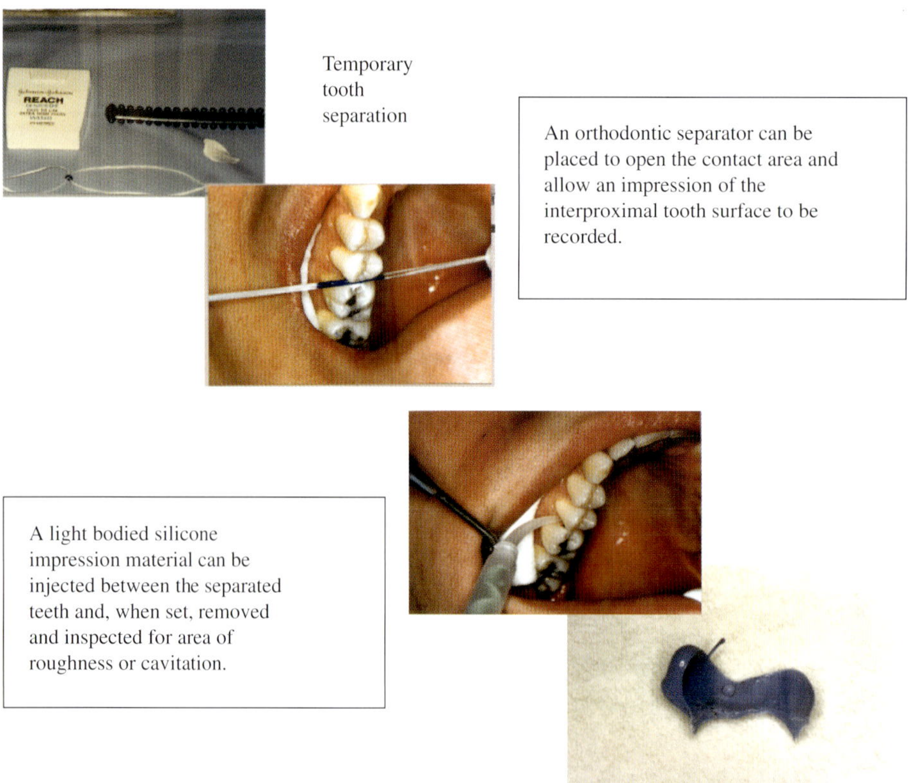

Figure 6.3 Diagnosing an interproximal cavity can be demanding and is best done by separating the teeth and recording an impression of the tooth surfaces. *Source:* Printed by kind permission of Dr L.V. Foster.

There are a number of clinical techniques that can be used to place a direct restoration in a tooth with interproximal caries. These include the traditional two or three surface restorations incorporating an occlusal key. Alternatively, self-retentive boxes or tunnel restorations may be used where there is no involvement of caries in the occlusal fissures.

Tunnel Restorations

Tunnel restorations maintain the marginal ridge of the posterior tooth, and this prevents weakening of the tooth and perhaps future loss of cusps. The caries is approached from the occlusal surface or sometimes from the buccal or lingual side. Adhesive materials are used in the restoration of these tunnel preparations, and the polyalkenoate cements are favoured because they are naturally adhesive and leach fluoride, which may be cariostatic. The tunnel restoration is limited to use in relatively small lesions that do not undermine the integrity of the marginal ridge, otherwise the technique can result in its fracture. It has been suggested that the remaining marginal ridge should be at least 1.5 mm in width and depth to provide sufficient strength. There is also the added complication of creating iatrogenic damage to the adjacent tooth during preparation of the tunnel. The use of dental loupes is required to prepare these minimal cavities.

Removal of the Marginal Ridge

Access to a carious interproximal lesion through the marginal ridge is still the most commonly used method of managing class II caries. The astute clinician will ***pre-wedge*** the area by inserting a wooden wedge between the two teeth. This has the added advantage not only of holding the rubber dam away from the cavity preparation; it also aids in achieving a tighter contact point when the restoration is inserted and the wedge removed.

Access to the caries is gained by placing the bur on the inner aspect of the marginal ridge at the centre of the contact area. In this way, a thin sliver of tooth structure can be kept to avoid damage to the adjacent tooth. This thin sliver of enamel can be fractured out subsequently using a sharp enamel or gingival margin chisel. The buccal and lingual walls and gingival floor of the cavity should be free of unsupported enamel because these could fracture during placement of the restoration or during function. This would result in leakage and a short life expectancy for the restoration. It is vital to be conservative of tooth structure to avoid weakening the tooth. If the tooth is free from caries in the occlusal fissures, the cavity design should avoid preparing an occlusal key and a self-retentive box should be employed. The width of the cavity is determined by the size of the carious lesion and the subsequent removal of unsupported enamel. This will usually leave the cavity margins clear of the adjacent tooth laterally and gingivally, which will leave these margins accessible to instrumentation by the dentist and cleaning by the patient. The buccal and lingual margins should not be extended more than necessary.

Class II cavities can be restored either using ***amalgam*** or ***composite resin***. Amalgam can be used with an adhesive technique, but it is more usual for the latter technique to be used with resinous materials. The advantage of bonding restorations into the cavity is to avoid the preparation of retentive features that weaken the tooth and are more likely to lead to a risk of subsequent tooth fracture.

Non-bonded amalgams require macro-mechanical features in the cavity design to achieve adequate retention. These restorations must have adequate retention to avoid displacement in an occlusal direction. This can be achieved by ensuring the cavity is undercut, although parallel walls will offer sufficient retention. Additionally, these restorations must resist displacement in an approximal direction, and this can be achieved by incorporating either an occlusal key in the fissure area or by preparing retention grooves in the lateral box walls.

The cavity design for adhesive restorations differs in that there is no need to prepare mechanical undercuts for retention because composite resin is bonded to the cavity surfaces using an acid etch technique. This produces micro-mechanical retention into the pores created in the enamel or into the opened dentinal tubules. However, a cavity that still has some features of resistance and retention is thought to be advantageous because this will protect the bond created by the micro-mechanical retention. Bonding composite resin to the cavity will also support any slightly weakened areas of enamel.

Lining

There is some diversity of opinion over the use of a base or lining material below restorations. Traditionally, they were placed to provide a thermal barrier below metallic restorations. Today, following the Minimata Agreement to limit the use of amalgam, more resin based filling materials are being placed, and this has led some authorities to suggest there is no need for lining materials because the bonding resin will flow into the dentine tubules and seal them to prevent both fluid movement and microleakage around the cavity margins. However, some authorities still advocate the use of linings because they can act as a visual warning that dentine is being approached when replacing old restorations. If a lining material is placed in a class II cavity, it is essential that the gingival floor of the box is not covered on its outer 1 mm to ensure good bonding and microleakage resistance is achieved. This will prevent sensitivity and recurrent caries. The thickness of dentine between the axial wall and the pulp is frequently less than below the pulpal floor of the cavity, so lining the axial wall is frequently promoted. It is important, though, to remember to round the pulpo-axial line angle to avoid imparting stresses in the restorative material that could result in fracture of the restoration across its isthmus. In addition, if a lining is placed it must not inadvertently block any features of mechanical retention.

Matrix Bands

It is difficult to form a tight contact area when restoring posterior teeth. The contour is dictated by the matrix band. When amalgam is used as the restorative material, it can be condensed into the cavity and the tightness of the contact improved. If composite resin is used, it cannot be condensed. Composite resin materials used in the restoration of posterior teeth are viscous, but their final shape will be dictated by the matrix system used.

A thin matrix should be used to aid the development of the contact point. These can be made from metal or clear plastic. A metal strip can be inserted more easily because it is more rigid and can be burnished against the adjacent tooth. A polyester strip, on the other hand, will allow light to pass though it and aid polymerisation. Both metal and plastic matrices can be flat or contoured in cross section. Obviously, the contoured matrix will produce a more anatomical surface.

Matrix bands should be wedged into position to avoid a gap forming between the gingival floor and the band. This would create an overhang of filling material and hinder plaque control. Either wooden or plastic wedges are available. Some plastic wedges can reflect light from their sides and aid in the polymerisation of the filling material near the gingival floor of the box.

Finishing the Restoration

Amalgam restorations are finished and polished in an entirely different way from those placed using composite resin.

When the cavity has been filled with small increments of amalgam, the marginal ridge is carved to the same height as the neighbouring tooth. This is done by running a dental probe around the inner aspect of the matrix band to create the correct occlusal embrasure. Thereafter, the matrix can be removed and the sharp side of an amalgam carver – such as the half-Hollenbach – is used to carve the excess material by laying the sharp side of the instrument parallel to the cuspal slopes and carving away from the marginal ridge to avoid fracture of the unset amalgam. Finally, the marginal Y shaped spillway is created to deflect food away from the contact area. The surface is then smoothed using either a wet or dry cotton wool pellet. At a subsequent visit, the hardened surface can be perfected with multi-fluted steel burs of various shapes and polished using impregnated rubber points and a slurry of zinc oxide powder and alcohol. This produces a highly reflective Beilby layer on the surface of the restoration.

The finishing and polishing of composite resin restorations differs in that polymerised excess material has to be removed using diamond or tungsten carbide burs in an air turbine handpiece. The danger is that the surface of the enamel is roughened by this process. The marginal ridge is perfected while the matrix band is still in place to help protect the adjacent tooth. After removal of the matrix, the anatomy of the occlusal surface can be accentuated using a range of diamond and tungsten carbide burs or a tapered white stone. Finally, the surface can be polished using a series of abrasive impregnated discs and points. These may contain alumina or industrial diamond grit. The surface of the restoration can be polished using a diamond polishing paste to bring it to a lustrous finish.

The Extensive Restoration

A large multi-surface cavity can result from the ravages of untreated caries that undermine marginal ridges and cusps or from the fracture of weak cusps in a heavily restored tooth. The problem with such large cavities lies in their successful restoration.

Such a tooth needs to be carefully assessed, and it should be '**PROVed**' that a new restoration is advocated.

P for perio: A BPE (Basic Periodontal Examination) of the mouth and a six point pocket measurement should be undertaken around the tooth. If the margins of the cavity are subgingival, some periodontal surgery may be advocated to make the margins supragingival.

R for restorative condition: The tooth should be assessed with a bitewing and periapical radiographs to see the extent of the caries and its proximity to the dental pulp. The periapical radiograph will show the number of roots and their curvature should root canal therapy be required.

O for occlusion: The way the upper and lower teeth meet in the intercuspal position and during lateral guidance should be studied and adjusted if necessary to avoid detrimental forces. Study models are useful for this purpose too.

V for vitality: Sensibility testing will show if the tooth has turned non-vital due to amount and extent of previous restorations or caries. A periapical radiograph should also be examined to see if there is any apical change in appearance or if the tooth has been previously root treated.

E for endodontics: The quality of any previous root treatment should be assessed using a periapical radiograph. The tooth should have re-root treatment if significant faults can be identified or if symptoms of an endodontic origin are associated with the tooth.

The old restoration should be removed by sectioning it into various pieces and elevating these from the cavity. This helps avoid unnecessary tooth removal that could occur if the restoration is drilled out. The caries is removed from the enamel dentine junction to render this area caries free. The deeper caries over the pulp should be treated carefully to avoid exposure. This can be done by removing the soft dentine, but, as demineralisation precedes bacterial penetration, stained dentine can be left if it is felt that its removal would result in an exposure. This area can be indirectly pulp capped using a setting calcium hydroxide cement that will positively stimulate the pulp to lay down reparative dentine.

The choice of restorative material should be carefully assessed, and if the cavity is surrounded by enamel, composite resin would be a good choice because it can use micro-mechanical retention to retain the restoration and support areas of slightly unsupported tooth structure. Otherwise an amalgam can be used using undercuts, slots, and grooves or dentine pins for retention. These materials can be further supported by covering with a crown.

The use of dentine pins has reduced markedly over the last decade because it has been found that many errors can be encountered during or after their placement. Generally, one dentine pin is used for each missing cusp, but these must be placed to avoid such areas as pulp horns or over furcation areas. The insertion of pins weakens both the remaining tooth and the restoration. The pin holes are made to a depth of 2.5 mm and should be placed at least 1 mm in from the enamel dentine junction. The diameter of the pin hole varies with the size of pin but generally ranges from 0.5 to 0.7 mm. The pin hole should be parallel to the outer surface of the tooth to avoid perforation of the pulp or periodontal membrane. The technique sensitive nature of placement and the high incidence of postoperative complications has resulted in clinicians preferring to use slots and grooves for retention as well as bonding to tooth structure.

Summary

- It is important to remove the contact point because this is the stagnation area where caries initiate
- The internal line angles in the cavity should be rounded to avoid stress concentrations and failure
- Unsupported enamel must be removed to maintain the integrity of the restoration in the longer term
- The adjacent tooth should be protected from damage during cavity preparation
- Always inspect the cavity design to ensure that there is adequate resistance and retention for the material that will be used to restore the tooth

Clinical Guide to Restoring an Interproximal Lesion with a Self-Retentive Box

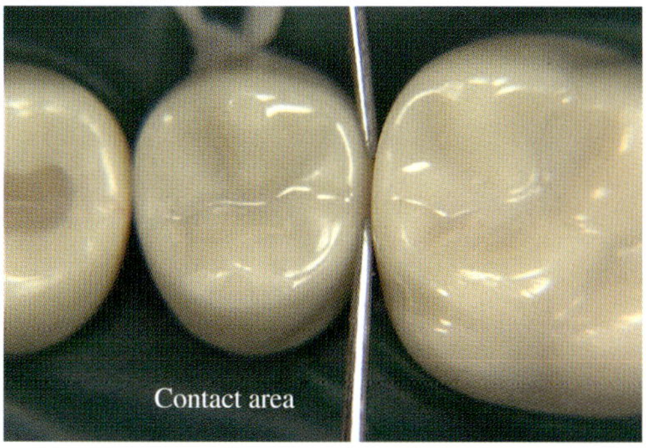

By placing a probe into the embrasure on either side of the contact area, the width of the contact can be seen clearly.
Caries initiate just below the contact area as a white spot lesion. The probes will help students to visualise where the initial lesion is likely to be within the stagnation area.

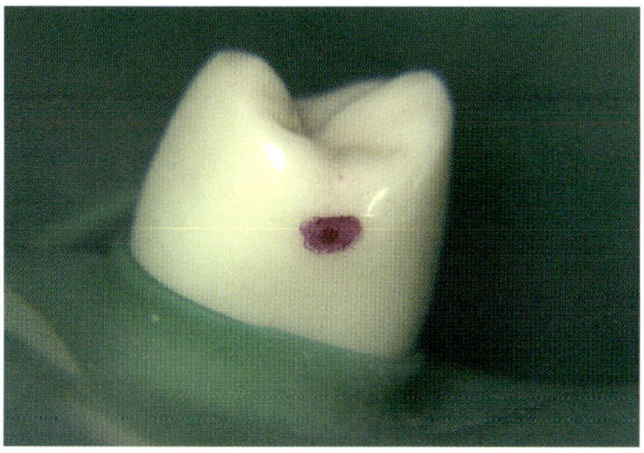

The shaded area represents the carious lesion. The lesion is 2 mm wide at the amelodentinal junction (ADJ) and is centred just below the contact point. The fissure in this tooth is completely free of caries.

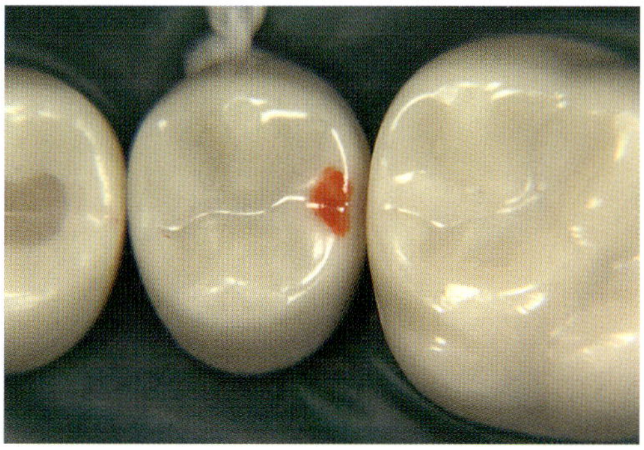

The shaded area in orange on the marginal ridge indicates the area of tooth structure that would need to be removed to gain access to the carious lesion lying immediately below.

Where fissures are not carious there is no need to remove them to provide access to the mesial lesion or for the retention of the filling material.

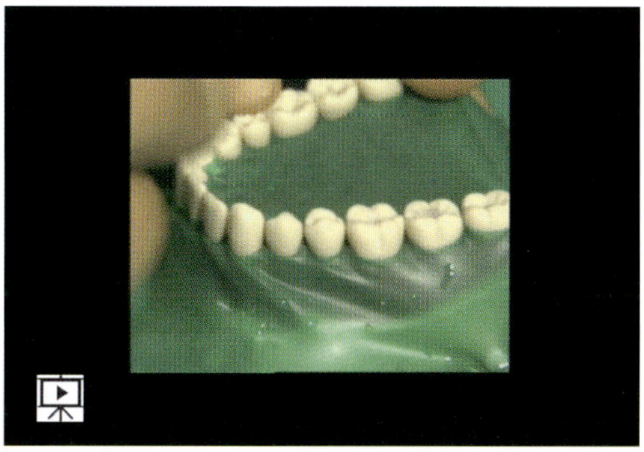

Video 6.1 and Video 6.2

The shaded area at the marginal ridge may be removed using a small round F/G bur. The bur shown is a tungsten carbide bur with cutting flutes but a diamond coated bur can be used equally well. This is used in the air turbine handpiece operating with a free running speed of 450,000 rpm.

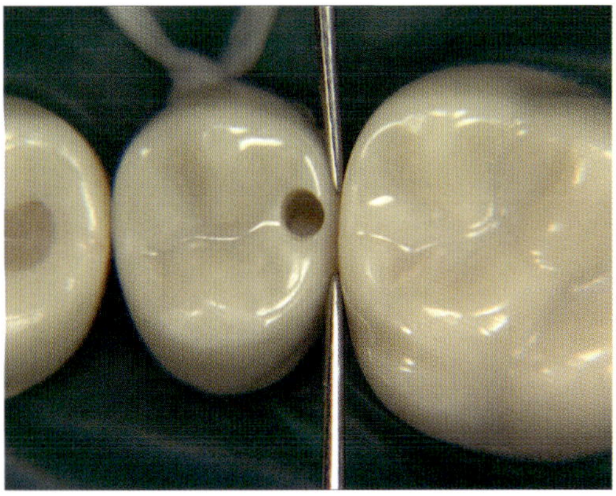

A small plunge cut is made into the middle of the contact area so that the bur will drop cervically to a level at the gingival aspect of the caries (~3 mm).

It is important that this cut is made within the marginal ridge area to avoid traumatising the adjacent tooth.

The initial penetration of the bur should extend to the level of the carious lesion.

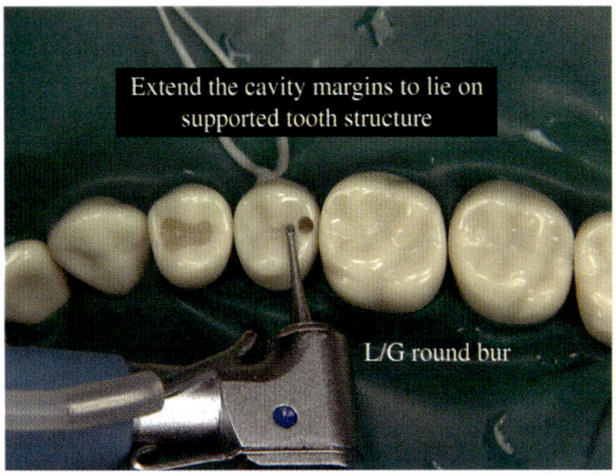

To avoid over-cutting the cavity, slower-speed rotary instruments are then used.

A round bur may be employed to move down into the carious lesion and also to thin the marginal wall until it is paper thin. In this way, it will be unsupported and easy to fracture using hand instruments.

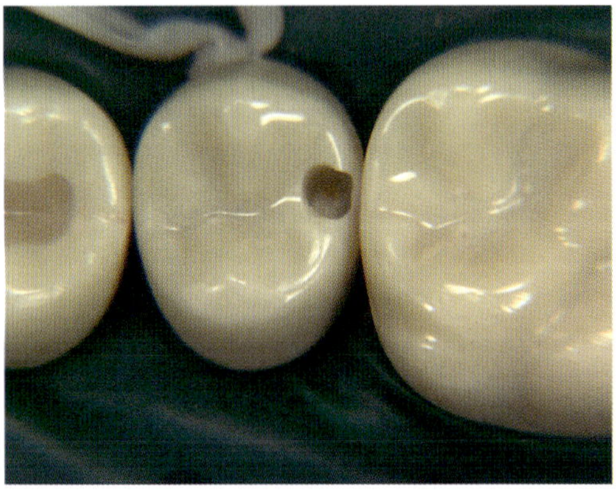

This slide shows the extension of the cavity towards the gingival tissues and the thinning of the marginal and distal enamel.

Clinically, if the lesion had cavitated, a small area of open cavity may be visible in the middle of the distal wall.

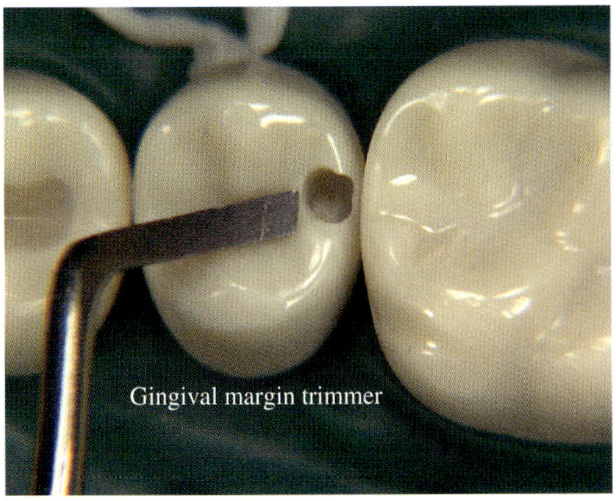

Unsupported enamel can be removed using a gingival margin trimmer to avoid damage to the adjacent tooth.

Should damage occur to this surface, a new carious lesion is likely to result quickly.

Some operators protect the adjacent tooth using a metal matrix band, but this can be easily damaged by rotary instruments.

Video 6.3

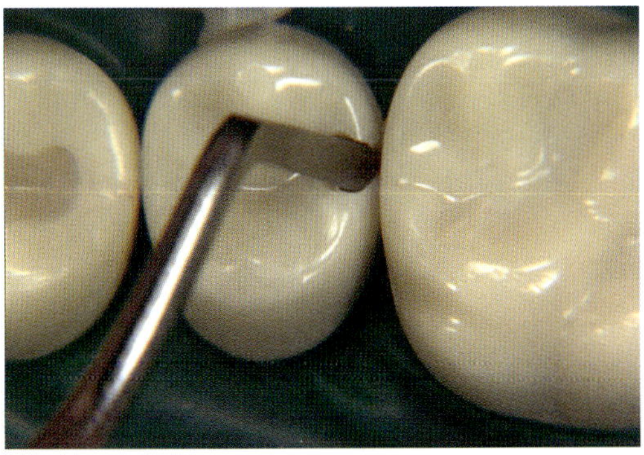

Some of the distal wall has been fractured out by applying a moderate finger pressure using trimmer.

The sharp leading edge of this instrument will fracture unsupported or thin enamel.

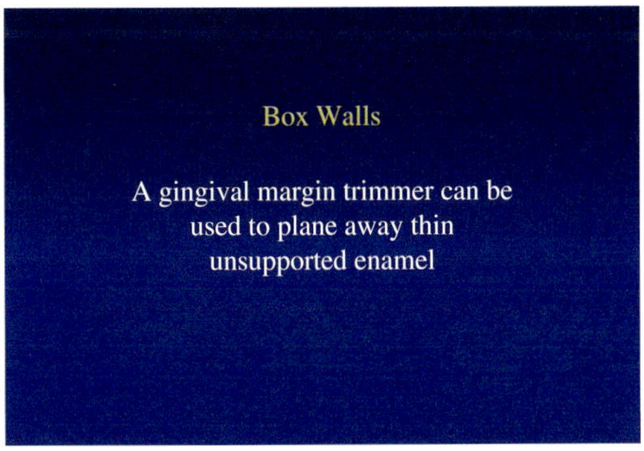

The use of rotary instruments in small boxes may result in damage to the adjacent tooth surfaces.

The unsupported enamel prisms can be planed away using the cutting edge of the gingival margin trimmer. The curve of the blade should be applied to the wall being prepared.

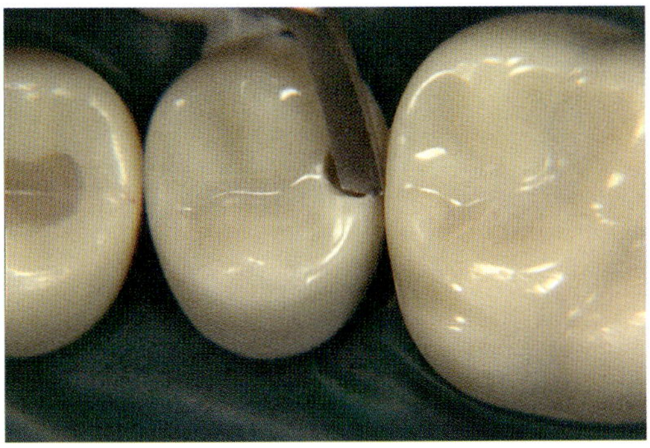

The other side of the instrument is then applied to the opposite box wall.

The longer side of the cutting edge is always placed towards the outer surface of the tooth, and the curve of the blade always faces the surface being instrumented.

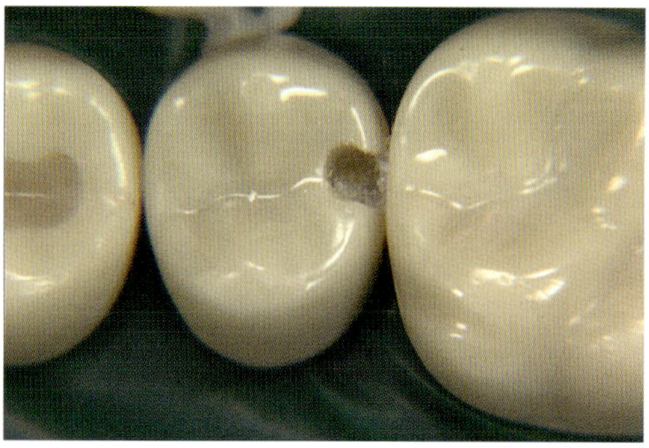

This should result in a narrow box with almost butt joints onto the approximaltooth surface. The cavo-surface angle should be approximately 90° to ensure no unsupported prisms are left at the periphery of the cavity.

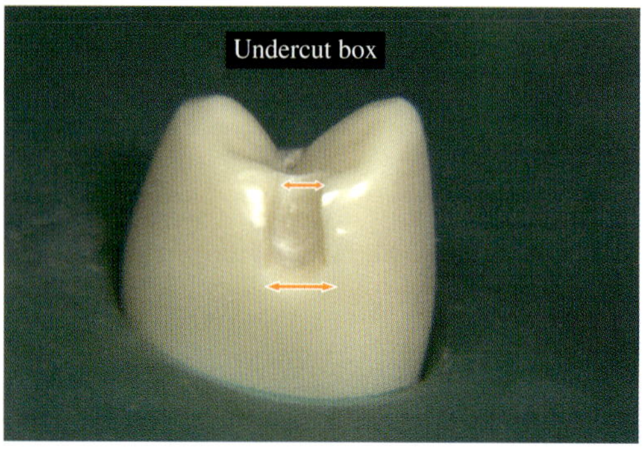

This view of the tooth is from the mesial surface and shows the undercut on the box with its narrower dimension towards the occlusal surface.

The gingival floor of the box is rounded at this stage and represents the shape of the carious lesion that was present.

Decalcification may still be present along the base of the gingival floor at this stage.

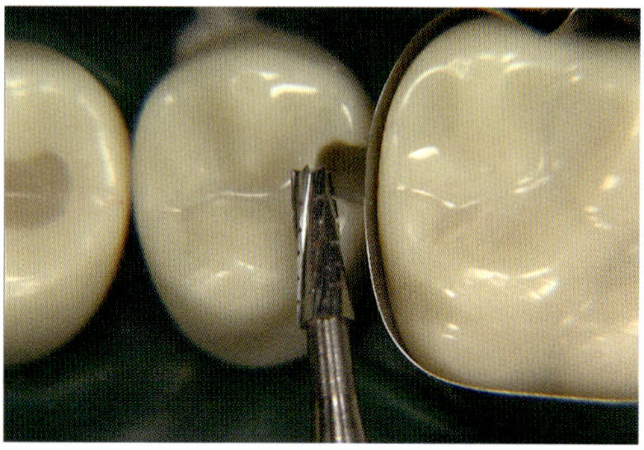

Some operators apply a stainless steel matrix band to the adjacent tooth to help protect it during preparation of the gingival floor.

To achieve a good seal of the filling material to the walls and floor of the cavity they should be smooth.

The tapering anatomy of the premolar crown means that the gingival margin is reasonably clear of the adjacent tooth. In the accompanying picture the tapered fissure bur is being used to smooth the floor of the box.

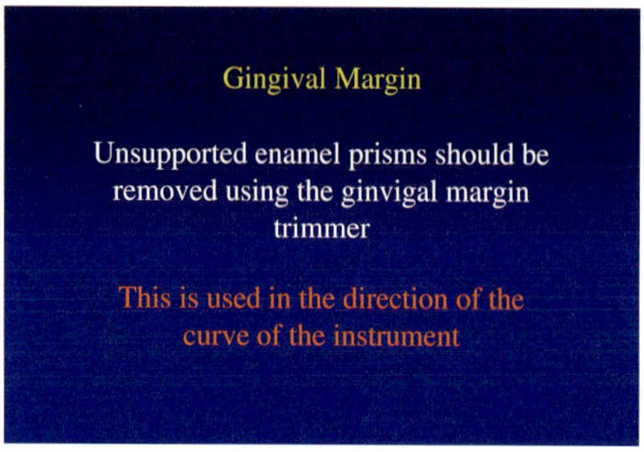

Due to the nature of the prism direction in the cervical third of the tooth, unsupported prisms will be present even when the floor is finished at right angles to the long axis of the tooth.

A gingival margin trimmer should be used with a sweeping action directed to accord with the curve of the instrument and ensuring that the point of the cutting edge is directed towards the soft tissues.

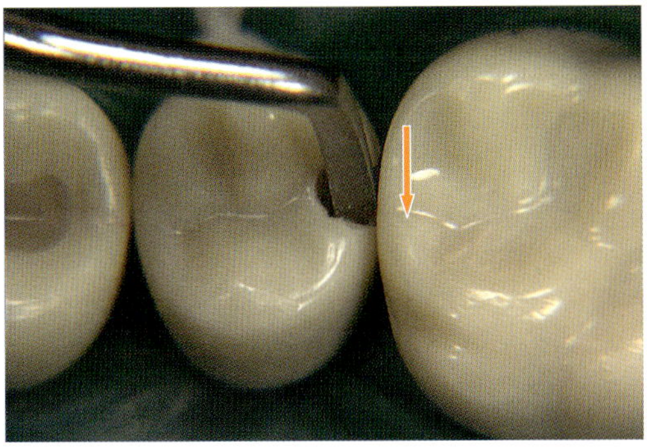

In this view the instrument is being swept towards the palatal side of the tooth, removing unsupported enamel prisms from the gingival floor.

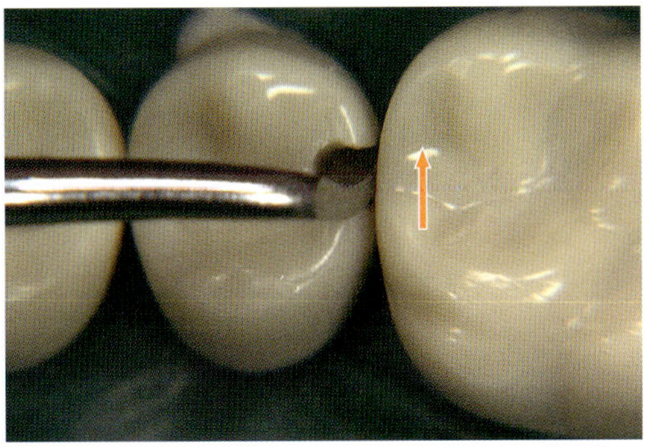

The other end of the instrument is curved in the opposite direction and can be used to sweep towards the buccal side of the box floor.

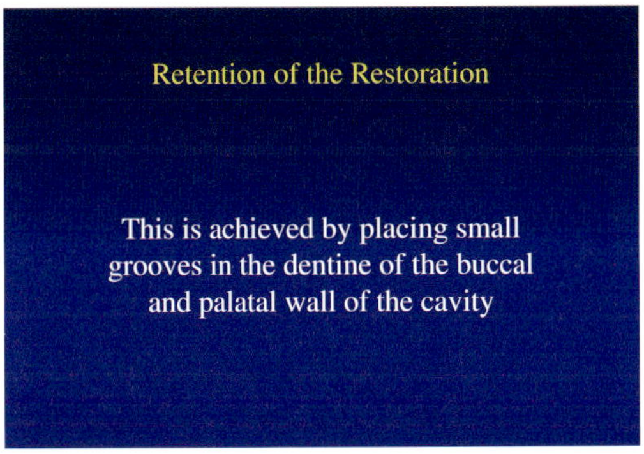

The cavity could be restored with either composite resin or compomer material, but if a non-adhesive material is being used in its restoration, retention factors should be considered for the cavity design.

Small grooves can be placed in the dentine on the walls of the box.

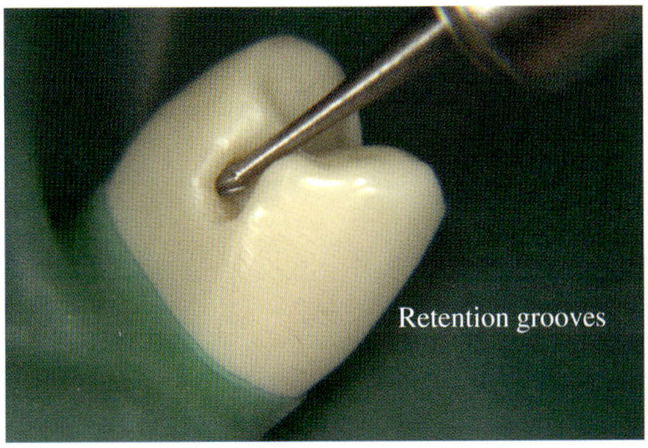

These are achieved by using a small round bur in the slow-speed handpiece.

The grooves are placed in the dentine, but care should be taken to ensure that their depth is not so great as to result in unsupported enamel at the box walls.

Video 6.4

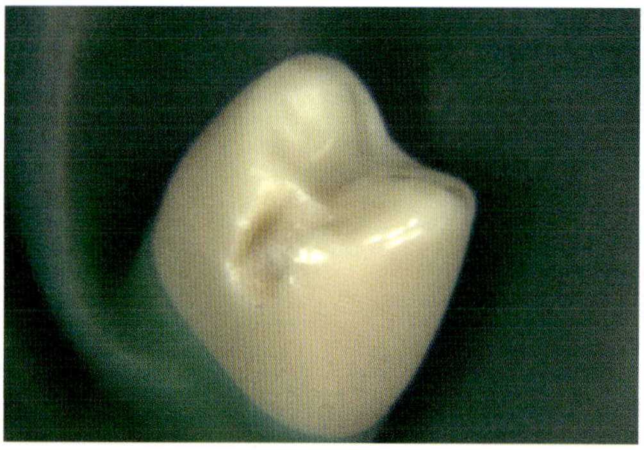

This view shows the position and shape of the groove preparation in the palatal wall of the box.

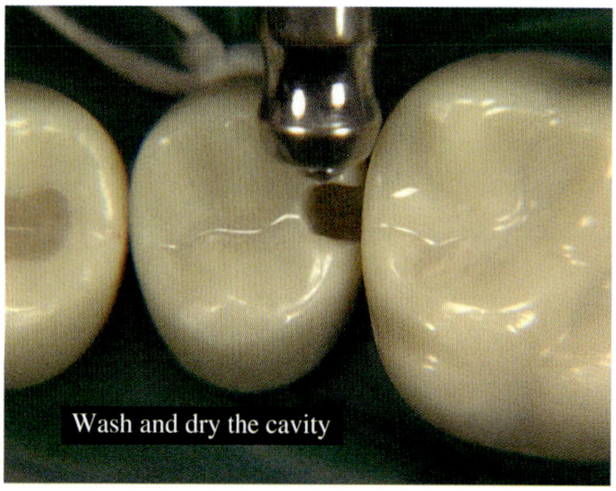

The last stage of cavity preparation involves a thorough wash and dry of the cavity with a careful inspection of the enamel margins and dentine surfaces for signs of decalcification.

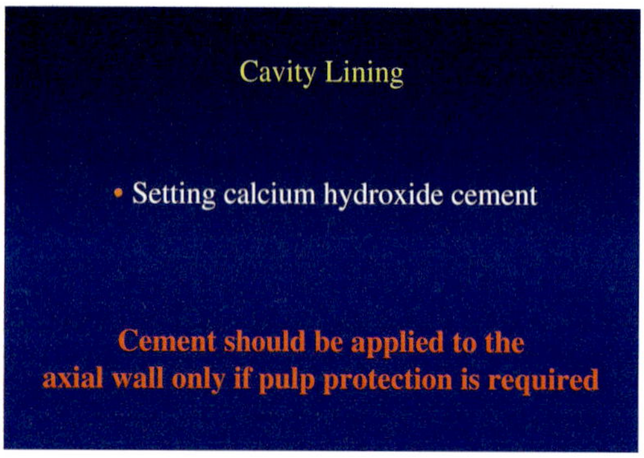

The cavity is lined to protect the pulp from chemical and thermal stimuli.

In this sequence a setting calcium hydroxide cement is used.

A light-cured polyalkenoate cement could be used as an alternative.

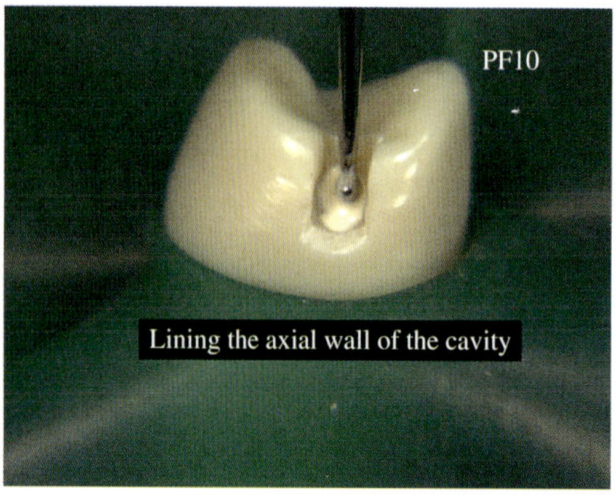

The cement is mixed and transferred to the cavity on the ball end of the PF10 instrument. The material is applied to the axial wall of the cavity only.

The enamel margins should not be lined because dissolution of the material will take place resulting in deficiencies at the margin of the filling.

This may give rise to sensitivity, secondary caries, and pulpal disease.

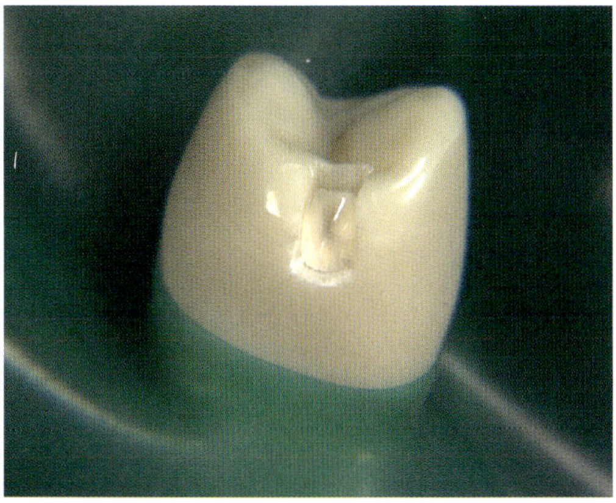

Any excess lining material that has spread towards the margins or into the undercut grooves must be removed using a sharp excavator.

This slide shows the material has been kept back from the enamel towards the occlusal surface.

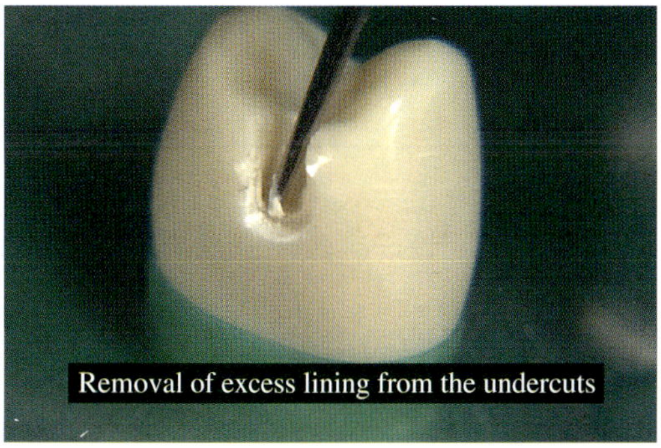

Excess material can be removed from the box walls, undercuts, and gingival floor using a sharp instrument such as this right angled probe.

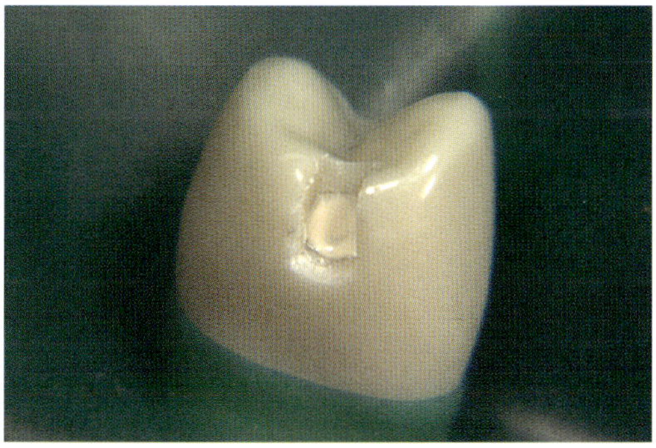

The gingival floor is now clear of excess lining material and is available for forming a hermitic seal with the filling material.

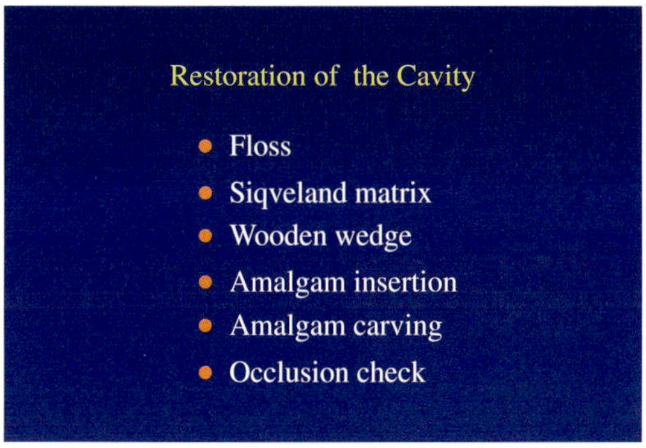

Shown here are the stages of the cavity restoration and finishing.

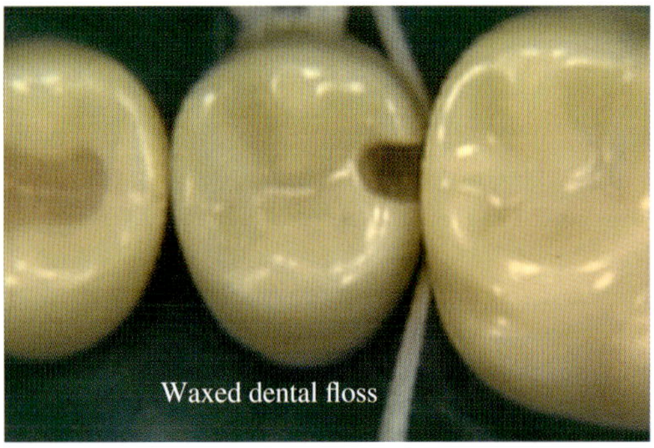

The floss has been inserted and its position is checked to ensure that it is below the gingival floor of the box preparation.

This will be used later to remove small amounts of excess amalgam from the gingival aspect of the restoration.

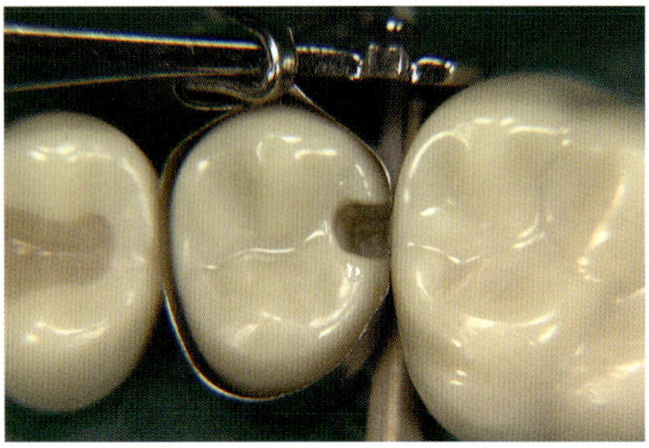

The Siqveland matrix band and holder (retainer) are applied to the tooth with the latch engaged towards the gingival aspect. This narrows the band to conform better to the flared tooth shape. A single use matrix band could also be used.

A wooden wedge has been placed from the palatal surface. This is used to adapt the band more closely to the gingival tooth structure and prevent excess material being packed past the gingival margin.

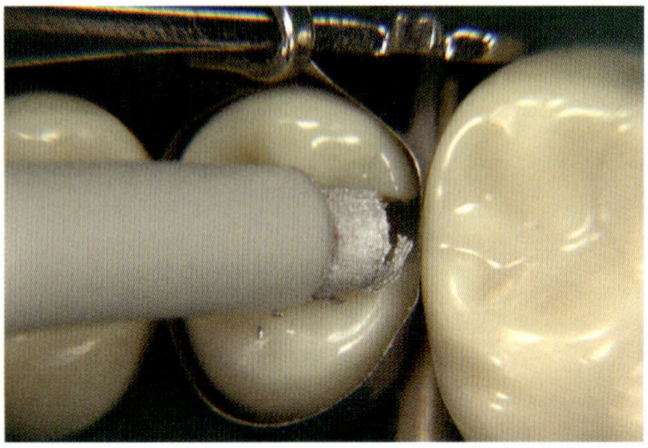

The first small increment of amalgam is transferred to the cavity using the carrier.

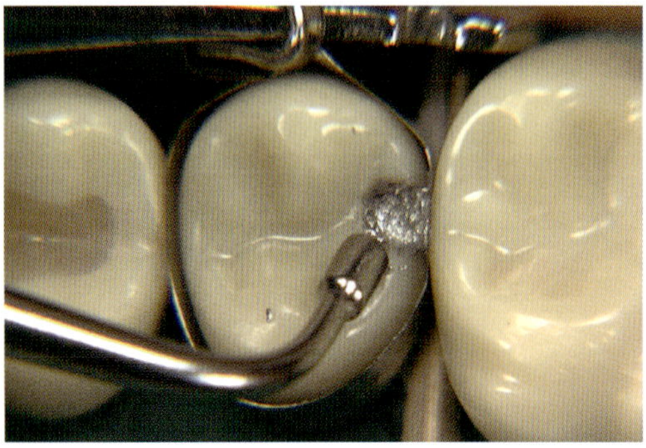

It is adapted to the gingival floor of the cavity using the amalgam plugger. An instrument small enough to reach the cavity floor must be selected.

It is used in two distinct actions:

- Vertical condensation
- Horizontal sweeping

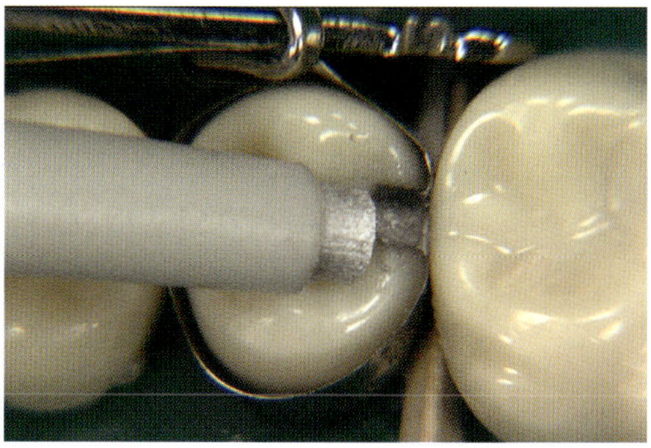

The mercury rich layer is removed, and further small increments of filling material are offered into the cavity.

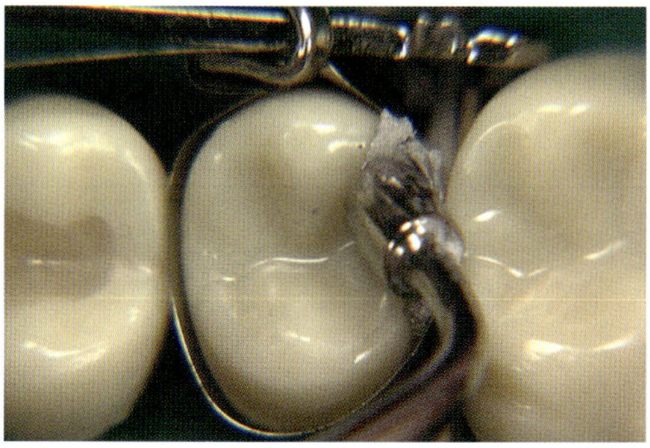

The condensation is repeated until the cavity is slightly overfilled.

The final layer of amalgam is condensed with the surface of the packing tip parallel to the cusp slopes. This commences the shaping of the final filling.

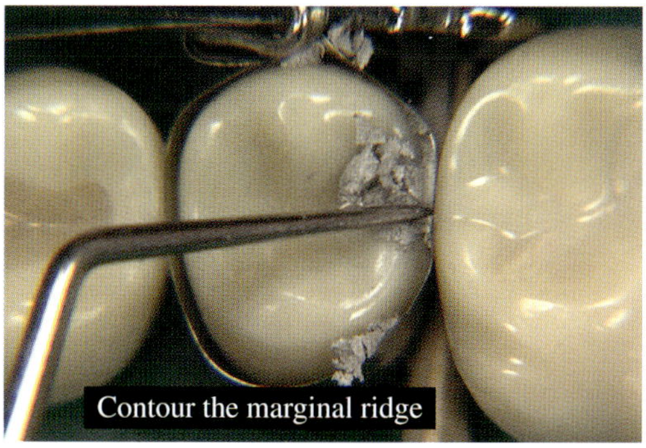

The marginal ridge is contoured using a right angled probe held at 45° to the matrix band.

Excess material is removed with a clean sweep of the instrument around the inner aspect of the band.

Ensure that the marginal ridge is placed at a similar height to that of the adjacent marginal ridge – avoid an upward step because this will be high in the occlusion and fracture during function.

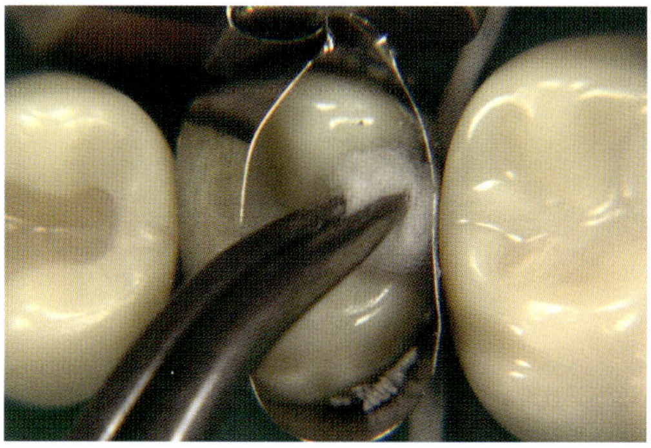

The wedge is removed and the band slackened.

The matrix is then removed carefully because undue pressure could fracture the amalgam before the material has had a chance to set.

If the marginal ridge of the filling is supported with a small pledget of cotton wool during this stage, the risk of fracture will be minimised.

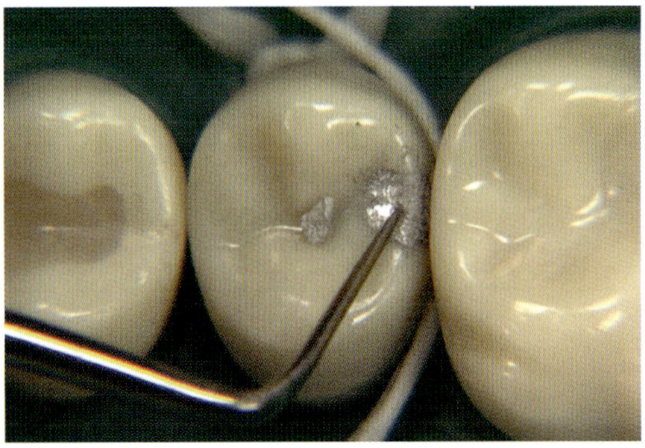

The occlusal surface of the filling can then be carved to conform with the surface anatomy of the tooth.

The half-Hollenbach amalgam carver is shown in this slide. The sharp side of the blade is laid parallel to the adjacent enamel surface and excess material removed by carving away from the marginal ridge.

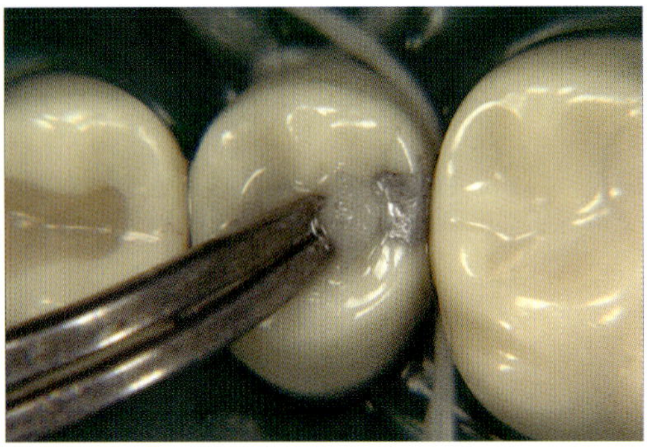

The surface of the restoration is smoothed using a small pledget of cotton wool.

There is some debate over the most appropriate manner to smooth amalgam surfaces after carving. Some operators prefer to use a wet pledget of cotton wool while others advocate a dry application. Some other workers have recently shown that a small piece of rolled up tissue paper works best.

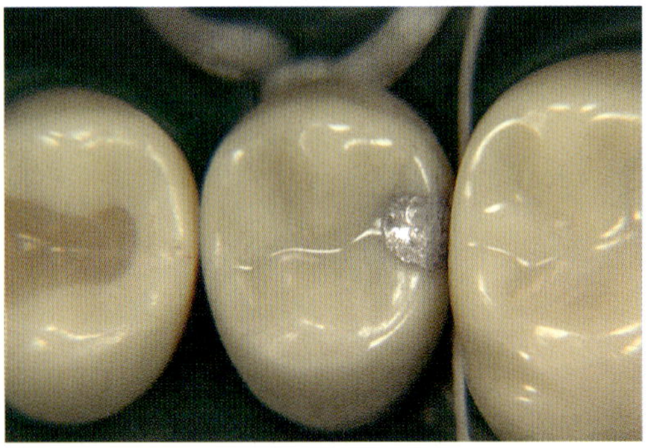

The floss can then be used to sweep across the gingival aspect of the restoration to remove excess material.

On no account should the floss be brought up through the contact point of the tooth as this may:

- Fracture the recently placed amalgam filling
- Result in a poorer quality of contact

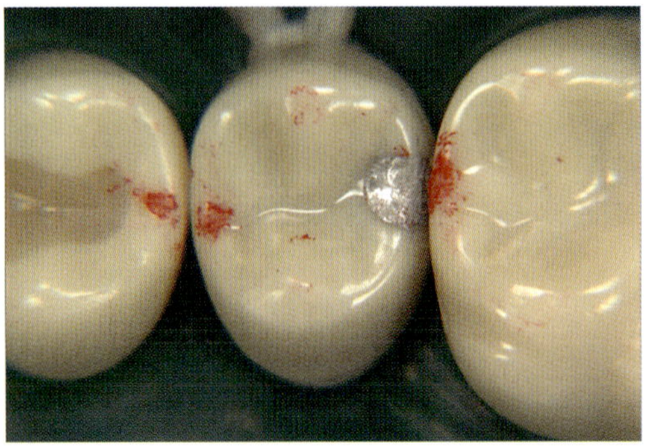

The occlusion is then checked using articulating paper.

Opposing cusps contact onto the marginal ridges so patient should be instructed to close gently until the first contact is reached.

In this way, fracture of the recently placed amalgam may be avoided.

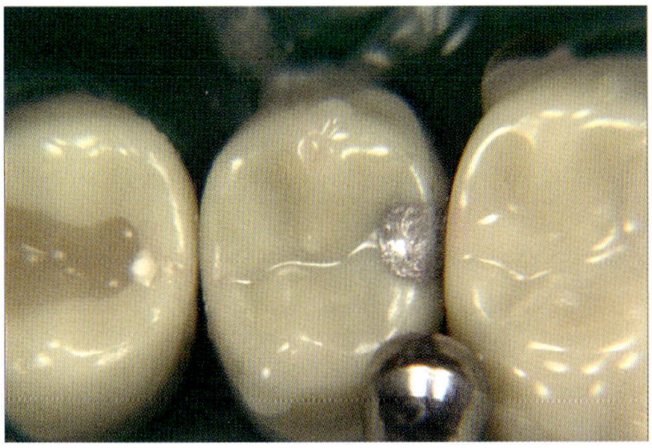

Wash thoroughly the contact area using the triple dental syringe.

This view shows the conservative restoration of an approximal carious lesion with no fissure involvement.

Clinical Guide to Restoring a Class II Lesion with Composite Resin

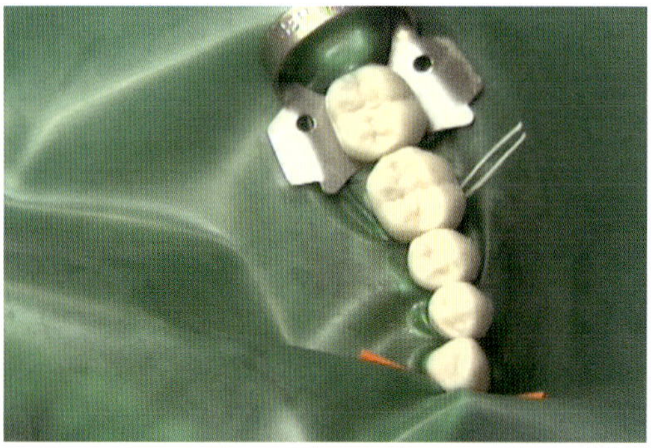

The mandibular first molar tooth has five cusps in total because there are three cusps on the buccal side.

The occlusal surface has a complex fissure pattern.

The marginal ridges of the adjacent teeth normally lie at a similar level unless the teeth are tilted following extraction of a tooth more mesial in the quadrant or if the tooth has over-erupted after the loss of an opposing tooth.

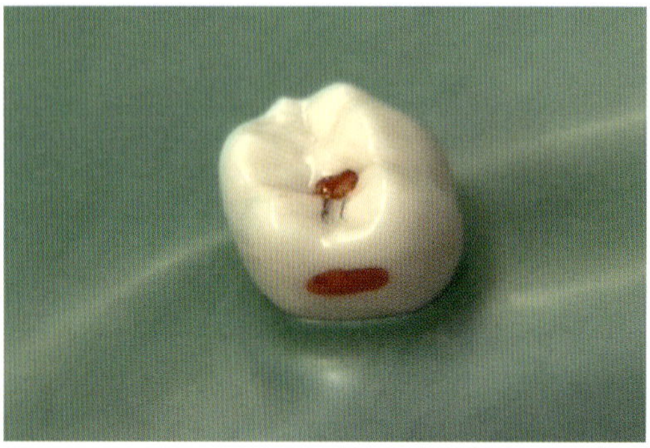

Superimposed on this tooth are the carious lesions at the ADJ.

The carious lesion on the mesial surface of the tooth has progressed about 1 mm into the underlying dentine.

The occlusal caries in the area indicated has also progressed into the dentine by about 1 mm. The caries in the fissure between the indicated area and the mesial marginal ridge has just reached the enamel dentine junction.

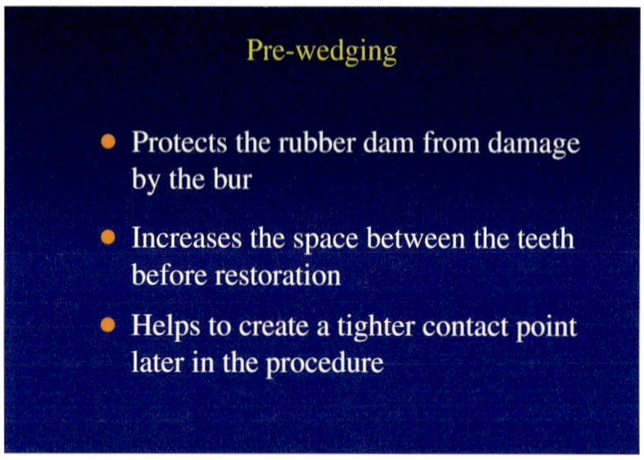

Placement of a wedge between the teeth has many advantages in that it will protect the rubber dam from damage during the cavity preparation.
It has also the beneficial effect of moving the teeth apart so that the contact can be over-built slightly, resulting in a tighter contact after the restoration has been placed and the wedge removed.

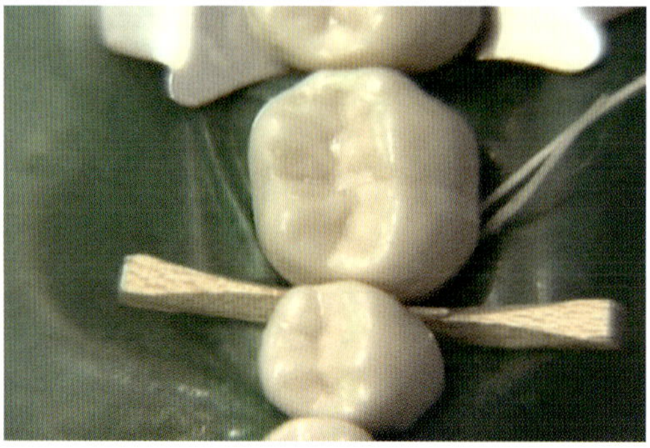

The insertion of a large wooden wedge from both the lingual and buccal sides is shown in this view.

This has the effect of creating a little space between the two molar teeth.

Each of these teeth can only move by the thickness of the periodontal ligament when the periodontium is healthy.

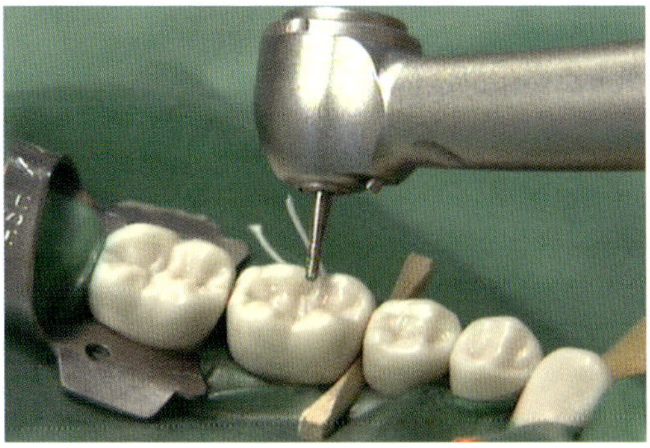

The bur used to prepare this cavity is the F/G dome-shaped cylindrical diamond bur used in the air turbine handpiece.

This particular bur is the 544, which has a diameter of 1 mm.

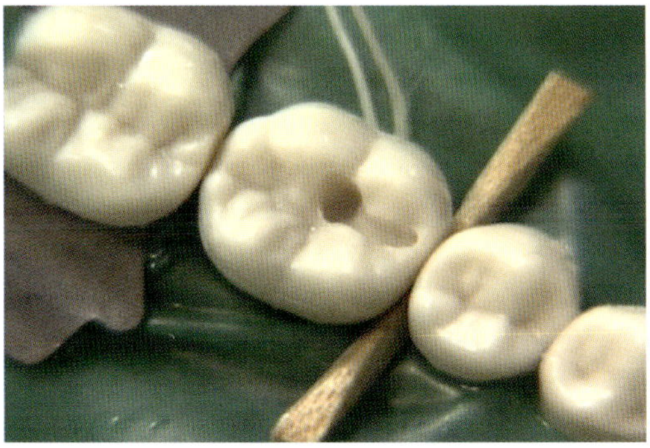

The initial cut is made into the main part of the carious lesion underlying the seemingly intact enamel surface.

The initial cut is then extended along the mesial fissure towards the marginal ridge where the interproximal carious lesion is present. At this time, the bur should be just into the dentine and should therefore be approximately 2 mm deep.

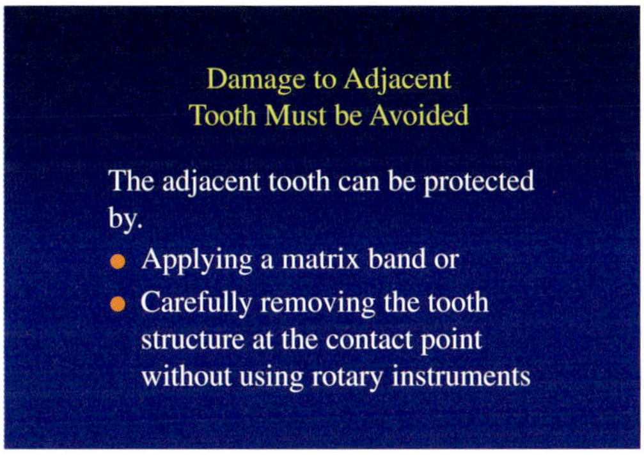

Fracturing out this surface by breaking the contact with a gingival margin trimmer is the best way to avoid adjacent tooth damage.

Placement of a matrix band will protect the adjacent tooth from only light damage with the bur if this method is used.

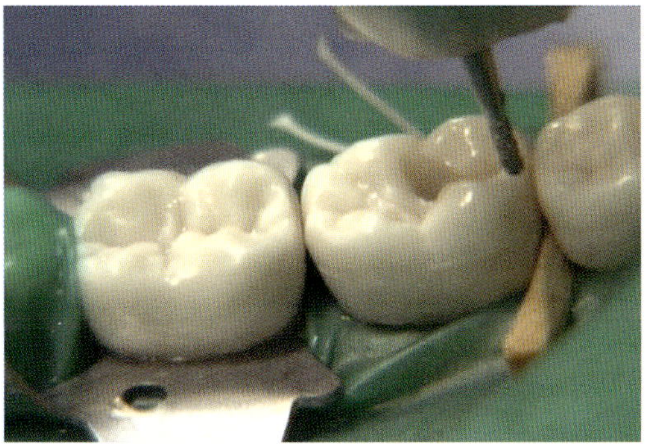

The bur is replaced into the mesial aspect of the cavity and extended towards the middle of the contact area where the caries is present. The tip of the bur will meet the carious lesion in this position and should be introduced through the caries onto the sound tooth structure found at a more gingival level.

The handpiece should then be moved using a short pendulum motion so that a rounded floor will be created and the walls of the box preparation will be undercut with a wider aspect near the gingival floor.

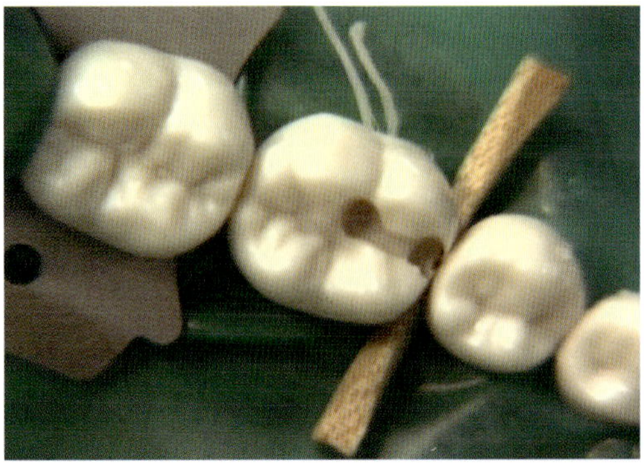

When the enamel surface is paper thin, it can be removed readily with hand instruments.

A gingival margin trimmer is useful for this purpose because it has a sharp leading edge to cleave enamel prisms.

In the adjacent picture the thin margin of mesial enamel has fractured away, leaving unsupported enamel to either side of the box. If this were left, it would fracture in function and leave a deficient restoration.

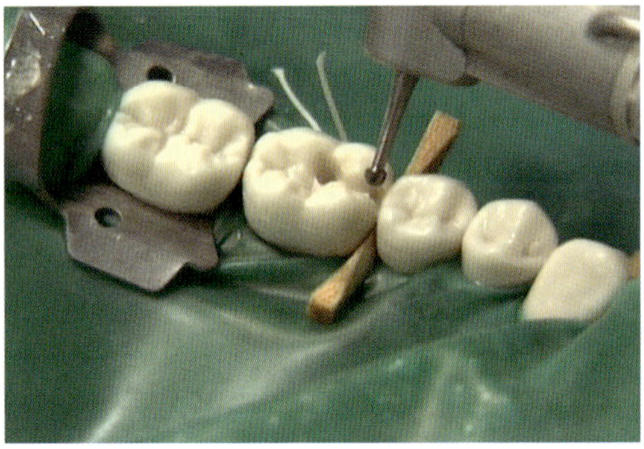

Caries is removed from the dentine at the enamel dentine junction along the gingival floor and from the latter aspect of the box walls.

Care must be exercised to ensure that the adjacent tooth is not subjected to iatrogenic damaged at this stage.

This stage may produce even more unsupported enamel at the buccal and lingual walls of the box.

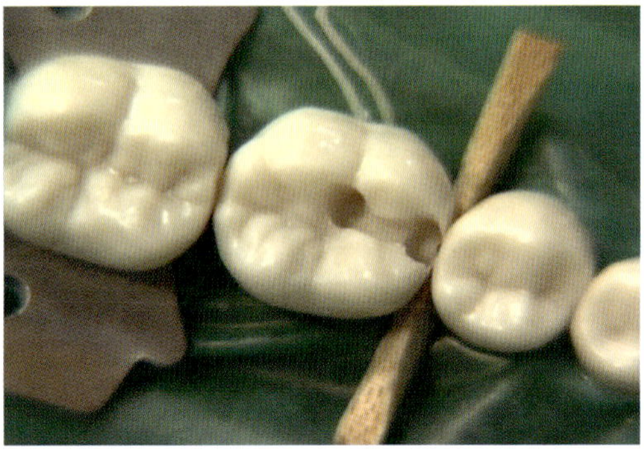

The caries has been removed but the unsupported enamel at the gingival floor and lateral walls of the box can be seen readily in this view.

These must be removed to produce a cavity with prisms that run perpendicularly to the surface of the tooth and produce a favourable cavo-surface angle for the material to be used in the restoration.

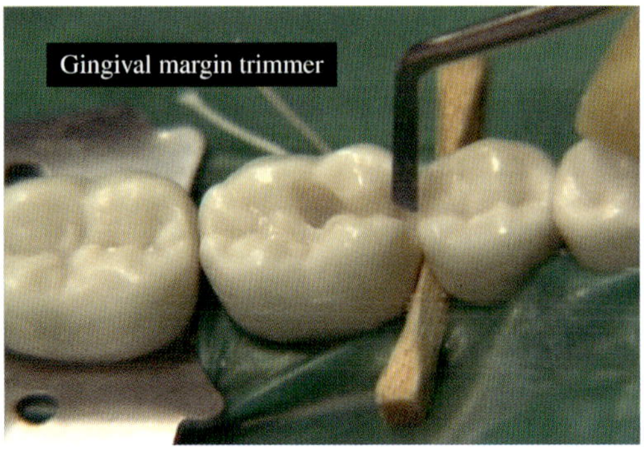

The sharp cutting edge of the gingival margin trimmer can then be used to remove the thin area of unsupported enamel.

Pressure applied to the prismatic enamel will remove this thin structure readily.

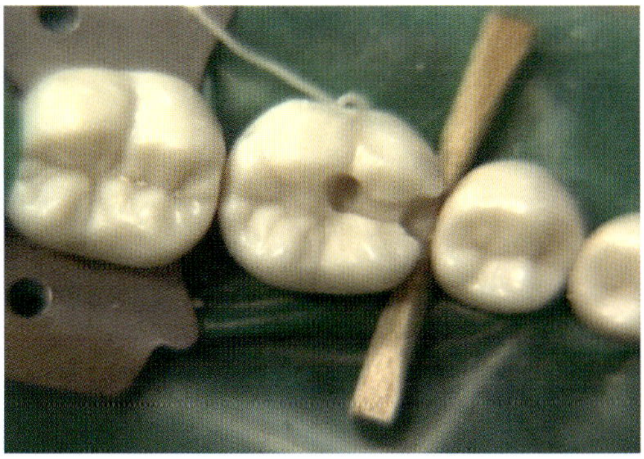

The unsupported tooth structure has been removed, and, in this case, this has taken the box walls to be clear of the contact area.

The box walls may be taken sufficiently lateral so that a toothbrush can clean the junction between the filling material and the surrounding enamel.

In this example, the size of the carious lesion has dictated that the box is slightly wider than the minimum width.

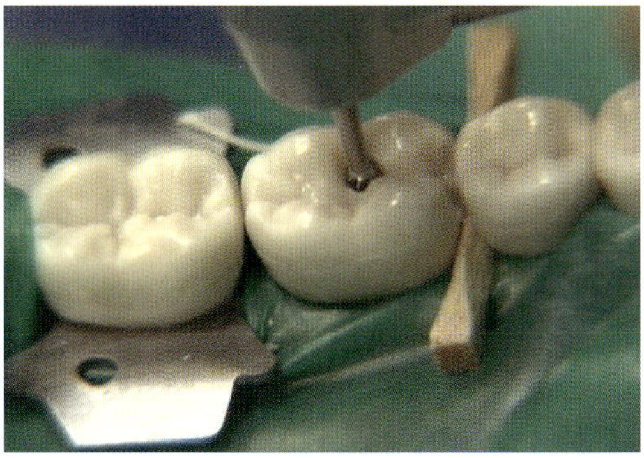

Caries is now cleared from the periphery of the deeper part of the occlusal lesion.

This can be achieved using a latch grip round bur operating at slow speed of approximately 3000 rpm. No water spray is required at this speed.

The ADJ should be left clear of staining and all areas of soft caries.

Frequent stops must be made to inspect the ADJ and ensure it is free from staining and is firm to probing.

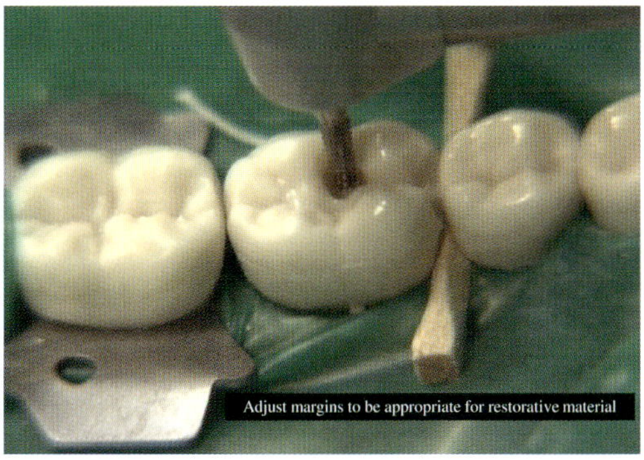

The outline of the occlusal cavity is then finished using the fissure bur shown.

This should ensure that the margin of the cavity is appropriate for the filling material that will be used to restore the tooth.

The margin of the cavity should be confluent in that it flows from one area to the next without sharp deviations.

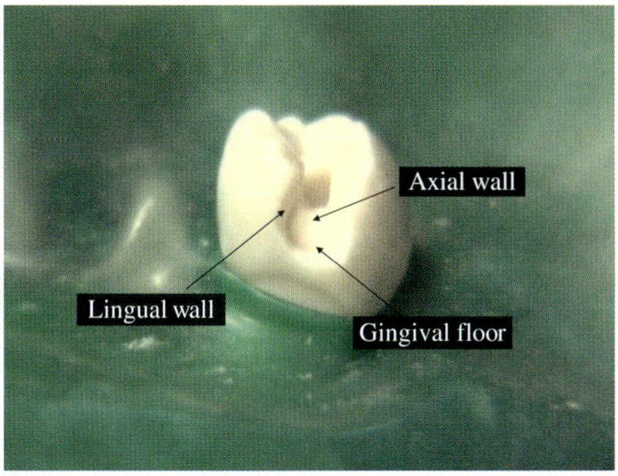

This view shows the box from the mesial aspect. The floor is rounded and the box is wider at its more gingival aspect, indicating that it would offer mechanical retention.

The axial wall joins the gingival floor to the pulpal floor of the occusal part of the cavity. This should be smooth and the junction between the above parts should be rounded to avoid stress concentration and maximise the thickness of the restorative material in this area.

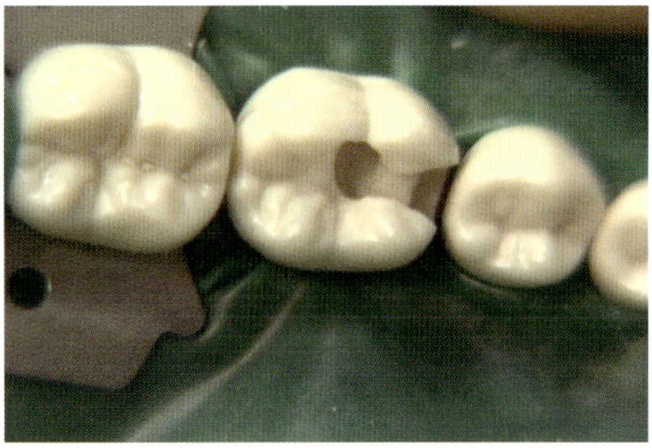

The outline has been smoothed and flows from one area to the next without sharp line angles that would concentrate stresses.
It is particularly important that sharp line angles are not present in the area of the isthmus–the narrower area between occlusal key and box. This area is under the most stress, and fractured fillings are often found in this area if they are too thin in cross section.
A lining is required only if the cavity is deep. The dentine bonding resin that will be applied next will seal the dentine.
Source: Dentsply Sirona.

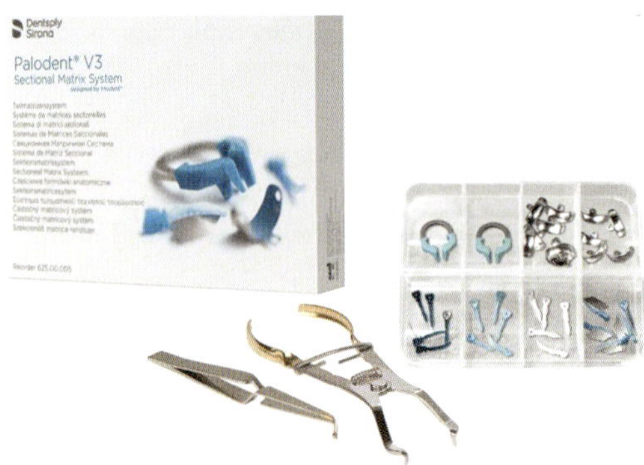

A matrix is required to contain the restorative material in the area where there is a missing wall of tooth.

The Palodent matrix system shown is a sectional matrix in which the small foil pieces are held in place using a spring steel BiTine ring.
This system provides a natural contour for better control of contact areas and embrasures.
Source: Dentsply Sirona.

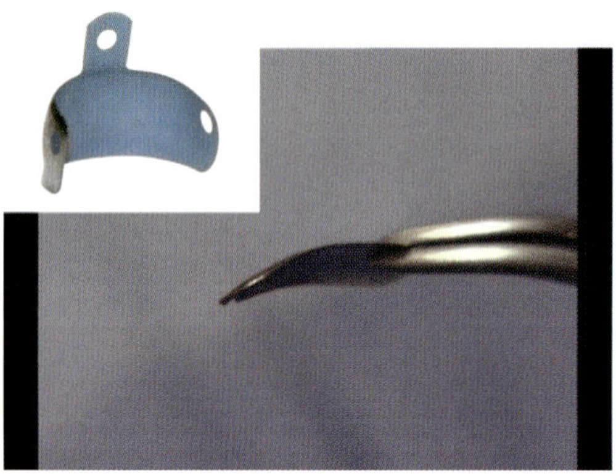

This picture shows the foil matrix of a sectional matrix system. The foil is held in place on the tooth using a BiTine ring. The operator can choose from five sizes of foil and two sizes of BiTine ring.
It has a convex contour both laterally and in an occluso-gingival direction. This allows the contact area to be re-established more easily and for the contour interproximally to be more anatomical.
The tab on the occlusal aspect can be used for ease of placement and adapted to the adjacent occlusal surface.
Source: Dentsply Sirona.

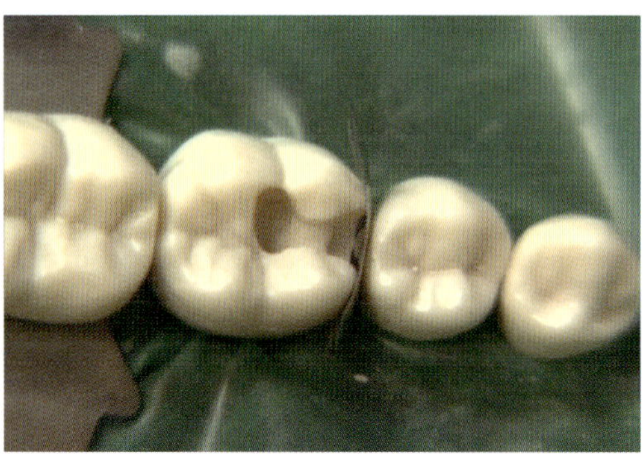

The matrix is inserted between the teeth immediately that the wedges used for tooth separation have been removed.

An appropriate size is selected that allows the matrix to be inserted to a position below the gingival floor. The upper aspect close to the occlusal surface should be positioned to form the marginal ridge at a level adjacent to that of the neighbouring tooth.
Source: Dentsply Sirona.

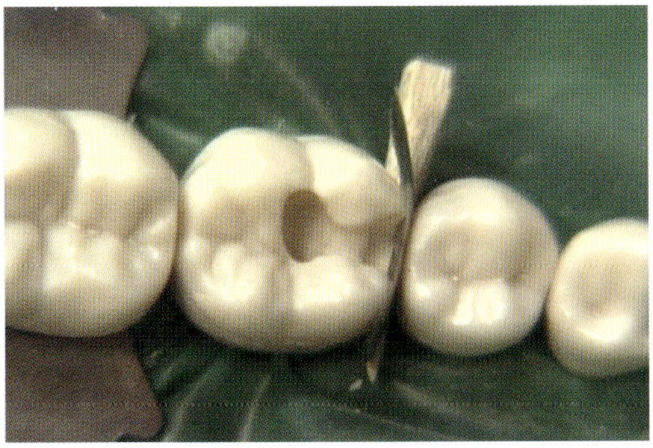

The sectional matrix is adapted at its gingival aspect by re-inserting a wedge while maintaining its correct position for the marginal ridge.
Source: Dentsply Sirona.

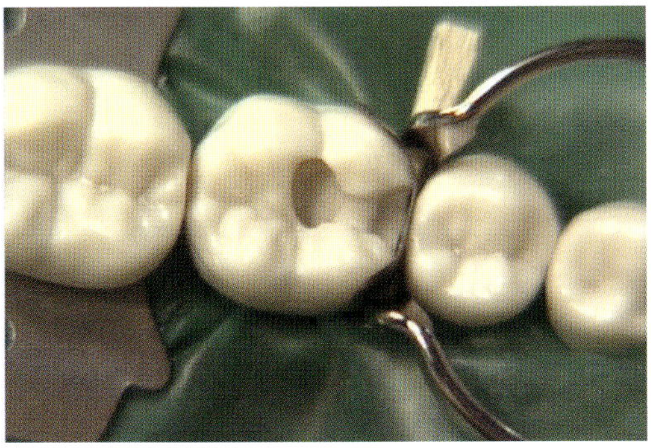

A BiTine spring ring is applied using the forceps. The vertical flanges on the ring adapt the sectional matrix laterally onto the tooth structure adjacent to the box preparation.
The contoured matrix should then form a good contact with the adjacent tooth while still maintaining a natural anatomical form.
If a three-surface MOD cavity is being restored, another matrix and ring can be applied. This is where the elliptical ring is most useful because it can fit over the circular ring.
Source: Dentsply Sirona.

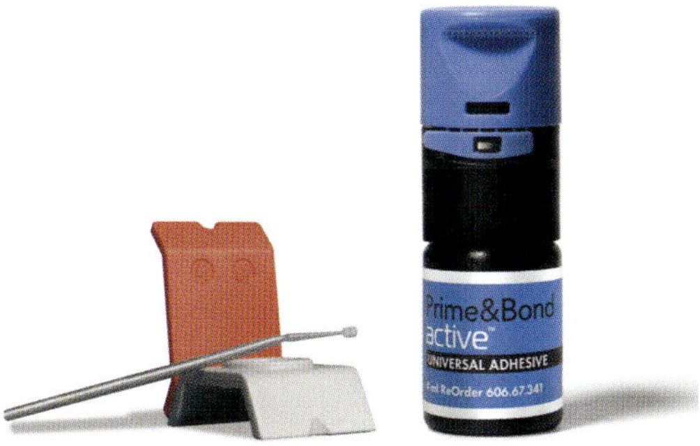

In this slide sequence a self etching primer will be used that etches enamel and dentine surfaces. It has the ability to penetrate the micromechanical pores that it creates in the enamel and also into the hybrid zone in the dentine.
Source: Dentsply Sirona.

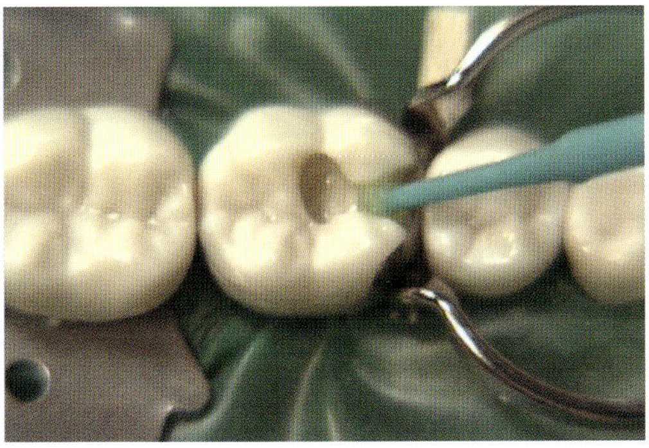

A self-etching primer is applied using a micro-brush. This will etch the enamel and dentine simultaneously and will penetrate the pores in the enamel and the hybrid zone on the dentine surface. It is left undisturbed for 30 seconds, after which the acidic content will have been neutralised but the attached resin component will have been carried into the micro-mechanical retention.
Source: Dentsply Sirona.

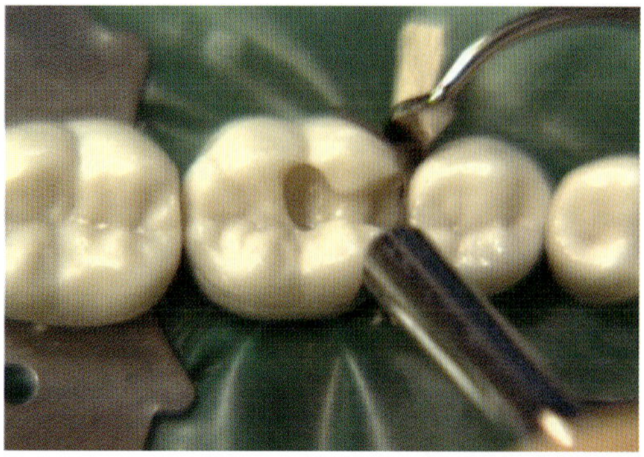

After 30 seconds, the solvent is evaporated from the acidic primer using a gentle stream of air from the triple dental syringe.

Xeno contains butanol as its solvent. This provides the material with a longer working time than other materials that use the more highly volatile solvent acetone.

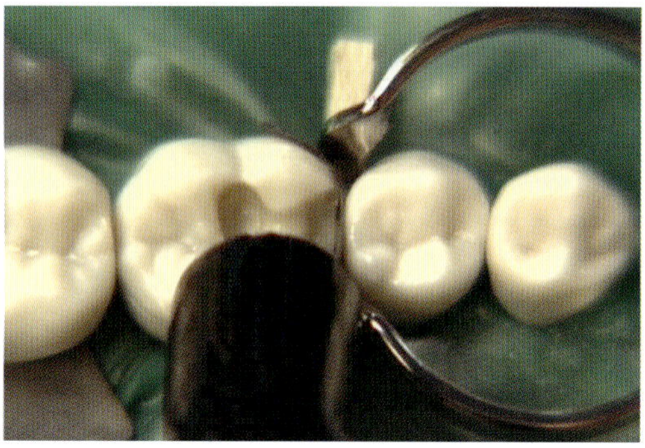

The bond is set by exposing the bonding resin to a 10 seconds application of the curing light.

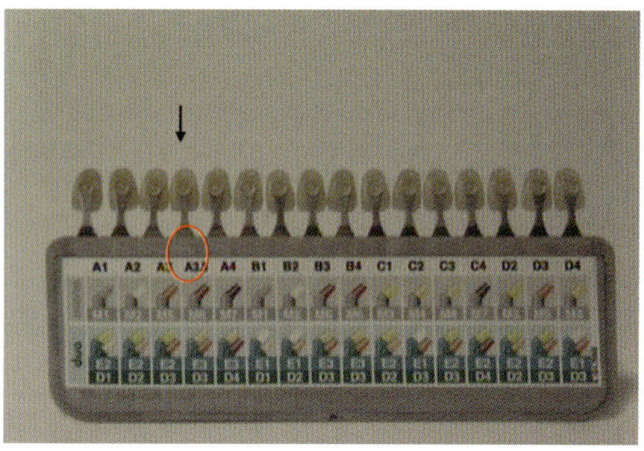

The shade is taken before the rubber dam is applied as teeth dry out under the dam and become lighter in shade.

The Vita shade guide can be used and the shade translated into an appropriate one for the Ceram X composite resin.

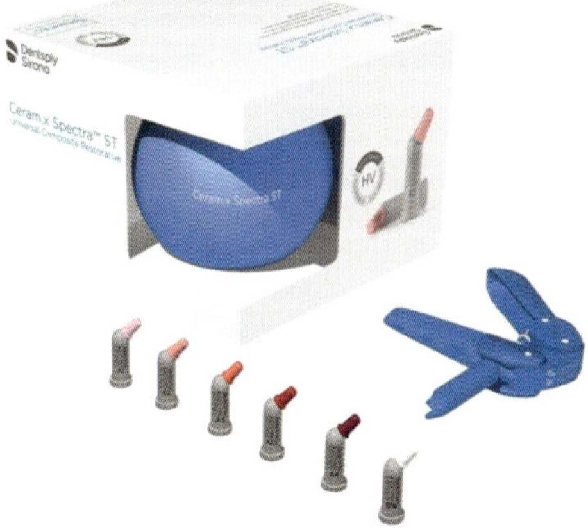

"Ceram X is a nano-hybrid composite resin with a variety of sizes of filler particles.

It is heavily filled and this imparts strength, wear resistance and minimal polymerisation shrinkage

Source: Printed by kind permission of Dentsply Sirona.

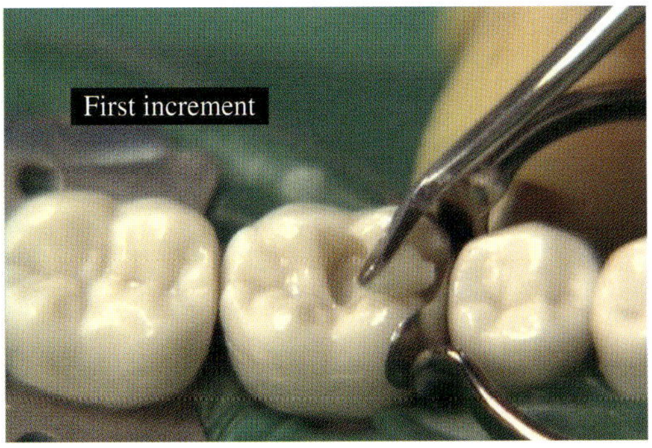

The first increment of material is transferred to the cavity on a plastic instrument or injected directly into the cavity from a compule.

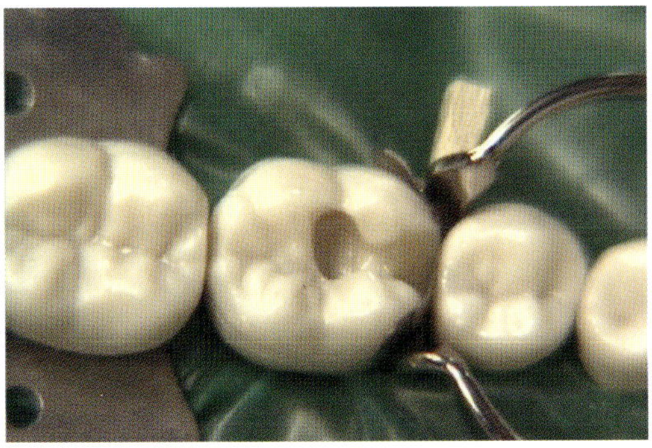

The composite resin is adapted to the gingival floor of the cavity using a ball ended burnisher.

It is vitally important that great care is taken at this stage to adapt the material carefully to the gingival floor. The rounded nature of this feature should ensure that this is more easily achieved.

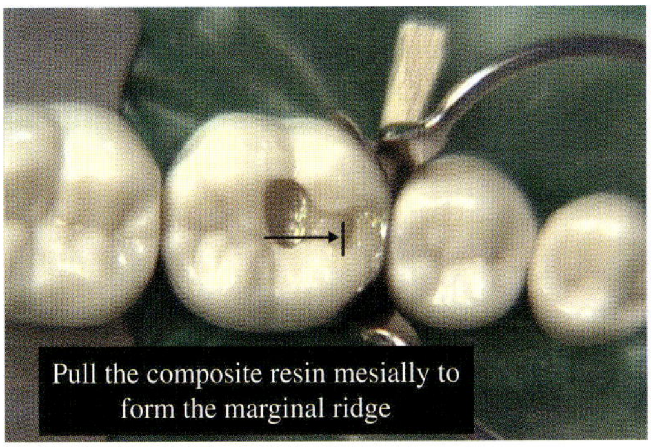

A plastic instrument can then be used to pull that material mesially against the sectional matrix so that it adapts to it and the marginal ridge is established at this stage.

It is important that it is at the correct level and harmonises with that of the marginal ridge on the adjacent tooth.

By pulling the material mesially, only an interproximal wall will be created with an empty void between it and the axial wall.

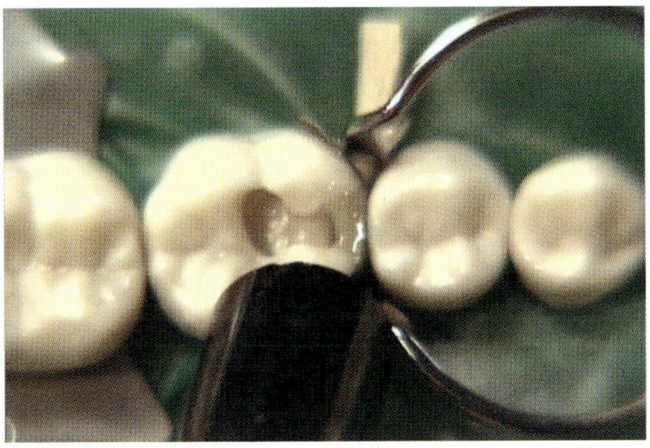

The first increment of composite resin is polymerised with visible blue light of 470 nm wavelength.

It is important to check curing lights regularly to ensure the intensity remains above 300 mW/cm^2.

As the material polymerises it shrinks towards the surface to which it has the greatest bond strength.

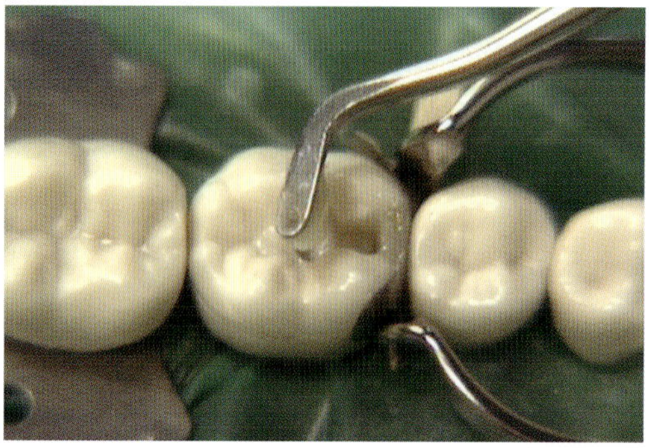

A second increment is then transferred to the cavity. The cavity should be built up in layers or increments of no more than 2 mm thickness to ensure full and effective cure occurs.

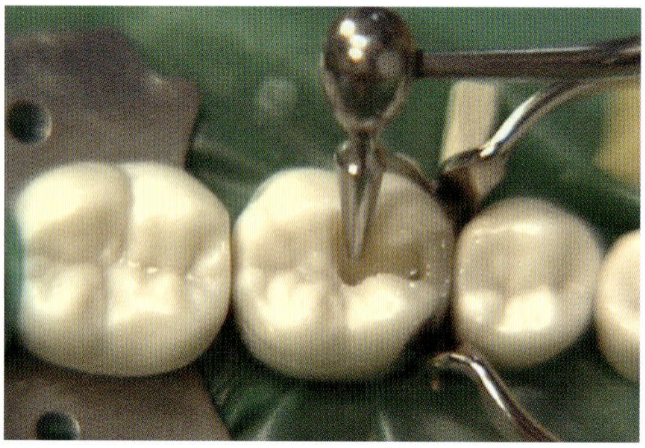

The P1 instrument is used to adapt this increment of restorative material in an oblique layer. The oblique layer should not contact the buccal and lingual walls of the cavity simultaneously to avoid the shrinkage pulling the two walls of the cavity towards each other and causing ‘cuspal bending’.

The composite resin should be adapted to the buccalwall and the pulpal floor only.

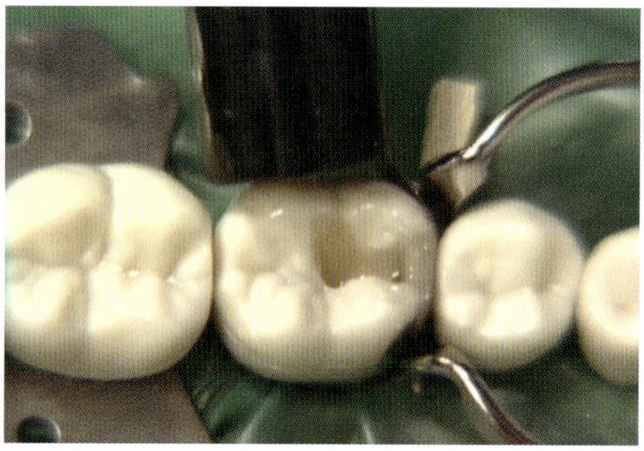

This is then polymerised from the buccal aspect first and then from the occlusal aspect. Both curing regimes should last for 40 seconds each.

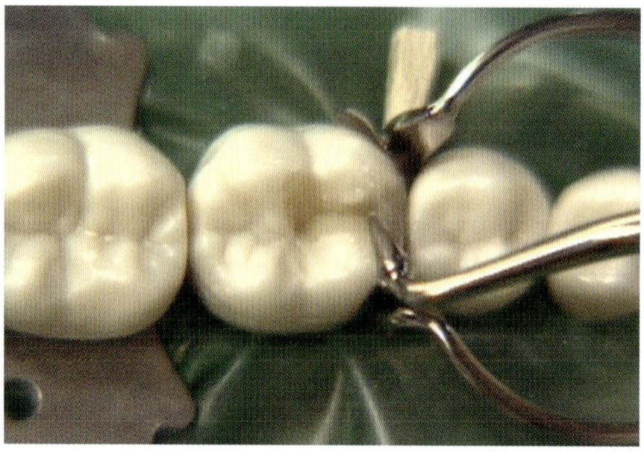

A third increment is applied that is adapted towards the lingual wall of the cavity and obliquely onto the second increment. In this way, the material cannot link the two walls of the tooth.

The tip of the P1 instrument is ideal to ‘scribe’ the fissure while the side of the instrument forms the cuspal slopes.

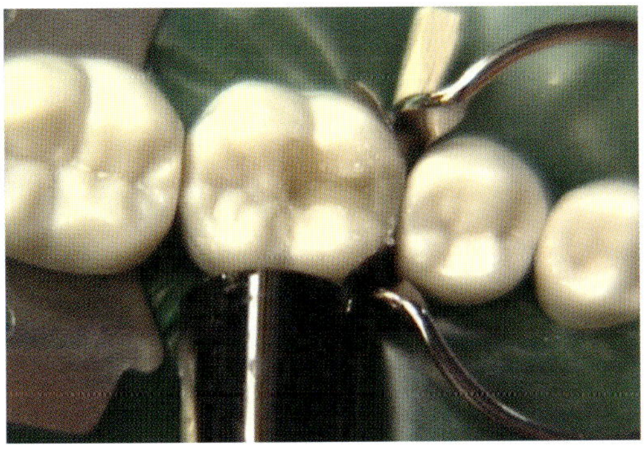

Another polymerising regime is followed, but, in this case, the first cure is from the lingual side.

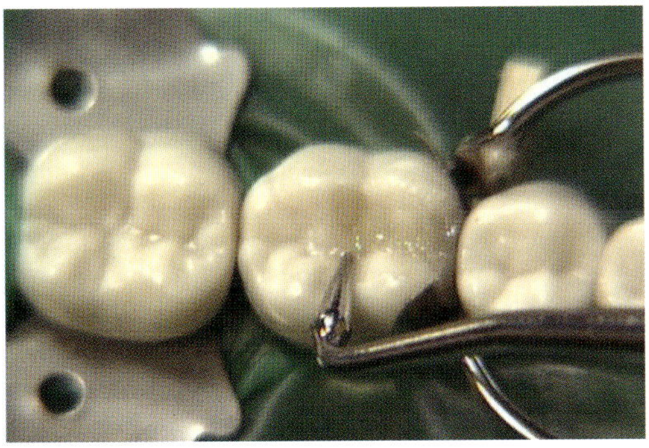

A final increment is applied so that the final shaping of the anatomy can be completed to return the tooth to its original shape.

The P1 hand instrument is ideal for this purpose.

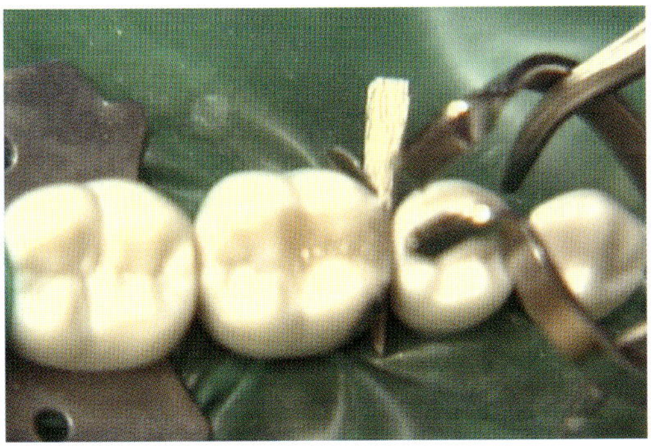

The forceps are used to remove the BiTine ring from the tooth. The flattened surfaces on the outer aspect of the forceps ensure that the ring does not slip from the grasp of the forceps.

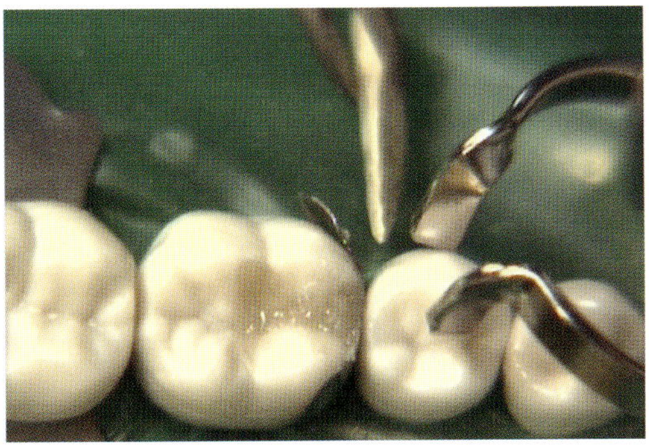

The wedge is removed from the interproximal space to leave the sectional matrix free.

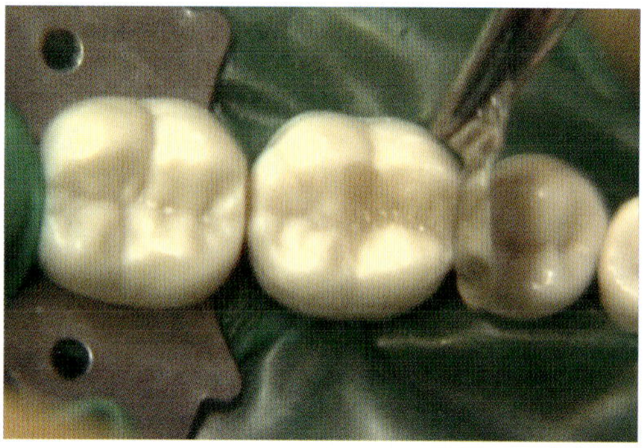

The freed matrix can then be removed easily by grasping with either college tweezers or mosquito forceps.

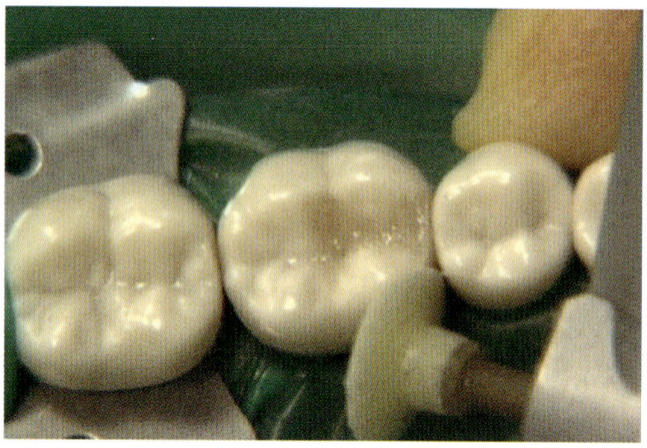

If care has been taken with the incremental buildup of the composite restoration, the final shaping will have been achieved.

An anatomical shape can be achieved using rotary burs, but this will leave the surface rough and require a great deal of polishing.

In this case, an good anatomical shape has been achieved so the finish simply requires a degree of polishing using the impregnated silicone points of the Enhance system.

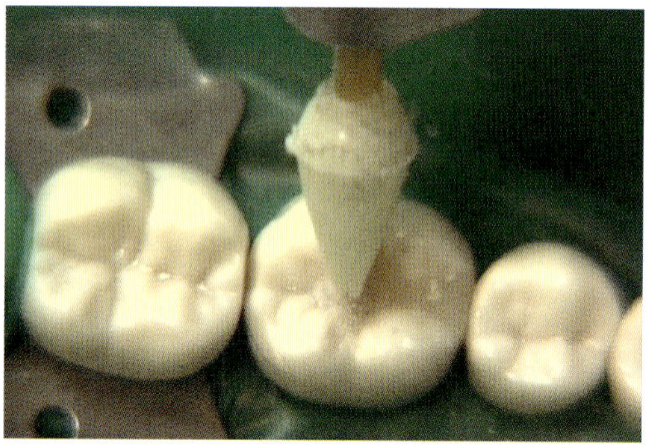

A cone shaped Enhance point is shown here. This is ideal to fit onto the cuspal slopes and into the fissures.

It should be used with a firm application initially and a more progressively light pressure as the procedure progresses.

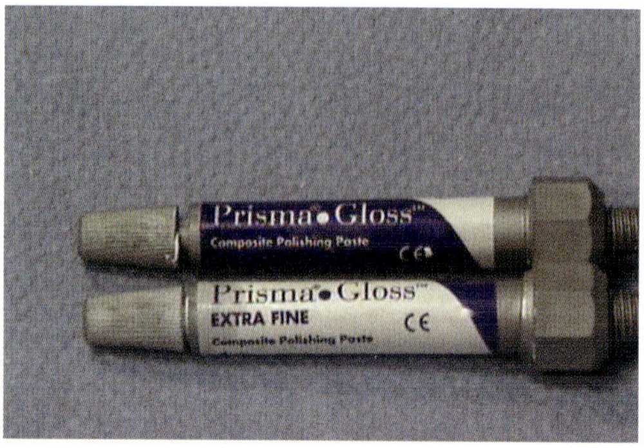

A final lustrous finish can be achieved by using the 'fine' and 'extra-fine' polishing paste.

Only a small amount is required, and this should be expressed from the syringe onto a paper slab.

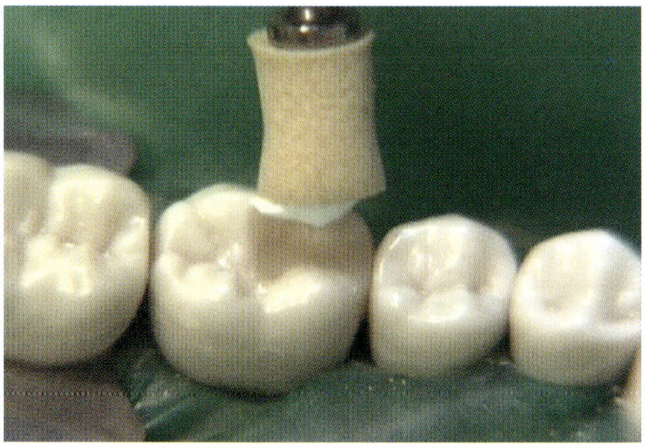

The polishing paste is applied to the tooth using the felt polishing cup mounted on its special mandrel.

The cup is disposable but the mandrel is not. The mandrel should be returned for sterilising between patients.

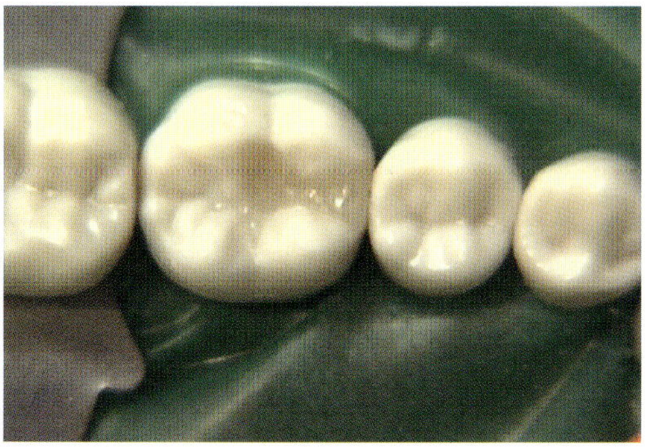

The completed restoration with its lustrous finish.

Note the quality of the contact point. This should be checked with dental floss to ensure it provides a resistance to insertion of the floss.

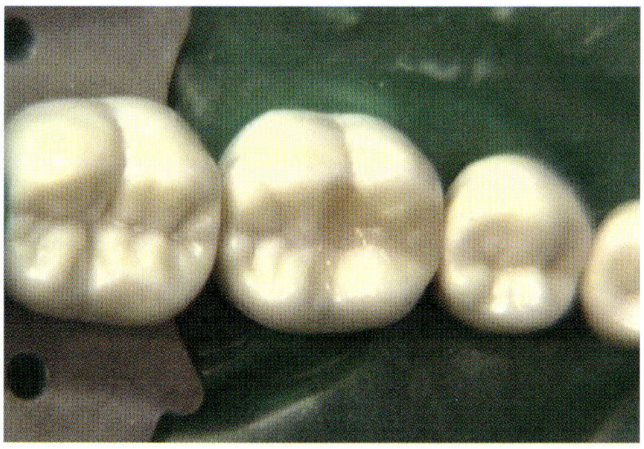

The completed restoration should have a smooth surface to resist plaque accumulation and have a good contact point to prevent food packing.

The anatomical features have been re-established–a fissure pattern and a marginal ridge to deflect food away from the embrasures.

A Clinical Case

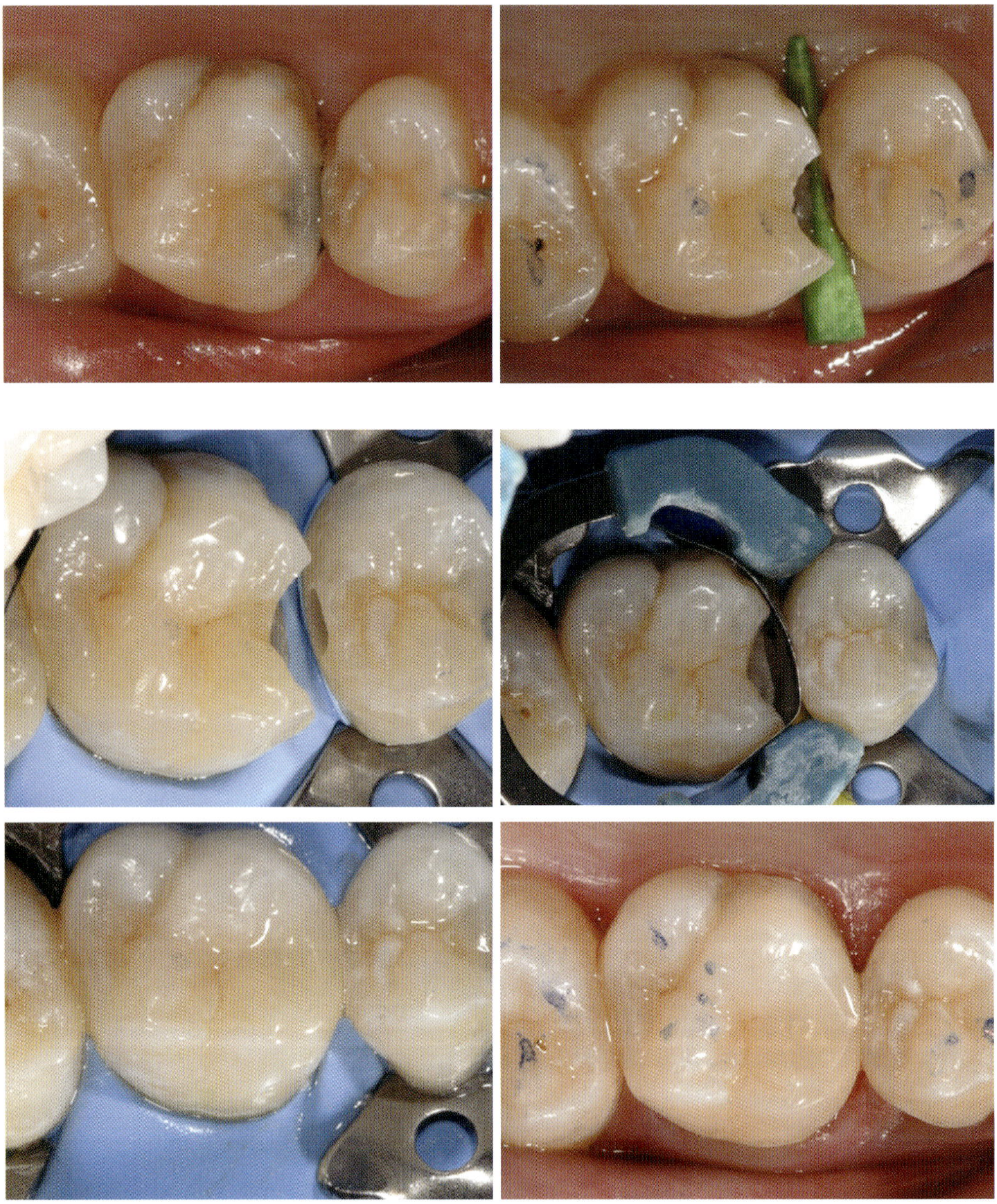

The above clinical case shows the preparation of a cavity in the maxillary first molar tooth giving access to a distal carious lesion in the premolar tooth. This has allowed the conservative restoration of these teeth.

Source: Printed by permission of Dr Osama Alkhatib.

Clinical Guide to Restoring a Class II Lesion with Amalgam

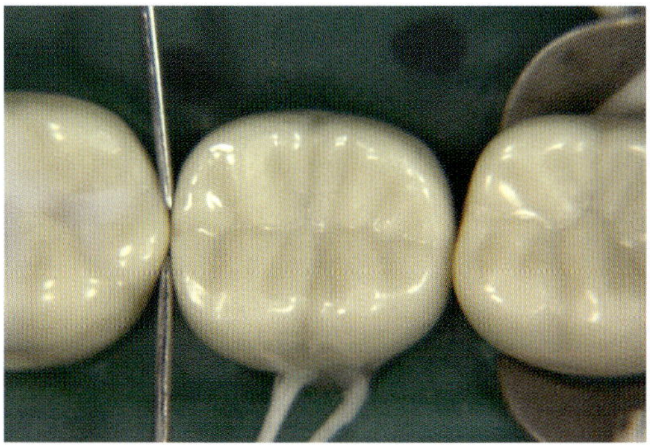

A class 11 cavity is required when the caries commences in the approximal surface(s) of a tooth at or below the contact point.
The two probes indicate the contact and stagnation area between the first and second molar teeth.

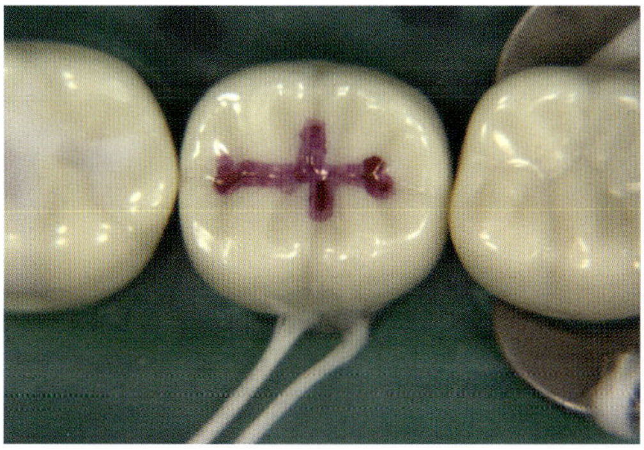

The area shaded in thee accompanying slide indicates the extent of the carious lesion at the enamel dentine junction in relation to the fissure caries. This has been superimposed on the tooth surface.

Note that the lesion also involves most of the fissure pattern in this instance.

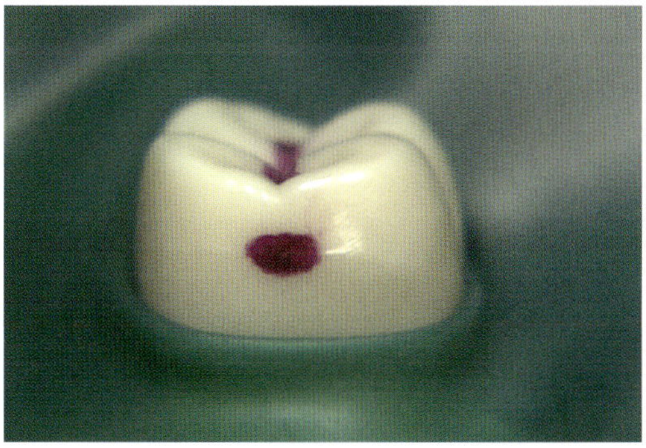

This slide indicates the extent of the carious lesion, just within the dentine, superimposed on the mesial tooth surface. The lesion occurs at or below the contact and clinically cannot be viewed directly. The caries mesially may communicate with the fissure caries.

If the adjacent tooth is missing the enamel may show some cavitation or appear white and chalky (white spot enamel lesion).

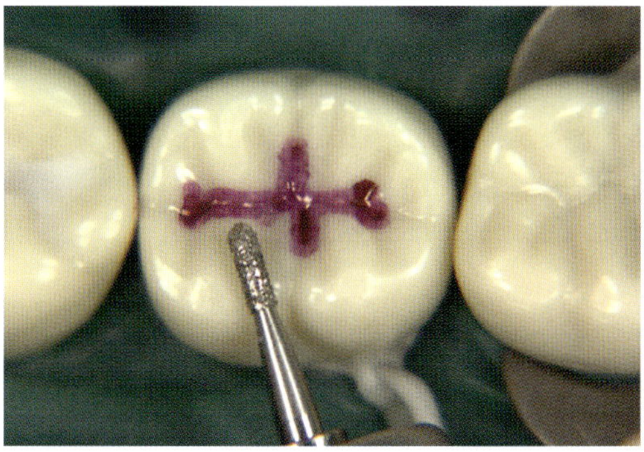

The initial preparation is carried out using a diamond coated domed cylindrical fissure bur in the air turbine handpiece.

Running at high speed this bur can grind away the tooth substance. This will generate heat, which should be dissipated with water coolant to avoid pulpal trauma.

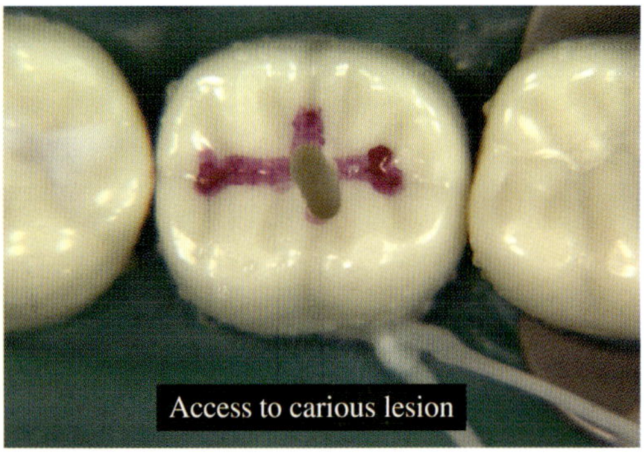

The initial access to the carious lesion is gained through the central fissure. The cut is extended just into the dentine (about two-thirds of the depth of the cutting part of the bur).

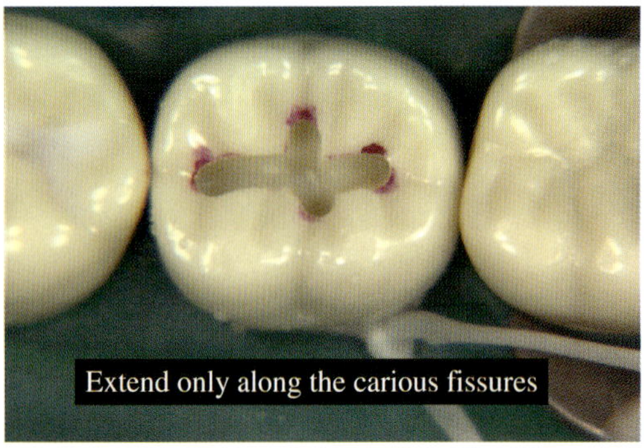

Video 6.5

The cavity should be extended to follow along the fissure pattern only as far as the caries extends.

Due to the angle at which the bur is held in relationship to the occlusal surface, some of the shaded area can still be seen. The outline of the occlusal part of the cavity should be smaller than the outline of the actual carious lesion in the dentine.

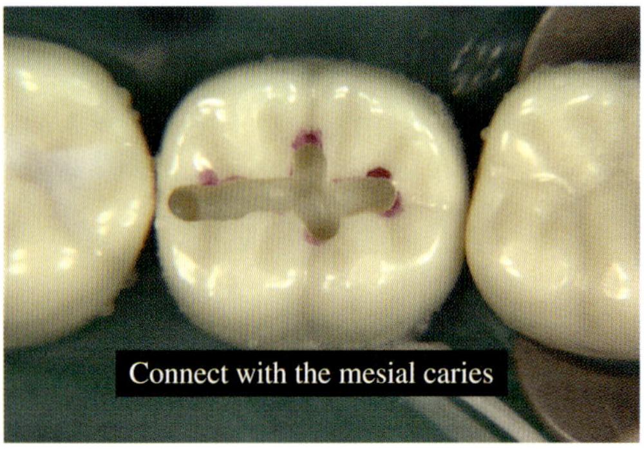

Video 6.6

The cavity is now extended towards the middle of the contact area on the mesial ridge under which lies the carious lesion that commenced at or just below the contact point.

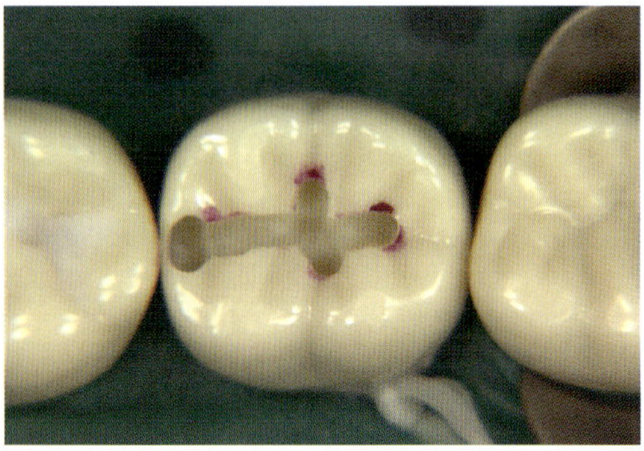

Clinically, when the tip of the bur meets the underlying soft carious lesion, it will 'sink' into the softer tooth structure.

The bur has cut a path into the carious dentine that is in line with the middle of the contact point with the adjacent tooth.

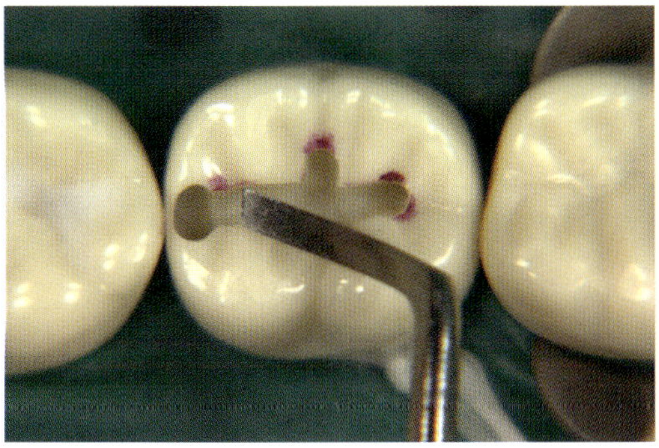

The mesial cavity can be seen to have been slightly widened with the bur. Note that a step can be seen between the level of the minimally carious fissures and the area involving the more deeply sited mesial caries.

The marginal area of enamel is reduced until it is paper thin. A gingival margin trimmer can be used to fracture out the contact enamel without damage to the adjacent tooth. If the marginal enamel wall is left too thic,k it will fracture at an angle and damage thc box margins.

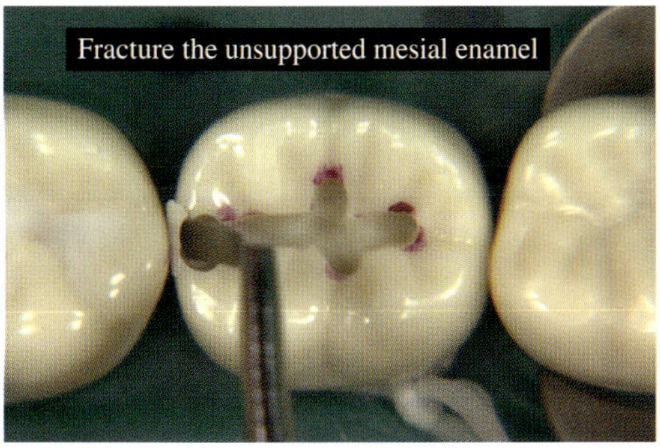

In the accompanying picture, the gingival margin trimmer has been placed in the deeper part of the cavity. Pressure is exerted mesiallyresulting in fracture of the thin unsupported enamel at the contact.

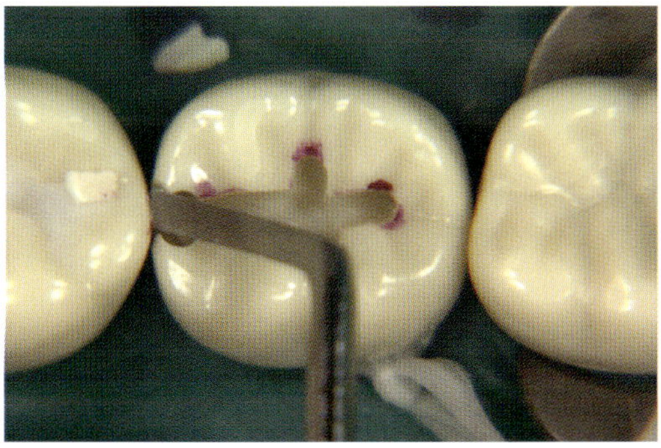

The fractured portion has been removed and it can be seen that there is no damage to the adjacent tooth.

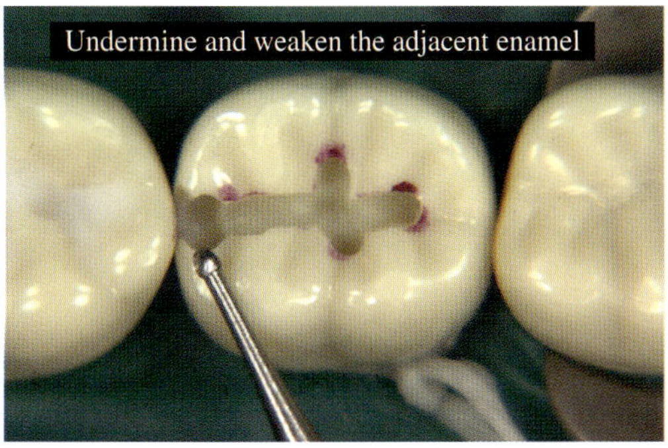

On the buccal side of the box, the mesial contact is not completely clear of the contact area and may still contain decalcified enamel.

A small round bur or the tip of a tapered fissure bur may be used in a slow handpiece to undermine the enamel on this buccal side.

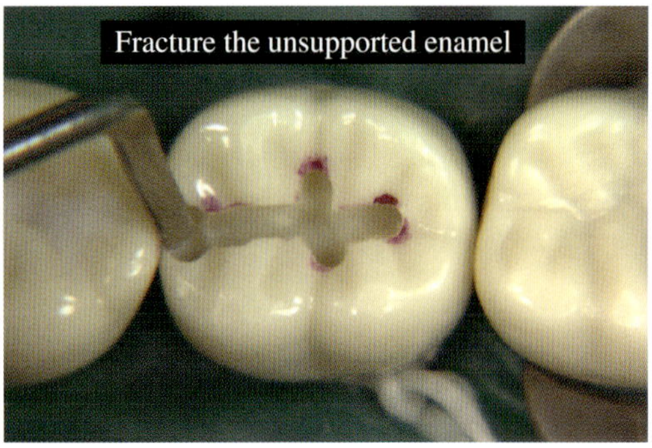

Once undermined, the enamel can then be gently removed using the angled tip of a gingival margin trimmer.

The cutting edge of this instrument has an oblique angle. The most pointed part of the cutting edge should be situated towards the outer surface of the tooth.

Video 6.7

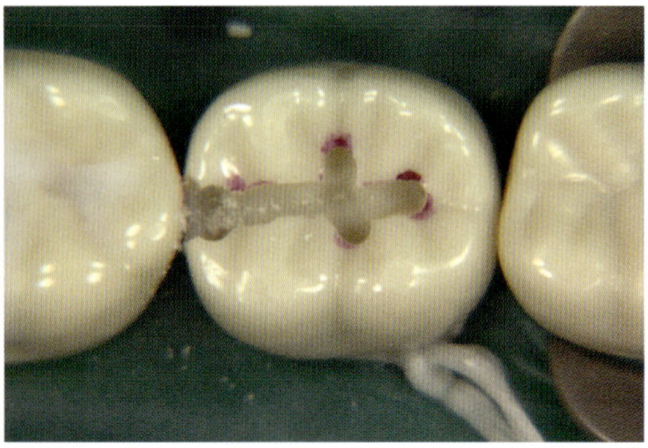

The width of the box is determined predominantly by the extent and size of the carious lesion.

According to the principles of cavity preparation, the marginal cavity wall should extend into an area that can be cleaned by the patient using either a toothbrush or dental floss.

Video 6.8

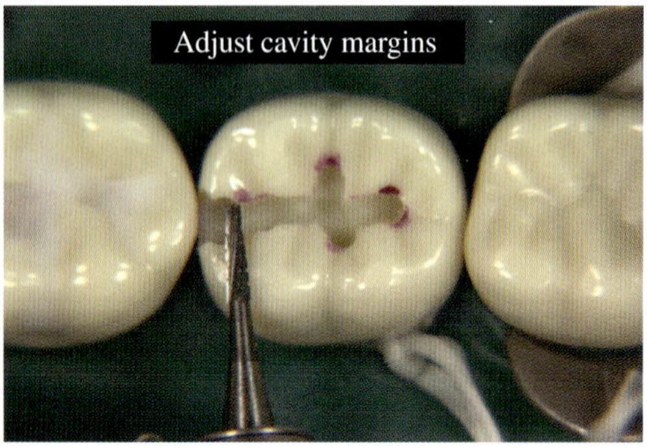

The walls of the cavity and the gingival floor are smoothed using a tapered fissure bur. The example shown is a cross-cut tapered fissure bur.

While smoothing the cavity please ensure that sharp line angles are not created between the walls and the floor of the box.

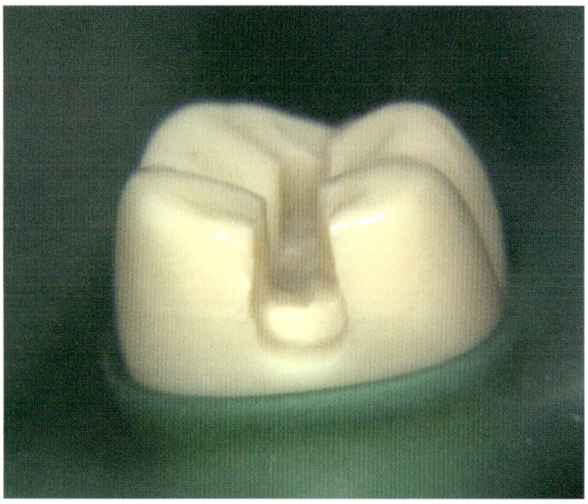

The cavity is now viewed from the mesial side. It can be seen that the preparation is slightly undercut such that the width of the cavity is wider gingivally than occlusally.

This undercut will provide retention for the amalgam restoration.

Identify the following:

-Gingival floor with step up to pulpal floor
-Axial wall
-Pulpal floor
-Pulpo-axial line angle

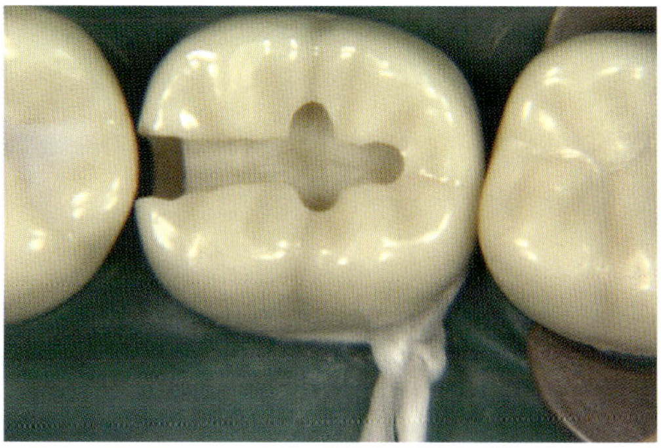

The almost complete cavity is now viewed from the occlusal surface.

Note:

- The box is just separated from the adjacent tooth contact
- The pulpal floor is smooth
- The outline is confluent
- The pulpal floor can be clearly differentiated from the deeper gingival floor

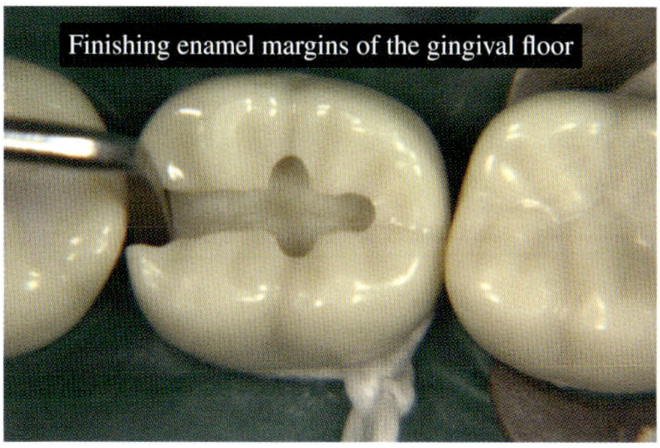

Unsupported enamel prisms can be removed from the edge of the gingival floor using a gingival margin trimmer.
There are two instruments – for any tooth one instrument will refine the mesial box and the other instrument will refine any distal box.
Each instrument is double ended and has an oblique cutting edge - the point of which should be directed away from the axial wall and towards the outer margin of the tooth.

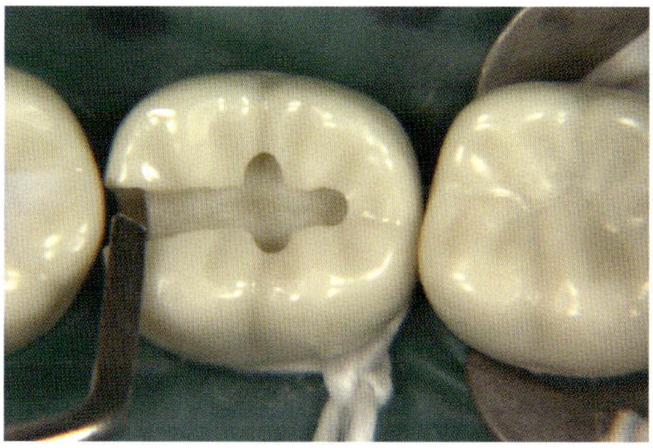

Note the curved blade and oblique edge of the instrument. The cutting edge of the instrument is shaped like a carpenter's chisel and should be used as a chisel to pare away the unsupported prisms.
The chisel edge is facing away from the camera towards the floor, and in this instance the instrument should be scraped from the lingual (top of the picture) to the buccal (bottom of the picture).

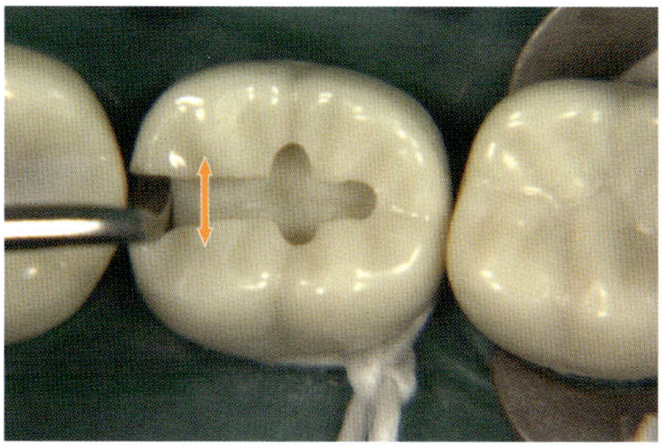

The curve of the instrument can be seen more clearly in this view. The instrument is being directed from the buccal to the lingual.
The arrows indicate the direction in which the instrument should be moved.

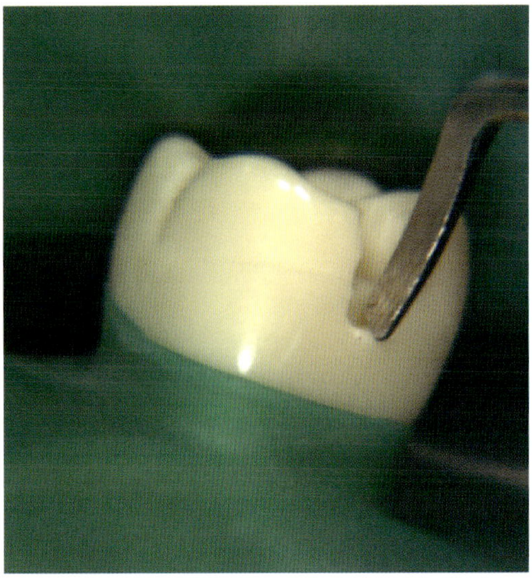

This mesial view shows how the chisel blade of the instrument lies on the edge of the gingival floor of the cavity and has been moved from the lingual towards the buccal (from right to left in this picture).

Video 6.9

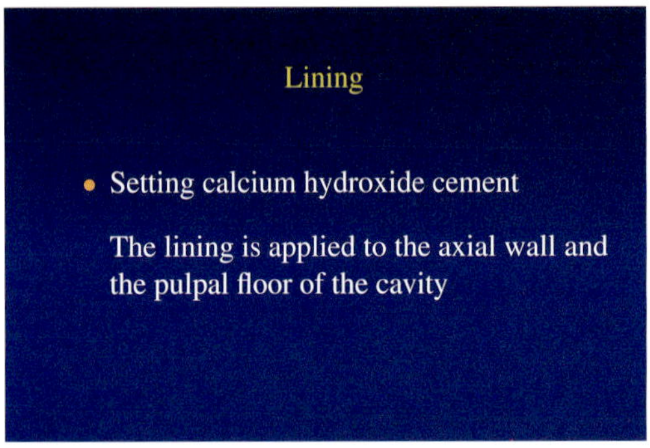

The lining is placed to protect the pulp.

Remember that, in this particular cavity, the pulp is closer to the axial wall than the pulpal floor because the cavity has only a minimal depth occlusally.

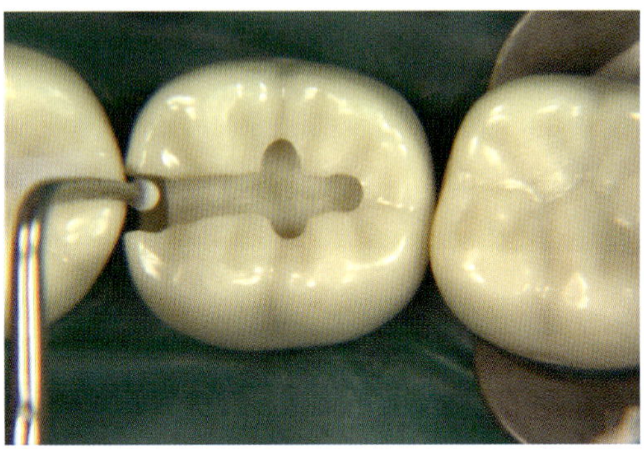

After mixing the base and catalyst pastes, the calcium hydroxide cavity lining is placed using the tip of a PF10 instrument.
Careful transfer of material should ensure coverage of the axial wall without the risk of applying material inadvertently to the walls of the box.

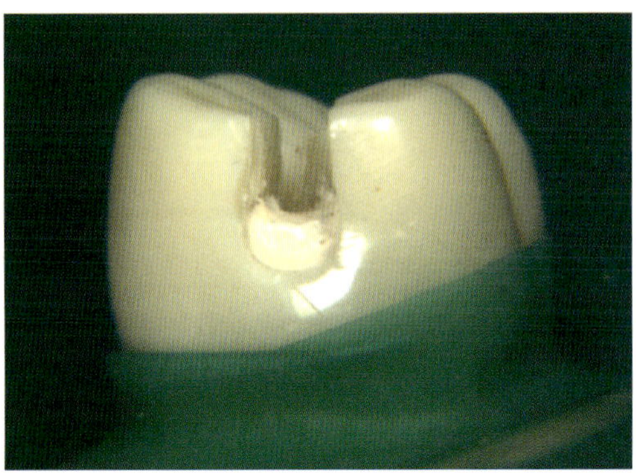

This mesial view shows that there is adequate coverage of the axial wall. The lining is carried up to (but not on to) the junction of the box walls (buccally and lingually) with the axial wall.

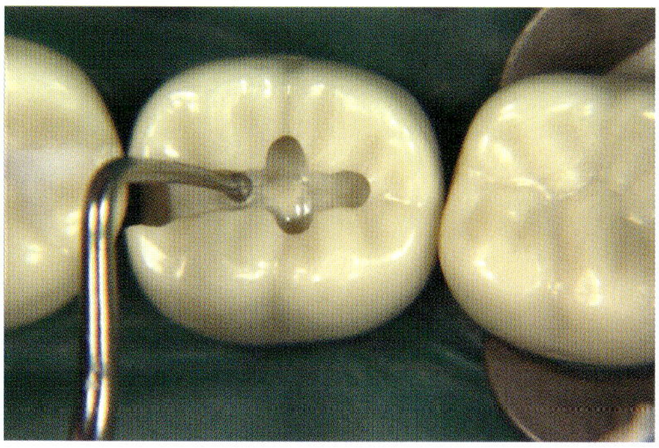

Occlusally, the material is placed using a similar technique to that described for the occlusal amalgam cavity.

The pulpal floor should be covered with a thin layer of this setting calcium hydroxide cement. To ensure smooth placement, endeavour to touch the material on to the floor of the cavity and maintain contact with the cavity floor as the instrument is moved, allowing the lining to 'flow' to form an intact layer.

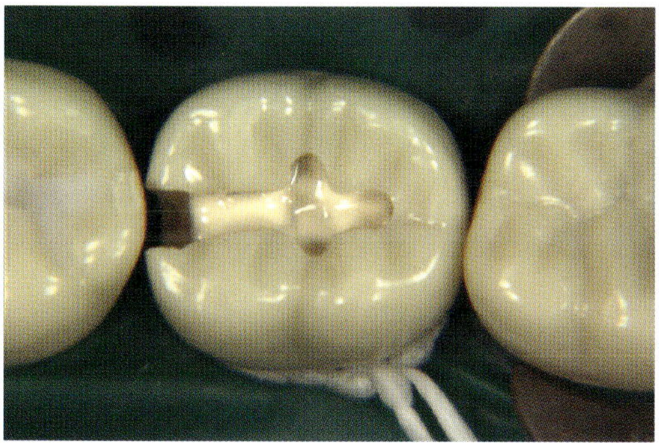

Careful application will ensure a smooth result. Remember to clean the PF10 instrument thoroughly if a further increment of material is required.

The pulpal floor and the axial wall are well covered with lining, but the cavity walls are clear of lining material.

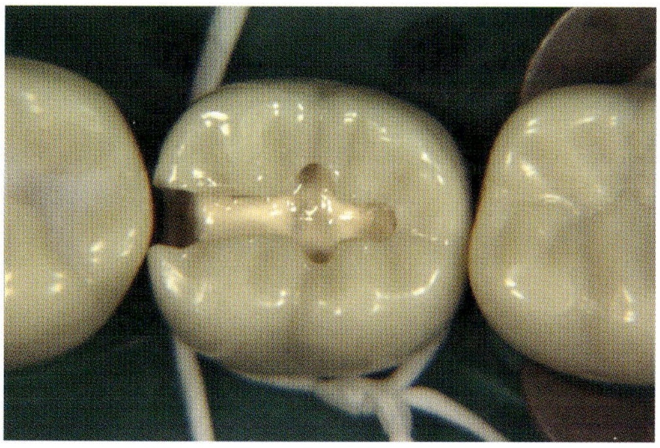

Now follows the placement of the restoration...

Firstly, place a length of waxed dental floss between the teeth, ensuring that it lies below the gingival floor of the cavity (the reason for this will become clear in later stages).

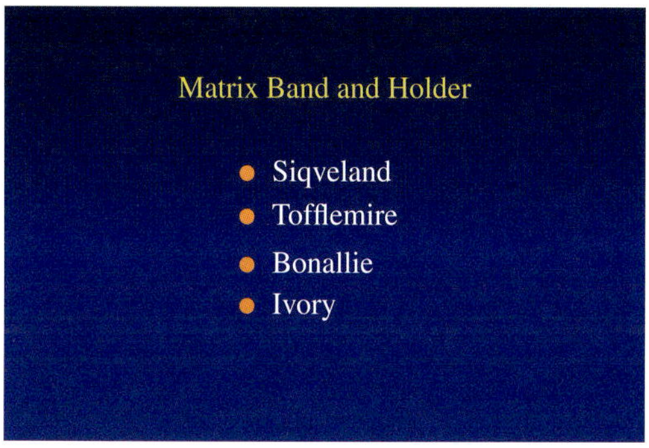

A matrix band is used to provide a surface for the filling material to be packed against in the areas where the natural tooth has been lost (in this demonstration the mesial wall has been lost).

The band is held in one of a number of holders.

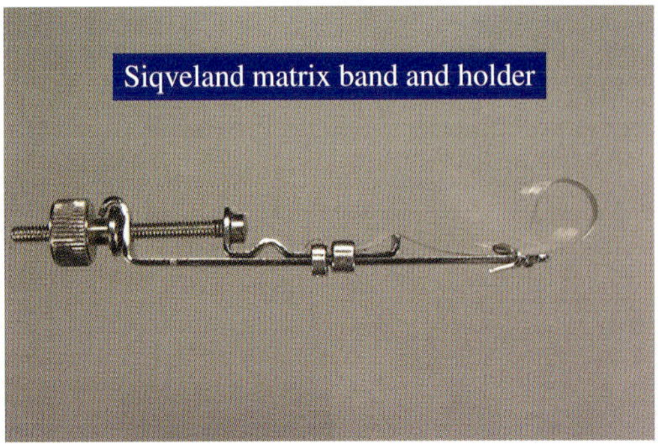

There are many varieties of matrix band holders. The two holders that will be used on this course are:

- The Siqveland (illustrated)
- The Tofflemire Junior

In this restoration a Siqveland will be used.
A Tofflemire will be used in later sequences.

Video 1.3

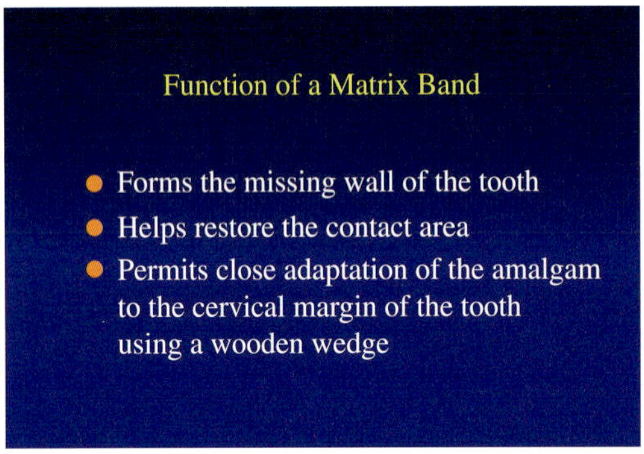

This slide summarises the functions of the matrix band.
Note that use of a wooden wedge will help to adapt the band onto the tooth structure gingival to the floor of the box.

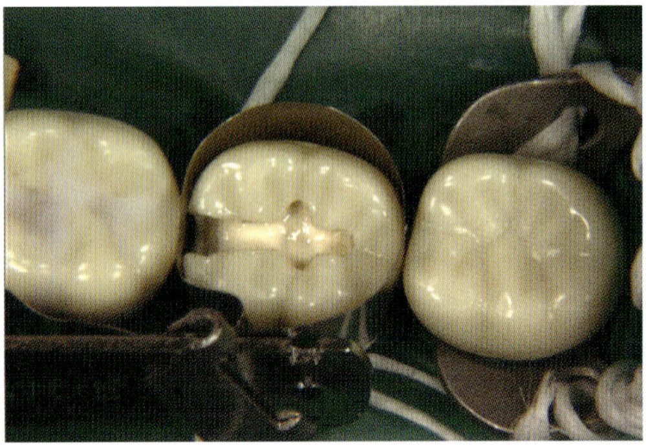

In this slide a matrix band can be seen in a Siqveland holder. It is important to use the band that has been manufactured for the holder.
Note that the floss is free of the band and lies outside the matrix.
There is a toggle latch at the end of the Siqveland holder that ensures that the circumference of the band is narrowed towards the cervical margin.
The toggle latch must be positioned correctly before the matrix is tightened on the tooth.

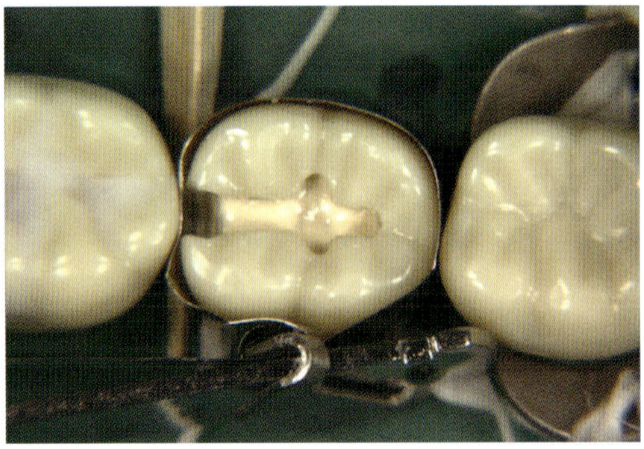

A wooden wedge is placed interproximally (in this case from the lingual side) to ensure a tight fit of the band in this inaccessible area.
Tight approximation of the band to the tooth can be confirmed by passing a dental probe along the cavity margin within the band.

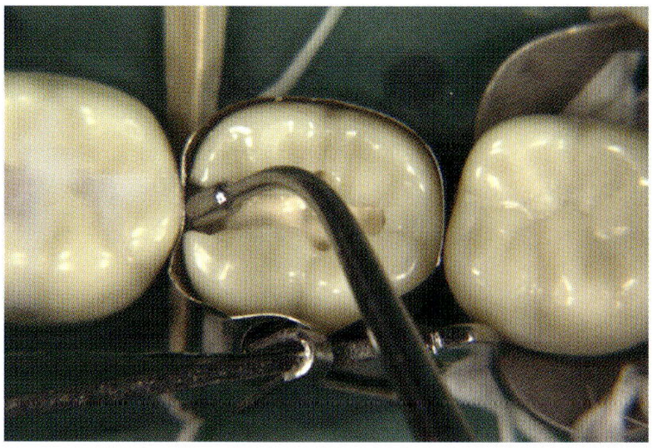

An amalgam condenser is selected that will pass into the base of the cavity, thus ensuring that the filling material can be condensed adequately without voids.

Close adaptation of the filling minimises:
- Marginal leakage
- Secondary caries
- Post operatively sensitivity

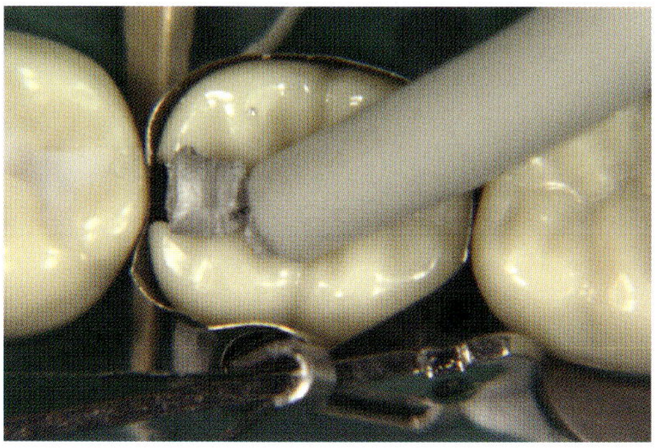

The first increment of amalgam is transferred to the cavity and placed in the mesial box.

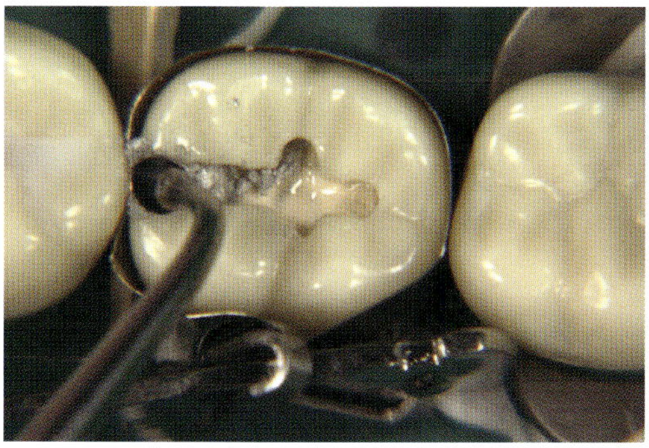

Following the technique described for the occlusal amalgam, initial condensation should be vertical followed by horizontal sweeping.

Such placement ensures amalgam is brought into close contact with the margins of the cavity.

Some operators perform angled packing into the corners of the box using a smaller condenser.

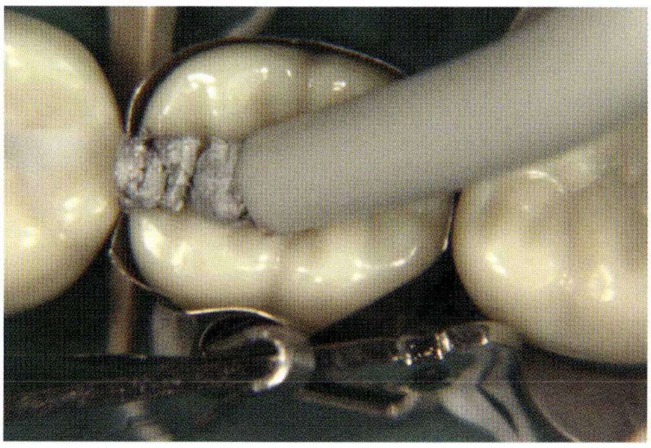

Further small increments of amalgam are packed into the mesial box area of the cavity in the same manner.

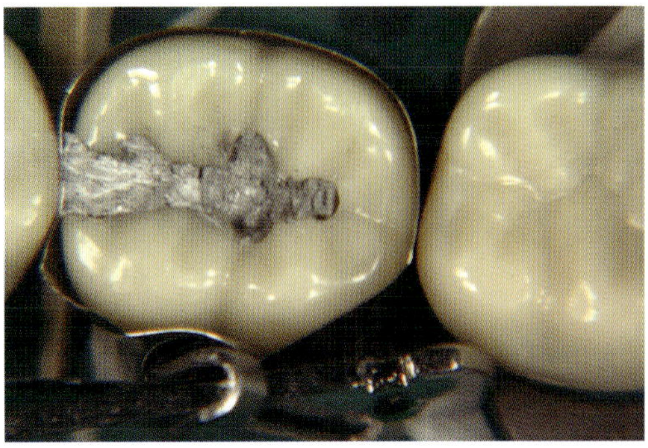

Once the box area has been filled, the amalgam is similarly placed over the pulpal floor in the occlusal portion of the cavity.

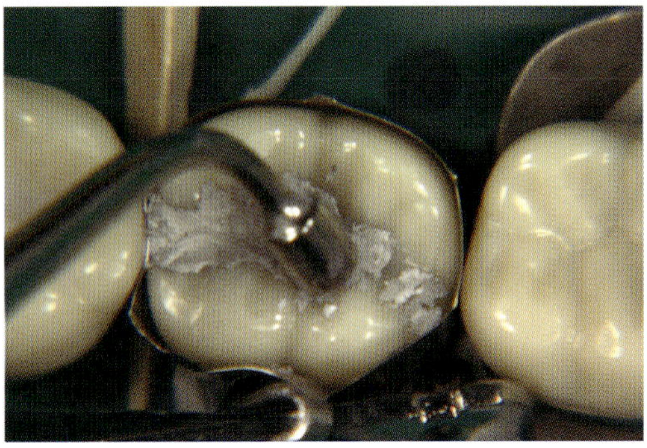

The cavity is filled to slight excess, and during the final condensation, the larger end of the instrument may be used.
The condensing point is held parallel to and just over the cavity margins.
Such condensation ensures that the cavity is well filled and begins the process of reconstructing some surface anatomy in the amalgam filling material

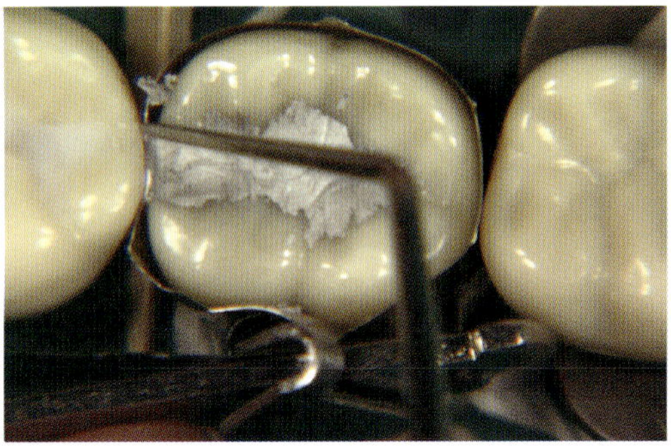

Once the cavity has been filled to excess, a right angled dental probe, held at 45° to the marginal ridge, is used to remove the unsupported excess, which is otherwise in danger of causing a fracture of the ridge as the band is removed.

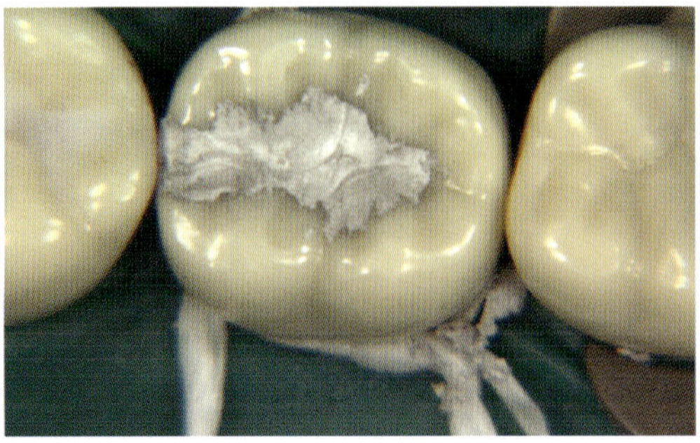

The wedge and band are carefully removed before any further carving is done, but note that the floss has been left *in situ* at this stage.

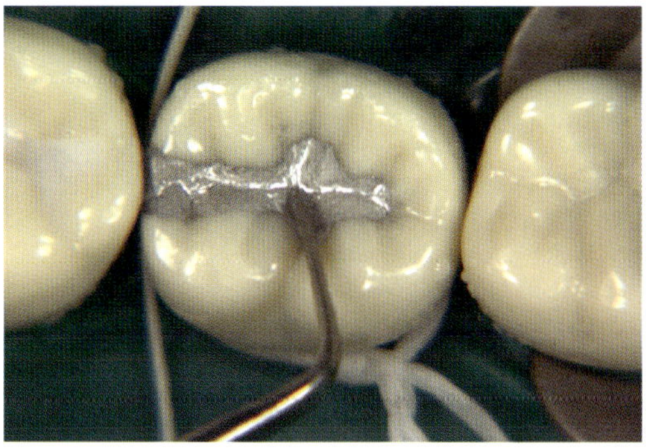

Using a carver (either a Ward's No. 5 or a half-Hollenbach instrument) the surface anatomy is recreated.
The sharp cutting edge should rest on the cuspal slopes while the tip of the instrument carves the fissure pattern. Take care to ensure that the tip of the instrument does not extend beyond the centre of the fissure.

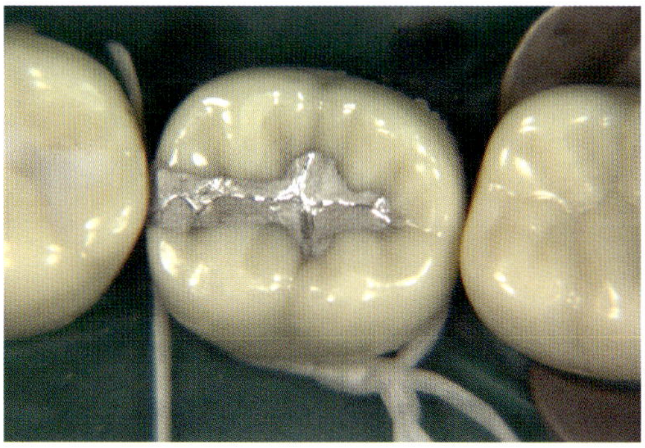

The finished contour can now be seen. The fissures and the marginal ridge should be clearly identifiable.
The floss can now be used to remove any inaccessible flash beyond the gingival cavity margins. The floss should then be removed in a lateral direction. On no account should the floss be pulled up through the contact because this may fracture the amalgam and compromise the quality of the contact.

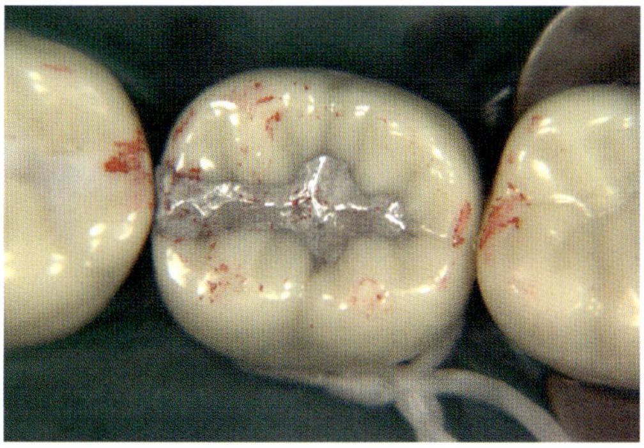

In the clinical situation, the rubber dam would be removed and the occlusion checked carefully with articulating paper as previously described, ensuring that contacts are evenly distributed. On no account should the amalgam be left with premature contacts.

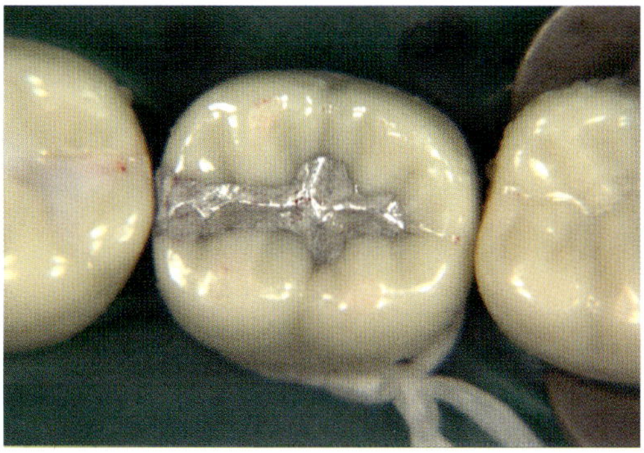

Finally, the restoration should be smoothed using a pledget of cotton wool.

Clinical Guide to Restoring an Extensive Class II Lesion

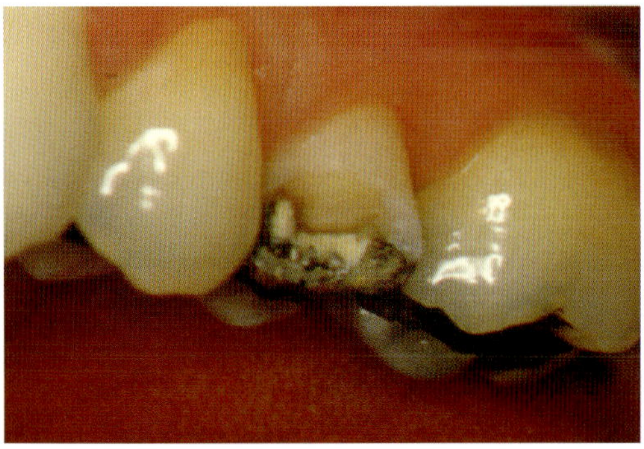

Where cuspalcoverage is not provided, an emergency visit by the patient may be necessary when the unsupported cusp fractures. Commonly, patients will report that the fracture occurred when biting into some relatively soft food.

Alternatively, patients may complain of sensitivity on biting. Testing the cusp by getting the patient to bite on a rubber point will indicate a cusp with a fracture. If this is left it will eventually fracture away, affording the patient some relief when biting.

The case seen here shows the loss of the buccal cusp from a heavily restored premolar tooth.

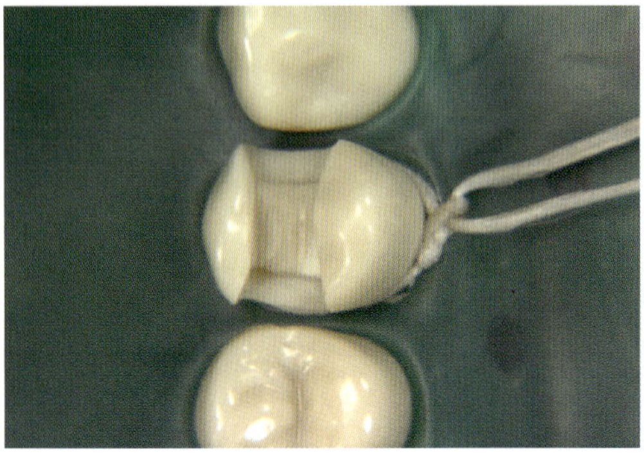

In this simulated restoration a large MOD cavity will be prepared. Note that the caries has been substantial and the width of the boxes and the occlusal preparation is commensurate with caries of at least 3 mm on the approximaltooth surfaces.

The thickness of the palatal cusp is still substantial, but notice the buccal cusp is unsupported – it has a lower bucco-palatal dimension than its gingivo-occlusal height. This predisposes this cusp to fracture in function. When this situation is apparent in prepared cavities, consideration should be given to providing cuspal coverage with a restoration such as a gold onlay.

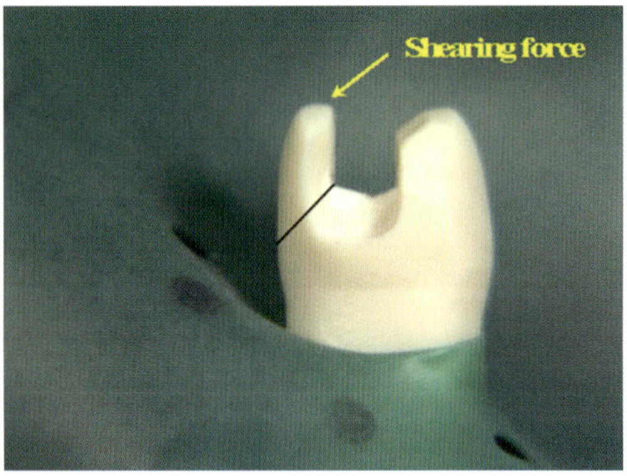

This view of the cavity shows that a force applied to the weak buccal cusp will result in its fracture leaving a sloped fractured surface. This will be at approximately 45°

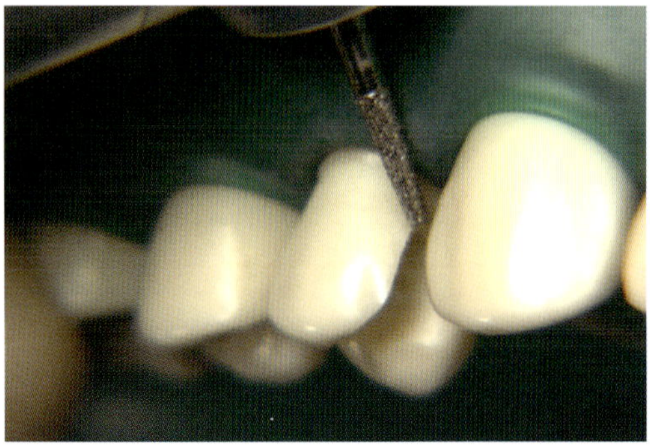

In this simulated procedure, the buccal cusp will be removed using a diamond bur held at a 45° angle towards the occlusal plane.

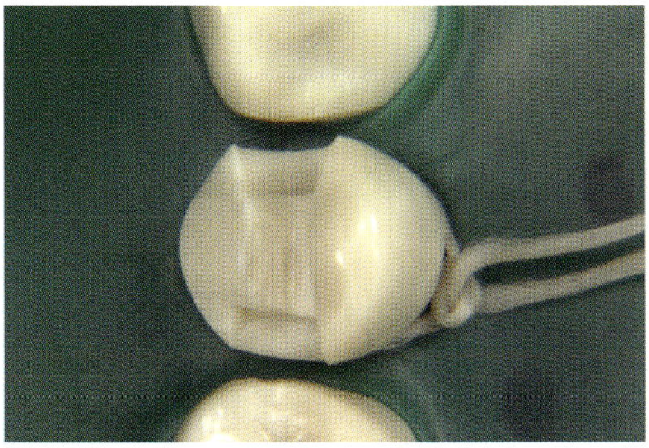

From the occlusal surface the fractured cusp slope can be seen to run to a knife edge finish along the buccal surface. This fractured edge will frequently be at a different level to that of the box floors.

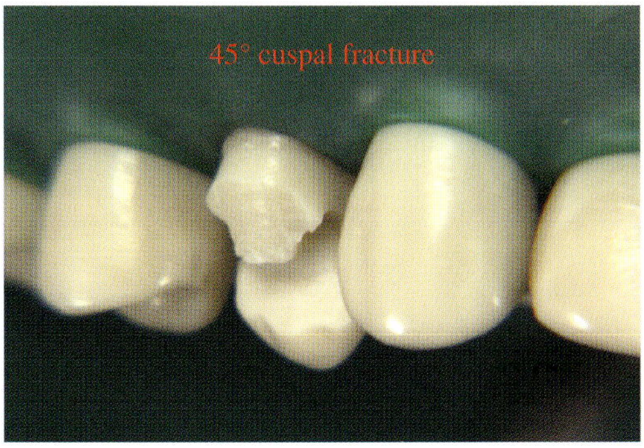

The ragged outline of the fractured surface can be seen more clearly in this view as can the slope of surface.

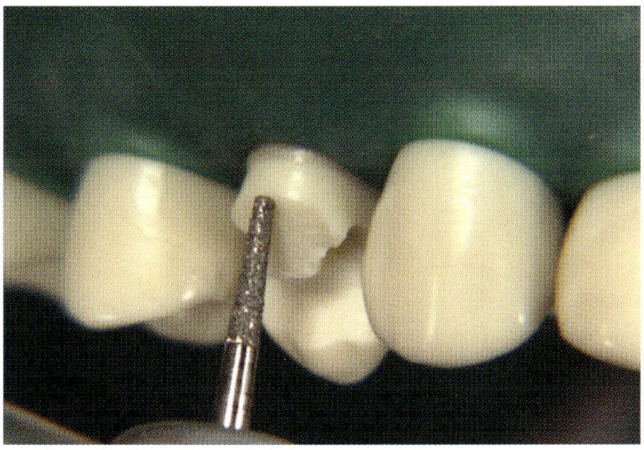

The ideal amalgam marginal angle is a but joint of 90°. This can seldom be achieved, but an angle of between 70° and 110° is acceptable.

In this case a 45° marginal angle would not be acceptable. A butt joint can be prepared by preparing a 1 mm wide shoulder along the fractured surface. This is not particularly destructive of tooth structure and will ensure a more lasting restoration.

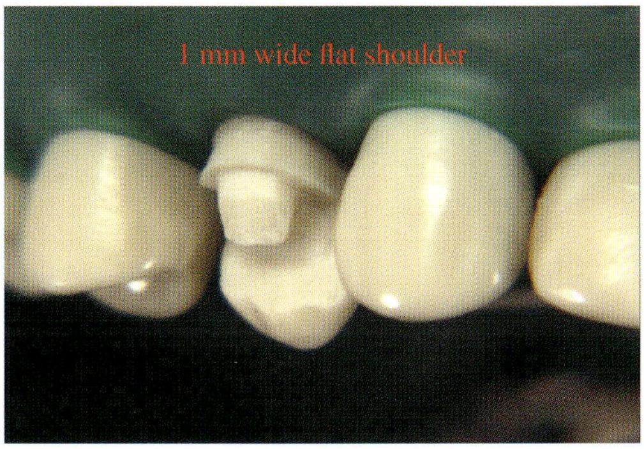

In this view a 1 mm shoulder has been prepared. In this particular case, the shoulder happens to be level with the floor of the boxes, but this may not always be the case. Tooth structure should not be sacrificed simply to achieve this goal.

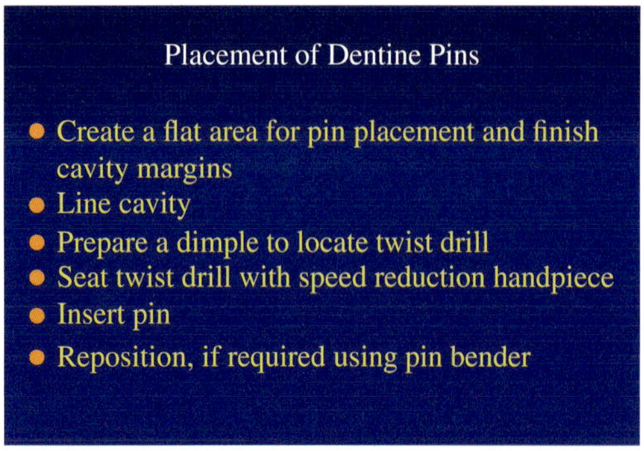

Pins should be placed into a flat surface and should be 1 mm in from the enamel dentinal junction (EDJ), ensuring that perforation of the periodontal ligament and the pulp is avoided. At least 1 mm of amalgam should be able to be placed around the pins.
It is for this reason that two dentine pins will be placed in this tooth to avoid the possibility of exposing the buccal pulp horn.

Once the flat areas have been prepared, the cavity is lined before the pins are inserted. If lining were left until after pin insertion, some problems of access may be experienced.

Let us now go through the sequence in a staged approach.

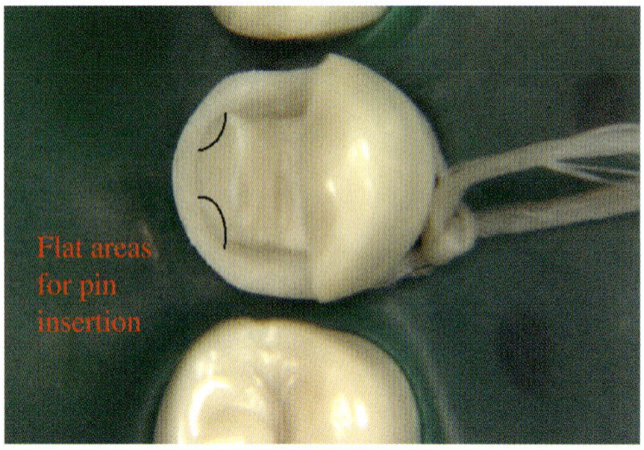

To achieve two flat areas with sufficient room around the pins for 1 mm of amalgam, some dentine must be sacrificed by removing two semi-lunar areas of tooth structure. These are highlighted on this slide.

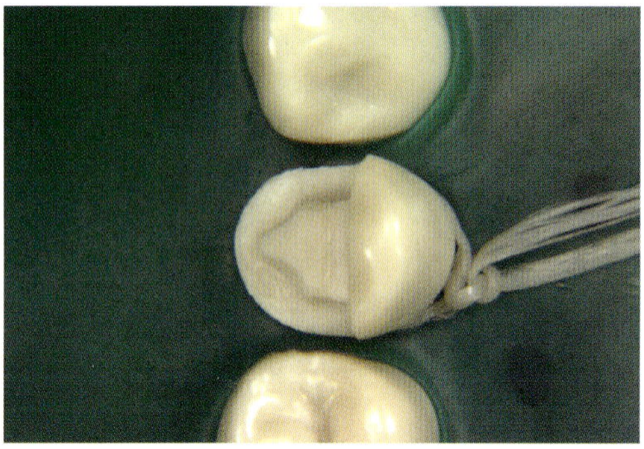

The removal of these areas now provides the flat surfaces required to insert the dentine pins.

Note the unsupported enamel along the shoulder and the box floors. Before continuing these should be removed.

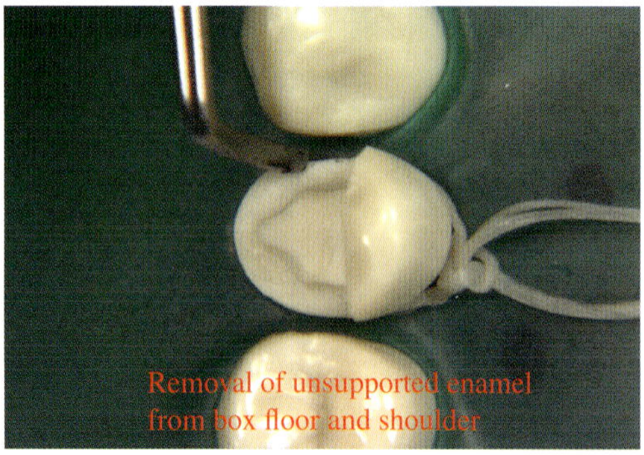

This is best achieved using the gingival margin trimmers. A firm sweeping action is required along the edges of the preparation to remove the brittle enamel. If they are not removed, they will fracture in function, leaving deficiencies along the amalgam tooth interface. In time, this will lead to secondary caries and sensitivity.

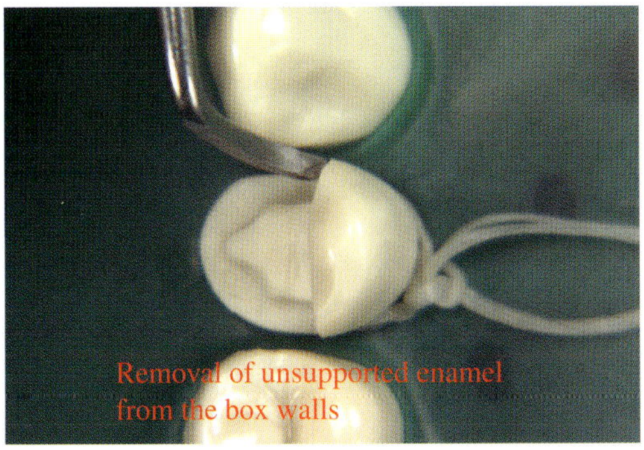

The gingival margin trimmer may also be used to cleave unsupported enamel from the walls of the boxes.

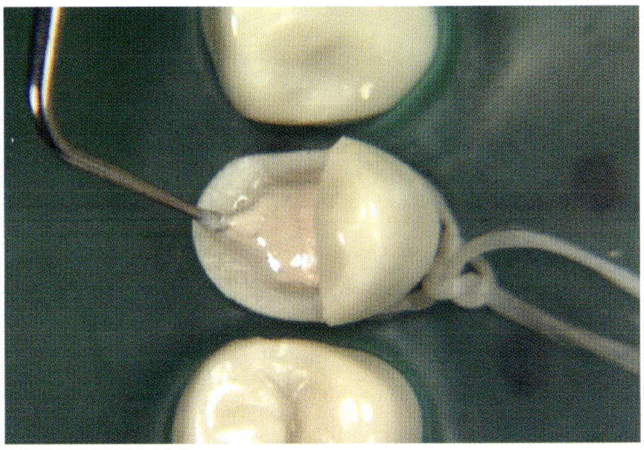

Both the horizontal pulpal floor and the vertical axial walls are lined. In this tooth a setting calcium hydroxide cement will beused. It seals the dentine surface, preventing fluid movement in the dentinal tubules. Even in thin layer, a calcium hydroxide cement forms an effective thermal barrier by preventing hydrodynamic fluid movement.

The axial walls are lined before dentine pin placement to facilitate adequate coverage of the surfaces deep to the pins.

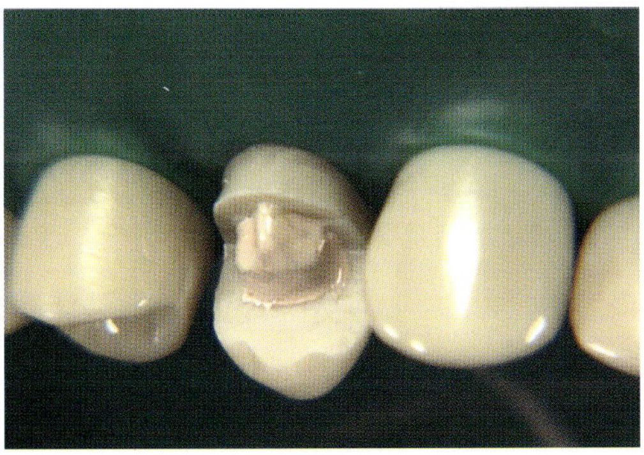

Excess cement on the walls and floor can be removed using a sharp excavator. Lining cement should not be placed on the shoulder or flat surfaces into which the dentine pins will be placed.

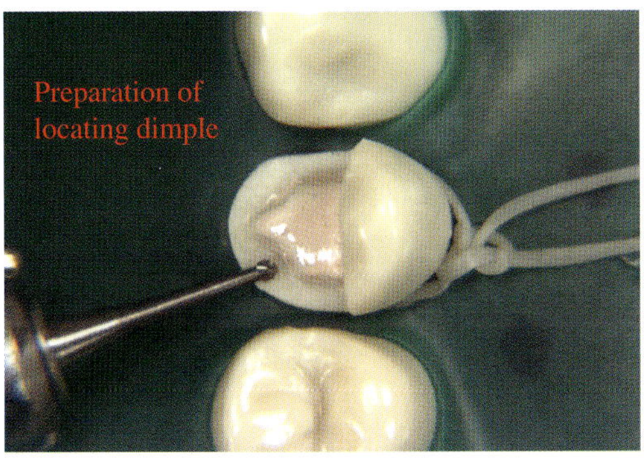

Video 6.10

To facilitate the preparation of the pin holes, locating dimplesshould be made using a number 1 round bur.

This bur should be used at slow speed and with the bur laid sideon to the dentine surface. In this way some degree of control may be exerted over the bur.

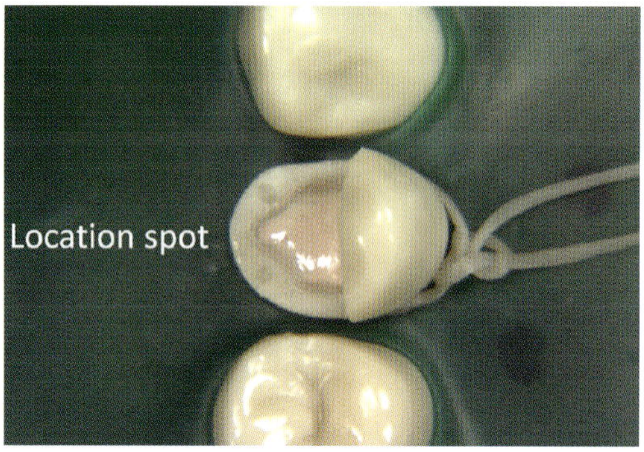

The small dimples in the dentine surface can be seen in this view. These will help locate the tip of the twist drill.
1 mm of sound dentine should surround the pin channel, and a thickness of 2.5 mm of dentine is a pre-requisite for pin placement. This thickness should be present to protect against pulpal or periodontal perforation. Remember that furcation areas should be avoided.
Pins should be placed at least 5 mm apart where possible.

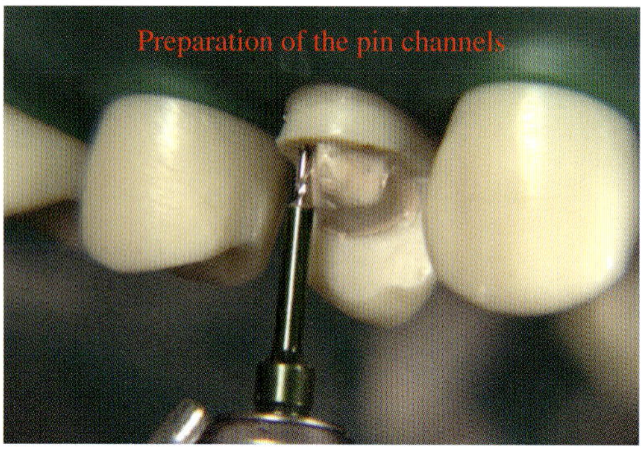

The twist drill should be placed into a speed reducing handpieceto provide lower speed but greater torque. The tip of the bur is placed in the dimple and the length of the bur aligned with the outer surface of the tooth.

Some operators use a plastic instrument to place against the outer surface of the tooth to judge the degree of taper towards the cemento-enamel junction (CEJ).

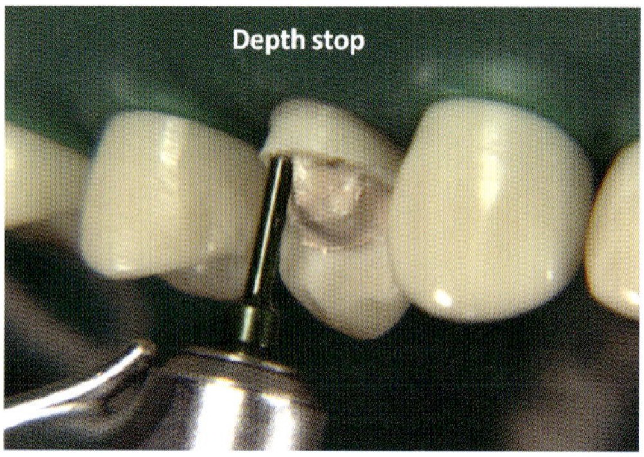

Video 6.11

The handpieceis operated and the bur pushed against the dentine surface to prepare the pin channel. Multiple attempts at cutting the cannel mustbe avoided as this will result in a channel that is too wide for the self-threading pin.

The depth stop shoulder on the twist drill is seated down onto the dentine surface in one firm movement. The twist drill is removed while still rotating.

Do not be tempted to try and re-seat the twist drill.

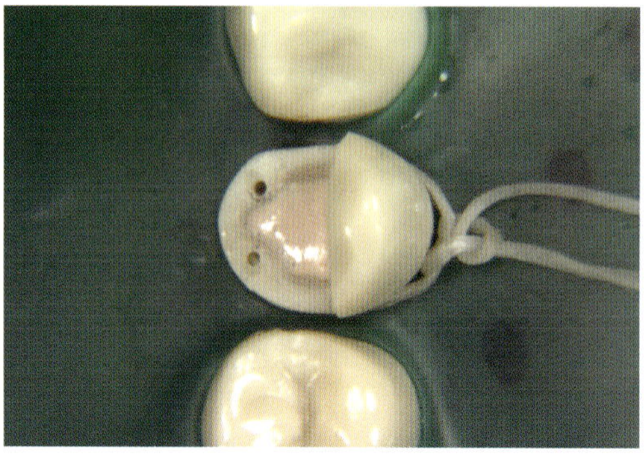

At this stage carefully wash and dry the cut swarf from the tooth surface.

The pin channels should appear as parallel holes in the dentine without a flared orifice. If flaring of the orifice is present,this indicates over-preparation and compromised retention of the pin.

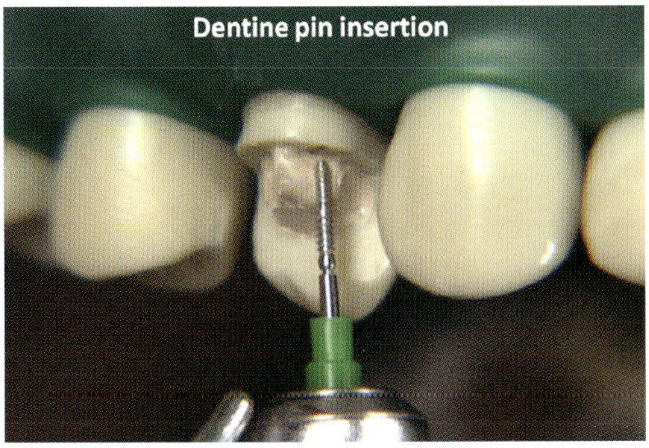

Video 6.12

The dentine pin comes presented in a plastic chuck. This shouldbe placed into the speed reducing handpiece.
Note that mid-way along the threaded pin a widened seat is present. This should sit onto the dentine surface when the pin is inserted.
The retention of a pin is related to its diameter, but the retention of the amalgam is not improved by having a length greater than 2 mm protruding into the cavity.
The long axis of the pin should be aligned with the direction ofthe pin channel in the dentine.

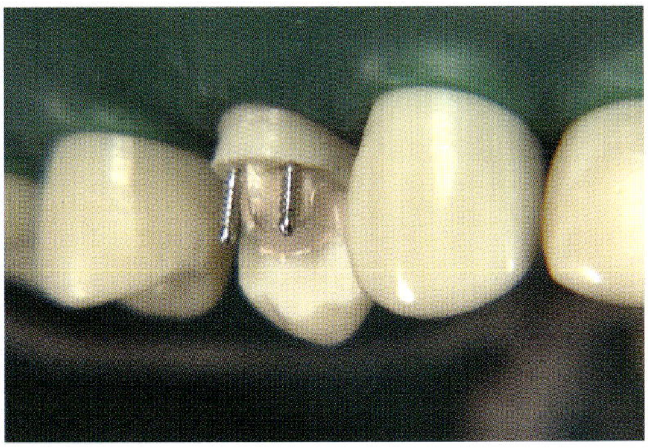

The pins are offered up to the pin channels with the handpiece operating at a moderate speed only.
The flutes on the pin will thread themselves into the elastic dentine walls until the pin has threaded into the depth of the pin channel.
The narrowed area of stainless steel above the pin will shear when the torque rises. This should only occur when the pin has fullyseated. If operated at too high a speed, the threads will stripfrom the dentine wall and retention will be compromised.
Incorrect placement speed or angulation of the pin may result in fracture of the tooth structure.

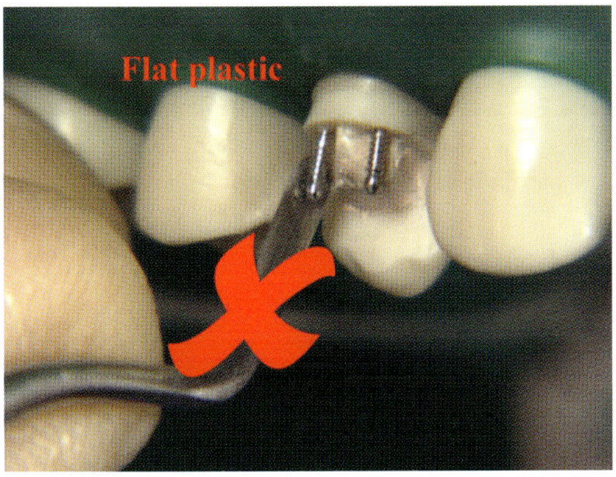

If the pins are not ideally placed and need to be bent over slightly, a flat plastic instrument is not recommended to bend them into a more suitable position. This will stress the surrounding dentineand may result in peripheral tooth fracture.

Pin height above the dentine surface should allow them to be overlaid with 2 mm of restorative material.
Occasionally, it maybe necessary to reduce the height of the pins. This should be done using the air turbine and a diamond coated bur while the pin is held firmly with mosquito forceps. If the pin is not supportedduring this procedure, the pin may be de-rotated and removed from the pin channel.

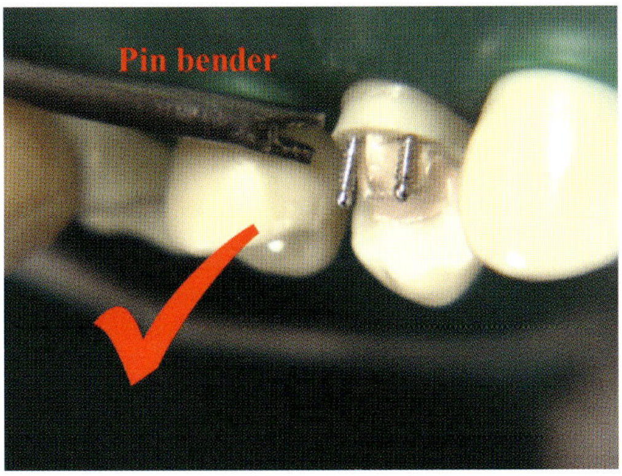

Video 6.13

A “pickle fork” shaped pin bender should be used to bend pins because this instrument supports the pin on one side while the other side of the instrument applies a counter force to bend the pin over. This avoids stressing the dentine and risking fracture.

The height of the pins should allow 2 mm of amalgam to be placed over the top of the pins.

The location of the pins should not interfere with any subsequent tooth preparation for a full coverage crown.

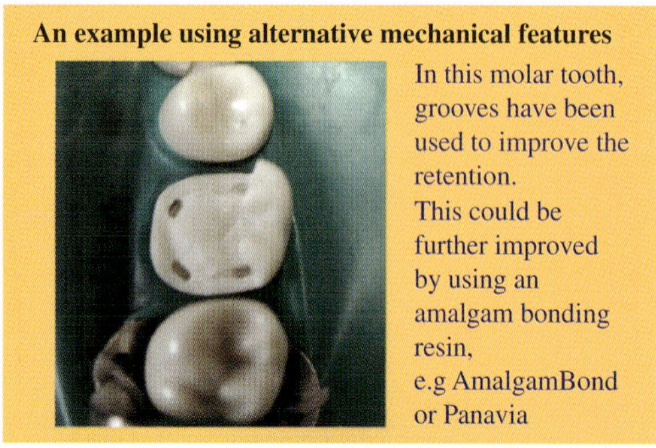

The placement of dentine pins can be fraught with adverse sequelae such as fracture of surrounding tooth structure or, perforation into the pulpal or periodontal tissues. In addition, postoperative sensitivity can be a problem.

It is for these reasons that fewer dentine pins are used today, and operators are recommended to place slots and grooves in the remaining tooth structure to provide resistance and retention. An example is shown in the accompanying picture.

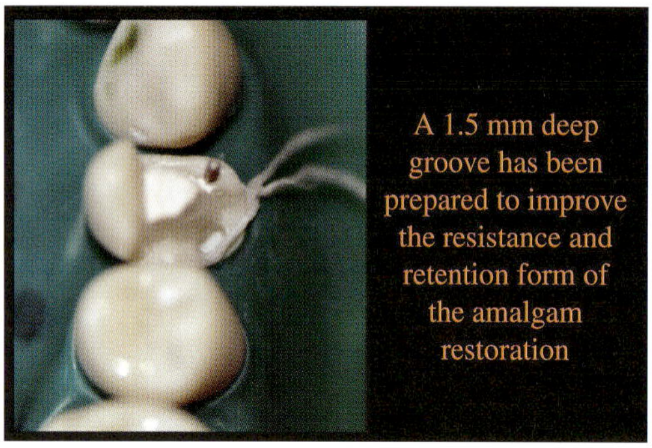
A 1.5 mm deep groove has been prepared to improve the resistance and retention form of the amalgam restoration

From this occlusal view it can be seen that one pin has been placed. Pins aid the resistance form of the cavity rather than the direct retention. Note that 1 mm of space exists around the pin for amalgam to be condensed in the next stage of restoration of this tooth.

In place of the second pin, a slot has been cut with a small tapered fissure bur – this should be 1.5 mm deep.

It would be unusual to use a pin and a groove in the same tooth. This is a simulated technical exercise only.

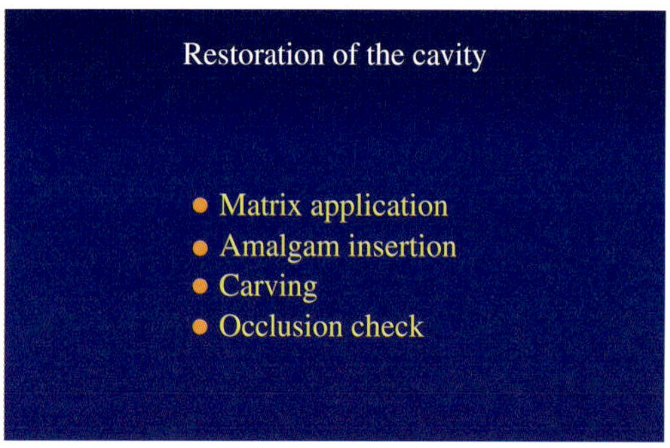

In the final stage of this restoration, the cavity will be restored.

Selection and placement of a suitable matrix system is challenging in many cases. A range of matrices are available and must be tried individually to assess their suitability for individual cases.

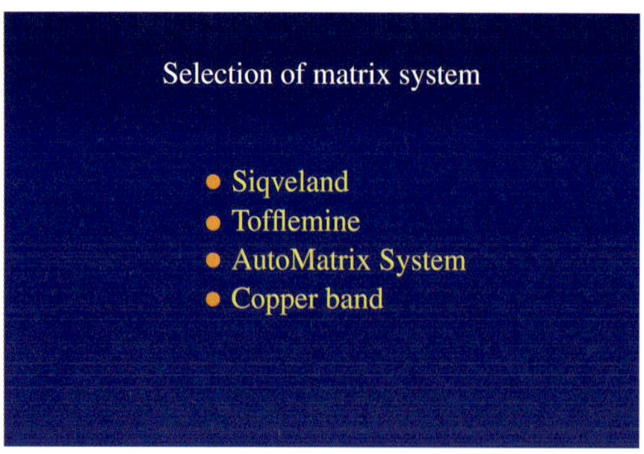

The matrices that can be used include those that remain attachedto their holder during all stages of the filling procedure (Siqveland) to some where the holder can be removed, leaving the band in place. This allows the operator to maniplulate its removal more easily with less risk of fracturing the newly placed, and only partially set, amalgam.
Some newer matrix systems are free standing and have no holder to interfere with the placement of the filling. The adjustable AutoMatrix allows such manipulation. A copper band is a rather old fashioned alternative but one thatstill has a place in restorative dentistry.

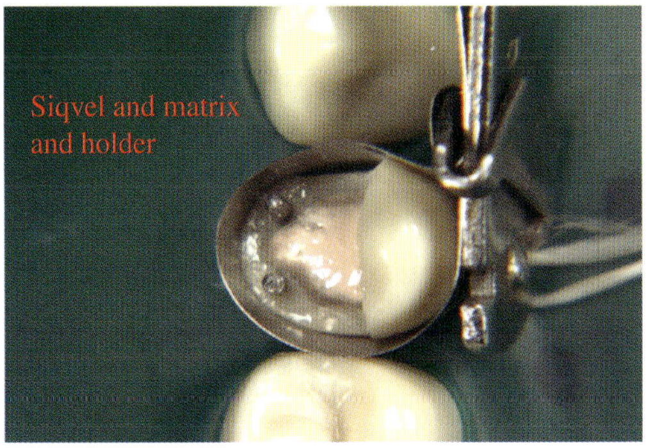

In this view, the Siqveland is in place with the latch engaged to the gingival side. This narrows the band towards the gingival floor of the cavity to simulate the natural narrowing of the crown of the tooth.

The disadvantage of this system is that the band cannot be removed from the holder while still attached to the tooth. Thishinders removal and risks fracturing the amalgam while trying to remove the band.

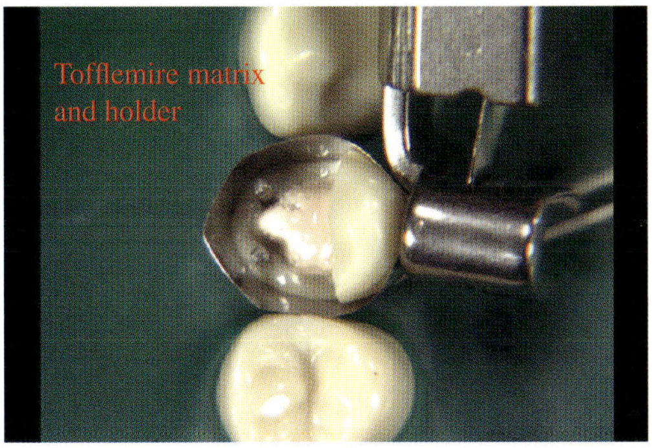

The Tofflemire matrix band and holder is more user friendly in that it allows the band to be teased gently from the tooth after the holder has been removed.

The band is boomerang shaped so that when it is inserted into the holder it will automatically adopt a flared shape similar to the flared nature of the crown of the tooth. It is important that the open end of the holder always faces the gingival tissues. This allows the holder to be removed more easily.

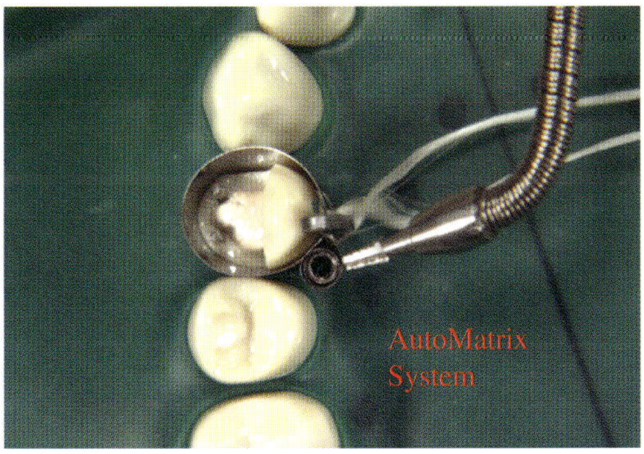

The AutoMatrix is an adjustable stainless steel band that can be tightened using a hand wrench. This system is also tapered to conform with the anatomy of the tooth.

After the insertion of the amalgam, the band can be removed by cutting the top from the retaining flange. This is done using a cutting tool similar to Maun's cutters but with a protective plastic sheath to avoid trauma to the soft tissues and to retain the removed tip and prevent accidental inhalation.

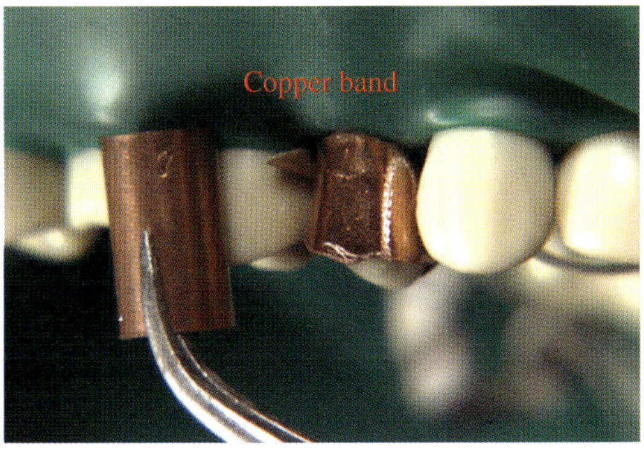

Copper bands come in a wide range of diameters but a standard height. A band of suitable diameter can be adapted to the tooth and the upper surface adapted with rotary instruments to conform to the occlusion.

The disadvantage of this system is that the band is not flared and cannot be adjusted easily to provide a snug fit over the marginsof the cavity. It is also thicker than all the previously mentioned stainless steel bands. This means that the contact point will not be tight when the band is removed.

One advantage that this system offers is that the band can be left in situto support the filling until the patient returns.

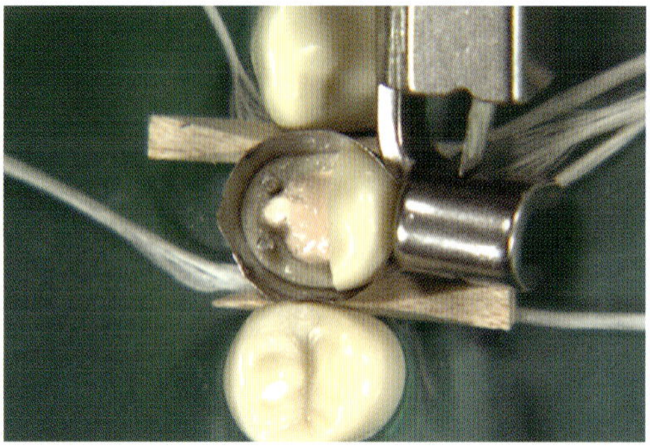

In this slide sequence, a Tofflemire band and holder will be used during the restoration of this premolar tooth. Two pieces of floss have been placed before the matrix band was applied. Wooden wedges have been inserted subsequently to adapt the band more closely to the gingival margin of the cavity. In this way overhanging margins of amalgam can be minimised or removed with the floss. Occasionally, the floss may become trapped between the band and the gingival floor of the cavity. Always check to ensure this has not happened.
In larger cavities, the placement of wedges frequently compromises the tightness or quality of the contact. The band should be burnished outwards against the adjacent tooth.

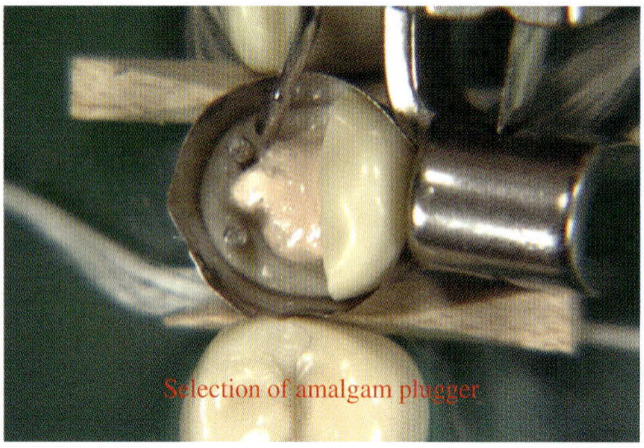

An amalgam pluggershould be selected that will allow the operator to condense amalgam firmly around the dentine pins and onto the narrowest areas in the gingival floor of the cavity.

If too large a pluggeris selected, the condensation of the amalgam will be compromised and may be porous. This will allow leakage and reduce the life expectancy of the filling.

The operator should also ascertain that the pluggercan condense the filling material into any prepared slots and grooves.

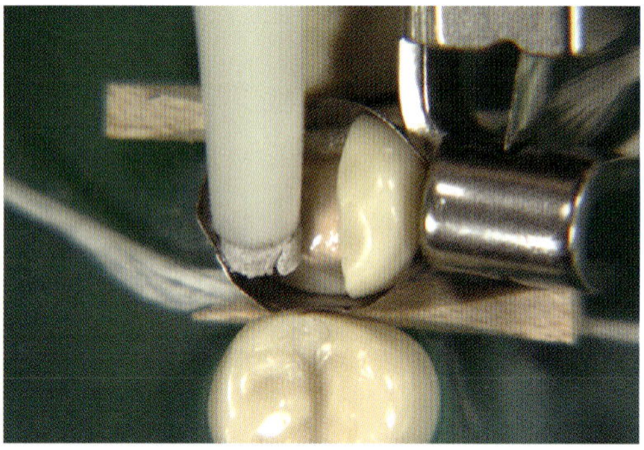

The first increment of amalgam is transferred to the cavity and placed close to the gingival floor. It is now ready to be condensed using the selected size of amalgam plugger.

Condensation of the amalgam should take place in two distinct actions:

- Vertical condensation
- Horizontal sweeping motion to bring the amalgam into intimatecontact with the box wallsAfter

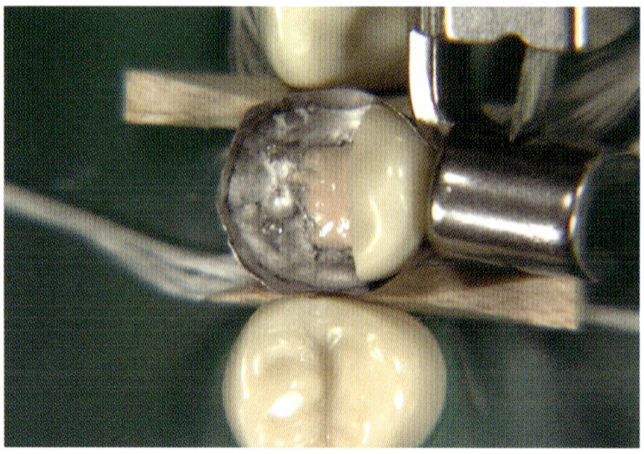

After a few increments of filling material have been placed, therestoration should be built up to around the top of the pins andthe occlusal aspect of the axial wall.

Note how the amalgam has been condensed firmly around the dentine pins and along the gingival floor.

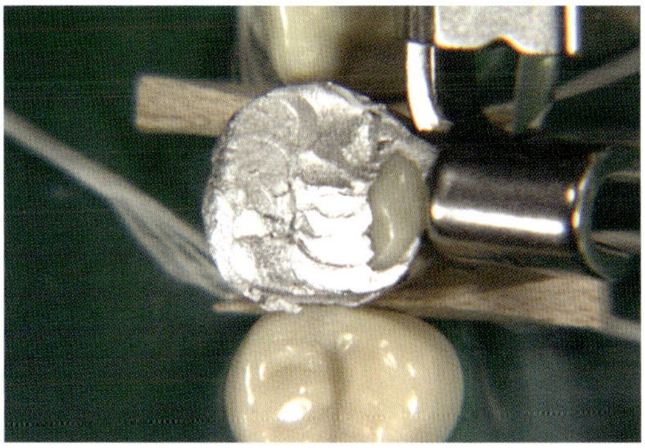

Further increments are added and condensed with a larger size of plugger. This is continued until the filling material has been built up to the same level as the lost area of tooth structure.

A slight excess will be present over the margins at this stage.

In the last stage of condensation, the pluggers should be used to try and shape the cusp slopes as the filling material is being condensed. To achieve this they should be used parallel to the cusp slopes and not used with vertical packing action.

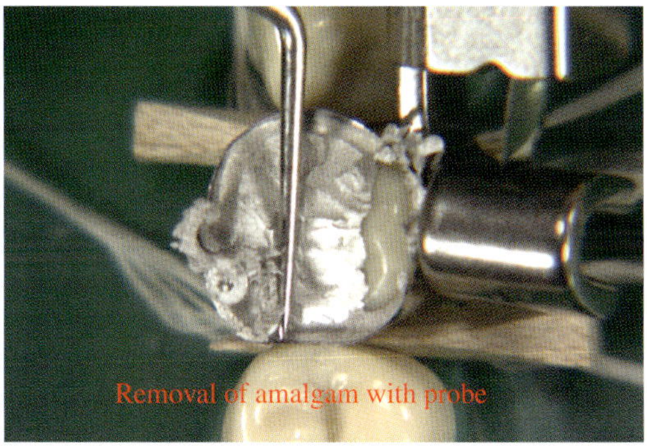

The amalgam from around the margins of the band should be removed by using a right angled probe at 45° angle against the inner aspect of the matrix band.

This removes the small fragments of weak material from the margin that would readily fracture during matrix band removal. In addition, it correctly shapes the interproximalmarginal ridge areas that form the contact point. Contact points commence about 1 mm below the marginal ridge area and NOT at the very edge of this anatomical feature.

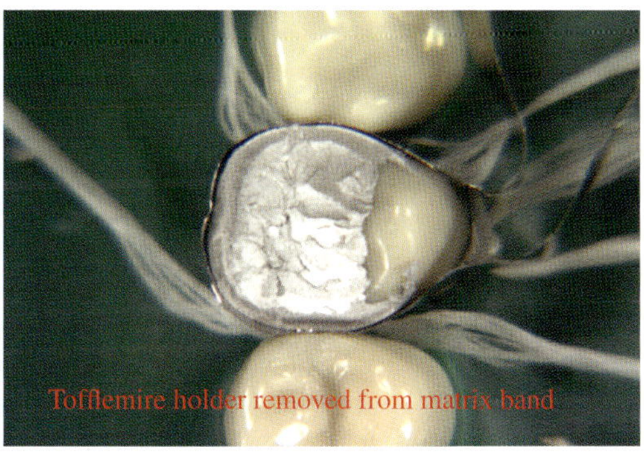

Once this has been completed, the wedges are removed and the Tofflemire matrix holder is removed from the band. This leaves the band loose but still in place around the tooth.

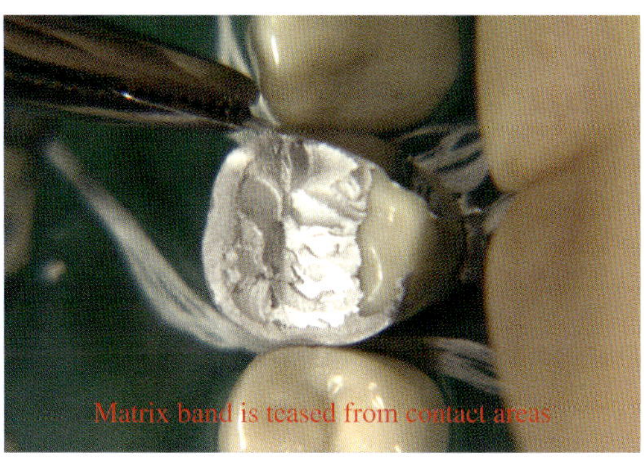

The boomerang shaped matrix band can now be removed by teasing it from the contact areas. In this view, the band is being held in the tip of mosquito forceps to facilitate manipulation.

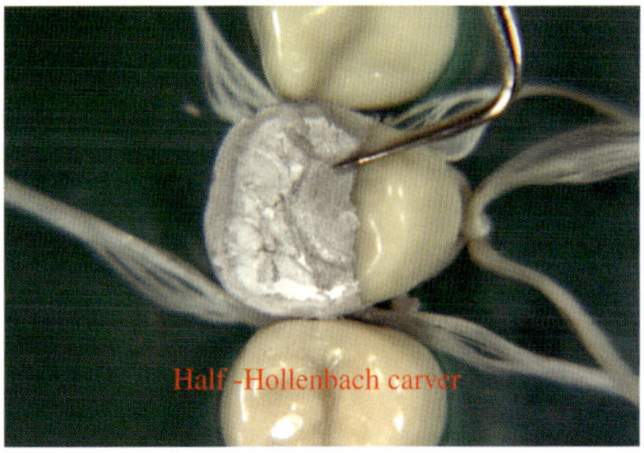

The half-Hollenbach carver can now be used to shape the amalgam accordingly. The side of the carver is laid on the enamel slopes and dragged along while the point of the carver is kept towards the mid-line of the tooth. In this way the appropriate shape of filling is produced.

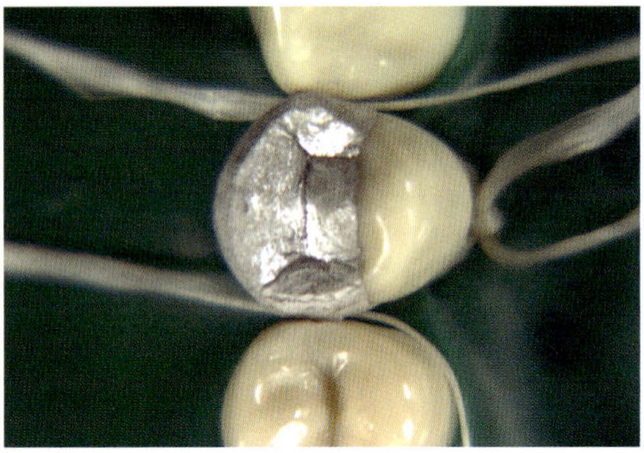

In this view of the carved occlusal surface, the following features have been reproduced:

- Missing buccal cusp tip
- Marginal spillways

These features are required in a good quality restoration to:

- Prevent over-eruption or drifting of the opposing tooth
- Direct food away from the interproximal areas where food packing would result

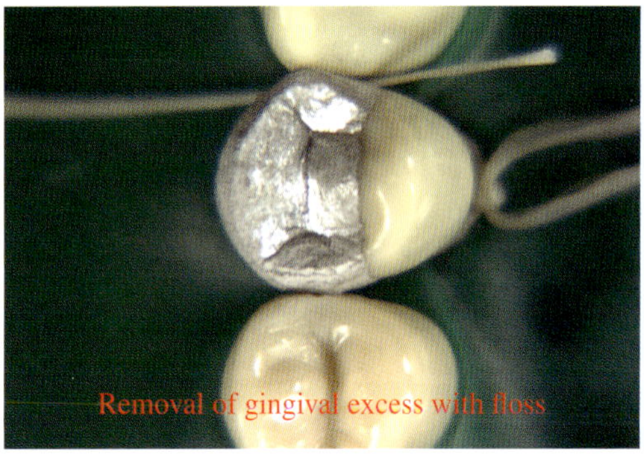

The floss that was placed previously before the matrix band can then be used to remove excess amalgam from the gingival areas.

Care must be taken to ensure that this floss is not brought up through the the contact points or the quality of the contact will be adversely affected.

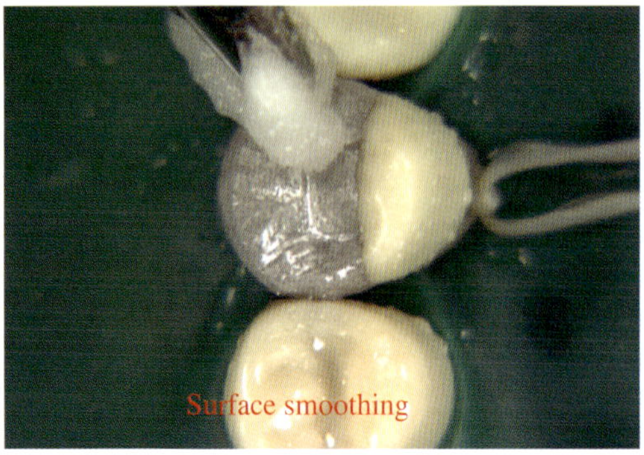

The surface of the filling material is then smoothed by wiping with a piece of damp cotton wool held in college tweezers. The smooth surface imparted is important in making the finishing andpolishing of the amalgam easier.

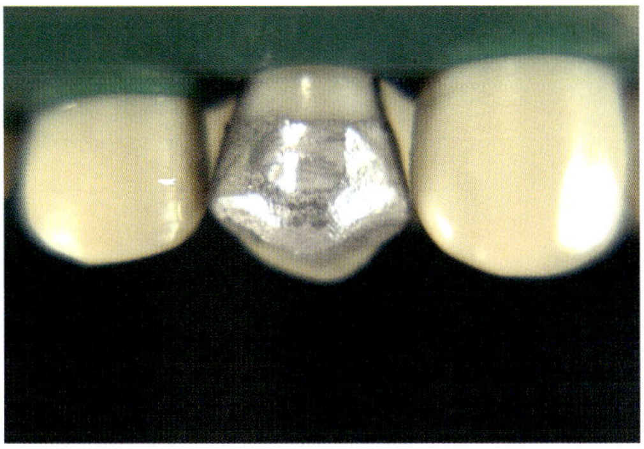

The contour of the filling should be inspected from various angles to ensure that it conforms with the natural anatomy. This view shows the absence of overhanging amalgam at the gingival margins and that the buccal cusp tip has been reproduced.

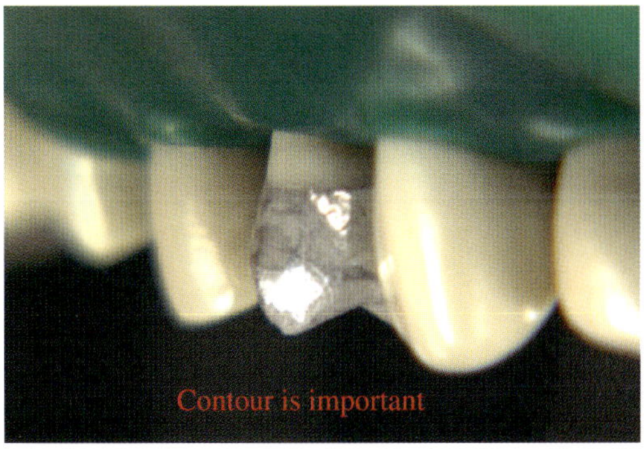

The more bulbous buccal surface has also been reproduced carefully. It is important that the cusp tip is not left in toobuccal a position. If this occurs patients will frequently complain of cheek biting and ulceration of the buccal mucosa.

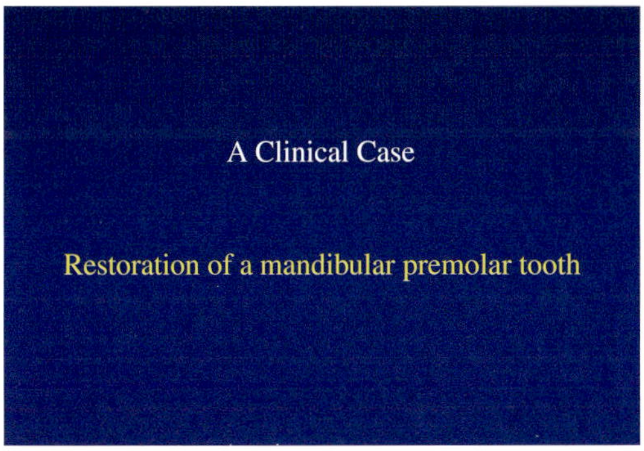

In the next two slides a root treated premolar tooth will be shown that has been built up prior to crowning at a later stage after the endodontic treatment has been reviewed for success.

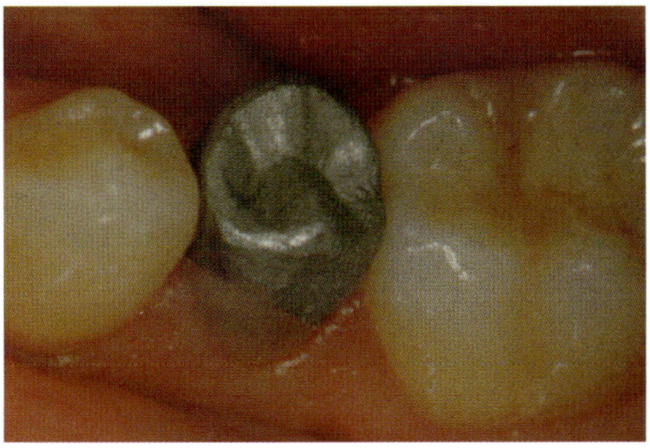

This mandibular second premolar tooth has been restored with a prefabricated post and dentine pin retained amalgam that was placed within an AutoMatrix.

While some nice anatomical features have been reproduced, it could be criticised for having only one lingual cusp when most lower second premolar teeth have two lingual cusps.

The lack of the correct anatomy will be important when this tooth is prepared subsequently for a crown.

Further Reading

Abdelaziz, K.M. and Saleh, A.A. (2018). Influence of adhesive-composite application modalities on their bonding to tooth structure and resistance of the performed restorations to failure. *Journal of Dental Sciences* 13: 378–385.

Baltacioglu, I.H. and Orhan, K. (2017). Comparison of diagnostic methods for early interproximal caries detection with near-infrared light transillumination: an *in vivo* study. *BMC Oral Health* 17: 130–137.

British Dental Association BDA Policy and Campaigns (2020) https://bda.org/amalgam

Bonsor, S.J. (2011). Bonded amalgams and their use in clinical practice. *Dental Update* 38: 222–230.

Bonsor, S.J. (2013). Are dentine pins obsolete. *Dental Update* 40: 253–258.

Chu, C.H., Mei, M.L., Cheung, C., and Nalliah, R.P. (2013). Restoring proximal caries lesions conservatively with tunnel restorations. *Clinical, Cosmetic and Investigational Dentistry* (5): 43–50.

Foster, L.V. (1998). Three year *in vivo* investigation to determine the progression of approximal primary carious lesions extending into dentine. *British Dental Journal* 10 (185): 353–357.

Gilboa, I. and Cardash, H.S. (2003). A conservative technique for restoring a tooth affected by interproximal root caries. *Journal of Prosthetic Dentistry* 89: 221–222.

Hurlbutt, M. and Young, D.A. (2014). A best practices approach to caries management. *Journal of Evidence Base Dental Practice* 14: 77–86.

Knight, G.M. (1992). The tunnel restoration - nine years of clinical experience using capsulated glass ionomer cements. *Australian Dental Journal* 37 (4): 245–251.

Llena, C., Folguera, S., Forner, L., and Rodríguez-Lozano, F.J. (2018). Implementation of augmented reality in operative dentistry learning. *European Journal of Dental Education* 22: 122–130.

Loomans, B.A.C., Opdam, N.J.M., Roeters, F.J.M. et al. (2009). Restoration techniques and marginal overhang in class II composite resin restorations. *Journal of Dentistry* 37: 712–717.

Lumley, P.J. and Fisher, F.J. (1995). Tunnel restorations: a long-term pilot study over a minimum of five years. *Journal of Dentistry* 23: 213–215.

Matvijenko, B.V., Milan, Z.V., Mitić, D.A. et al. (2012). Effect of irregular interproximal dental restorations on periodontal status. *Acta Stomatologica Naissi* 28: 1144–1154.

Olafsson, V.G., Ritter, A.V., Swift, E.J. et al. (2018). Effect of composite type and placement technique on cuspal strain. *Journal of Esthetic Restorative Dentistry* 30: 30–38.

Pintado-Palomino, K., Barros de Almeida, C.V.V., Gonçalves da Motta, R.J. et al. (2019). Clinical, double blind, randomized controlled trial of experimental adhesive protocols in caries-affected dentin. *Clinical Oral Investigations* 23: 1855–1864.

Politi, I., McHugh, L.E.J., Al-Fodeh, R.S., and Fleming, G.J.P. (2018). Modification of the restoration protocol for resin-based composite (RBC) restoratives(conventional and bulk fill) on cuspal movement and microleakage score in molar teeth. *Dental Materials* 34: 1271–1277.

Rajasekharan, S., Martens, L.C., RGCE, C., and Anthonappa, R.P. (2018). Biodentine™ material characteristics and clinical applications: a 3 year literature review and update. *European Archives of Paediatric Dentistry* 19: 1–22.

Roggendorf, M.J., Kramer, N., Appelt, A. et al. (2011). Marginal quality of flowable 4-mm base vs. conventionally layered resin composite. *Journal of Dentistry* 39: 643–647.

Vaught, R.L. (2007). Mechanical versus chemical retention for restoring complex restorations: what is the evidence? *Journal of Dental Education* 71: 1356–1362.

da Veiga, A.M.A., Cunha, A.C., Ferreira, D.M.T. et al. (2016). Longevity of direct and indirect resin composite restorations in permanent posterior teeth: a systematic review and meta-analysis. *Journal of Dentistry* 54: 1–12.

Wei, J., Zhi, C., and Frencken, J.E. (2009). Strength of tunnel-restored teeth with different materials and marginal ridge height. *Dental Materials* 25: 1363–1370.

Young, D.A., Nový, B.B., Zeller, G.G. et al. (2015). The American dental association caries classification system for clinical practice. *Journal of American Dental Association* 146: 79–86.

7

Restorations in Anterior Teeth

Restoration of incisor and canine teeth are most frequently performed using composite resin. Anterior teeth may require restoration due to caries on the interproximal surface, which Black described as a class III cavity, but, if these lesions are left untreated, they may progress and involve the incisal edge and, at this stage, are known as class IV lesions. Anterior teeth may also require restoration if they have been subjected to trauma resulting in their fracture or to mask unsightly developmental lesions. Wear of anterior teeth due to attrition, abrasion, or erosion may be restored using direct techniques (see Figure 7.1).

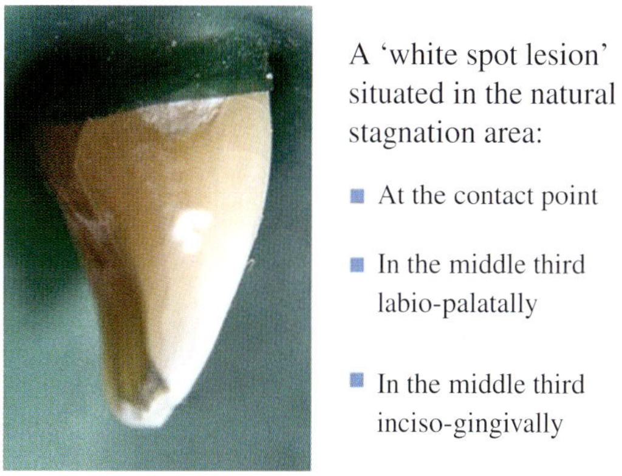

Figure 7.1 This extracted tooth clearly shows the central position of a white spot lesion.

An interproximal carious lesion commences at the contact point between teeth and may cast a shadow that can be seen clinically. This type of lesion is not seen on routine bitewing radiographs because they do not involve the anterior teeth, and panoramic radiographs fail to show adequate detail due to superimposition of the cervical spine. The only radiographic view that will show these teeth and lesions adequately is a periapical view. The incidence of class III cavities is lower than for similarly placed lesions in posterior teeth because anterior teeth are more amenable to plaque control measures and the natural stagnation area is smaller. However, the incidence can be raised in patients who have crowded or imbricated incisors because the size of the stagnation area is larger and access for cleaning is hindered. Patients who are mouth breathers may also have an increased incidence of caries due to the lack of adequate amounts of saliva and its buffering capacity.

A Practical Approach to Operative Dentistry, First Edition. Gordon B. Gray and Alaa H. Daud.

Companion website: www.wiley.com/go/gray/operative-dentistry

The diagnosis of interproximal caries can be made in a number of ways (see Figure 7.2). Diagnosis of the early white spot lesion is difficult, but once the lesion has spread into the underlying dentine, it may be diagnosed more easily.

Diagnostic Methods
- Probe
- Visual
- Radiograph
- Transillumination
- Shredding of floss

Figure 7.2 There are a variety of methods to diagnose interproximal caries in anterior teeth, and the relative merits of those are discussed below.

A Briault or Weston probe may facilitate diagnosis, but all probes should be used lightly because they can break down the surface of the white spot lesion and introduce cariogenic bacteria.

Good quality periapical radiographs are particularly sensitive in diagnosis because they will depict even early enamel caries.

Transillumination can be used as an aid to visual inspection, and this technique works well in thinner anterior teeth. The dental mirror can be used to reflect light from the operating lamp while the operator inspects the teeth from their labial aspect. Fibre optic transillumination (FOTI) may also be used as well as a newer digital technique (DIFOTI) where the images may be stored electronically for future comparison.

Dental floss may shred if inserted between the anterior teeth where there is a carious lesion present. The validity of this method of diagnosis is low because other such factors as the presence of calculus or sharp tooth or restoration margins can result in shredding.

Black classified interproximal caries in anterior teeth as a class III cavity where the incidence was found to be lower than that for pit and fissure caries or those lesions arising between posterior teeth. A newer classification was suggested by Mount and Hume in 1997, and this takes into account the site, size, and complexity of the carious lesion (see Figure 7.3).

A moderate sized carious lesion in an interproximal site of an incisor tooth may be referred to as a 2.2.

Mount Classification of Carious Lesions
- Site 1 – Pit and fissure lesions
- Site 2 – Lesions related to contact points
- Site 3 – Lesions related to gingival third

- Size 1 – Minimal
- Size 2 – Moderate
- Size 3 – Large
- Size 4 – Extensive

Figure 7.3 An alternative and contemporary classification for caries is shown.

Cavity Design

Isolation

The dental papilla occupies the space below the contact area, making this structure liable to bleeding during cavity preparation or seepage of crevicular fluid into the restorative material. Only where there is gingival recession is the papilla likely to be absent. It would be advisable, therefore, to use rubber dam to retract the papilla and ensure good quality marginal seal for the longevity of the restoration. A floss ligature will ensure the margins of the dam are inverted.

Accessing the Carious Lesion

Generally, access to the carious lesion is from a palatal approach so that a layer of intact enamel will be left labially to provide a good appearance. The cavity preparation removes the contact point via an access through the palatal marginal ridge. One of the dangers is that the cavity preparation will be overextended and show on the labial surface of the tooth. This would detract from the final appearance unless great care is exercised in the preparation. The cavity must be clear of the contact area, and, because it will be restored with composite resin, it should have rounded line angles and be devoid of unsupported enamel. The initial access cavity should be in the middle third of the palatal marginal ridge, otherwise the contact area will be missed in the cavity outline. In smaller to medium sized cavities that are not cavitated, a thin sliver of enamel can be kept to avoid damage to the adjacent tooth. This can then be removed using a chisel and the labial extent of the cavity adjusted until it can just be seen on the labial surface.

Caries Removal

The removal of caries should always be commenced from around the enamel dentine junction, where risk of pulpal perforation is low. The peripheral removal of caries onto sound tooth structure using a slow-speed round bur will make the inner aspect of the cavity larger than the access opening. This will generally make the cavity mechanically retentive. However, as the cavity will be restored with an adhesive restorative material, it is not necessary to actively prepare mechanical retention. Caries removal can then continue by removing the softened dentine from over the more central pulpal floor. In deeper lesions this can be accomplished using a sharp excavator where the risk of perforation is minimised.

Enamel Margins

Unsupported enamel should be removed from the periphery of the cavity and to provide an acceptable cavo-surface angle or between 70 and 110°. The cavo-surface angle is not so critical when composite resin is used as it would be for amalgam. This is due to the fact that bonding composite resin to the enamel using an acid etch procedure will support slightly weakened enamel prisms. A gingival margin trimmer is a very useful instrument in the finishing of the cavity preparation.

Bevelling the margin of the cavity is useful in areas where the tooth to restorative margin will be seen. This is because the composite resin can be blended into the surrounding surface in a more imperceptible manner. The majority of labial margins will be only just clear of the labial contact area, so this procedure should not be necessary and should be considered only for the more extensive cavity. The palatal margin will not be seen so the need for bevelling should not be considered due to the over-preparation of the cavity when the restoration is replaced in the future.

Use of a Lining Material

A lining material is generally used to provide additional thermal insulation below restorations. This is particularly important when metallic restorations are placed. The thermal conductivity of composite resin is very low, so if postoperative sensitivity is present, it is generally due to microleakage around the restoration margin or to movement of fluid in the dentinal tubules. The placement of a glass ionomer or setting calcium hydroxide lining will help protect the pulp from these effects, but the application of a dentine bonding agent to the etched dentine will also reduce sensitivity by penetrating the tubules and preventing fluid movement. There is a benefit to using a dental cement as a lining in that it will act as a visual barrier in deep cavities when restorations are replaced at a future time.

Summary

Cavity design features:

- The contact point must be removed
- The labial cavity margin should just be visible
- Internal line angles should be rounded to reduce stress
- Unsupported enamel must be removed
- Iatrogenic damage to the adjacent tooth must be avoided

Restoration of Anterior Interproximal Caries

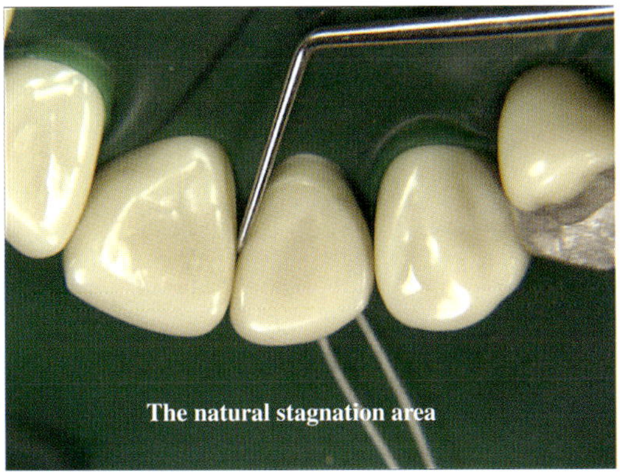

Maxillary incisors have concave palatal surfaces with distinct marginal ridges to the mesial and distal sides. A cingulum is frequently noted, and where present, a pit will be found.
A floss ligature will retract the gingivae and invert the margins of the dam, improving, the isolation. The probe indicates the natural stagnation area where this tooth contacts the adjacent central incisor. Caries may initiate just below this contact point unless oral hygiene practises are observed. Toothbrushing alone will not clean the interproximal tooth surfaces. The use of dental floss is required.

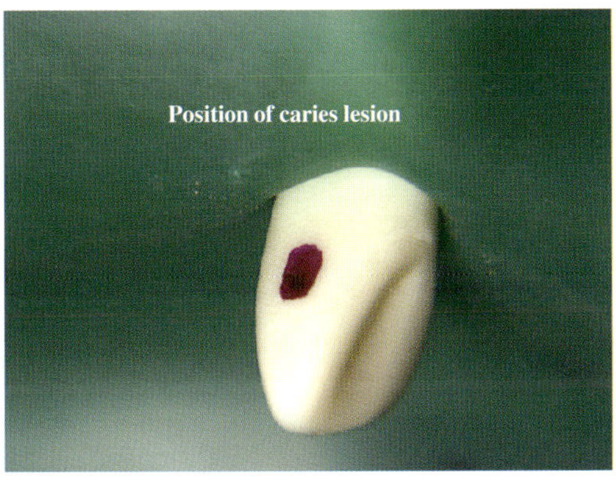

The shaded area on this interproximal surface depicts the area of the caries at the enamel dentinal junction (EDJ)
Note that it commences at and just below the contact point and is situated in the middle third of this tooth surface -in both a labio-palatal and an inciso-gingival direction .

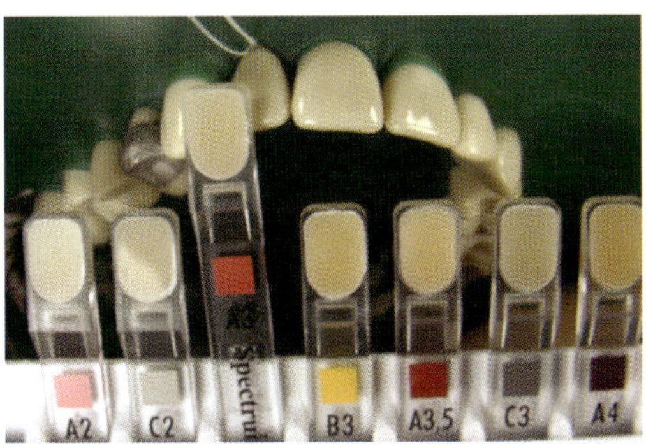

The appropriate shade of composite should be selected immediately before the tooth has had a chance to dry out under the rubber dam.
Many operators choose the shade before the tooth is isolated under the rubber dam because the tooth begins to lighten as it dries out.

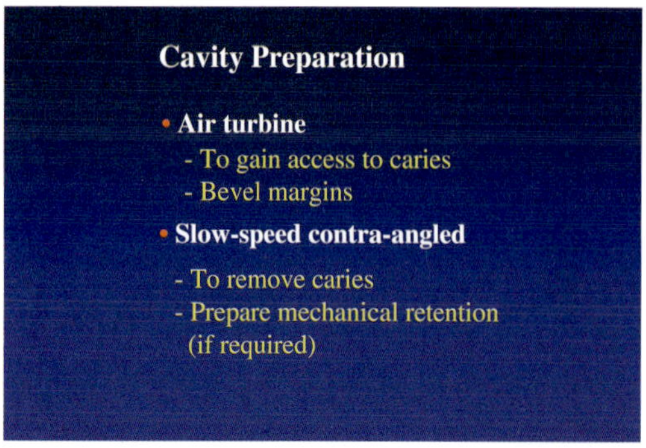

The air turbine handpiece is used only to gain access to the caries lesion.
Thereafter, the slow contra-angled handpiece is used to remove the caries from the cavity.
Most of the cavity preparation will be done using slow-speed burs.

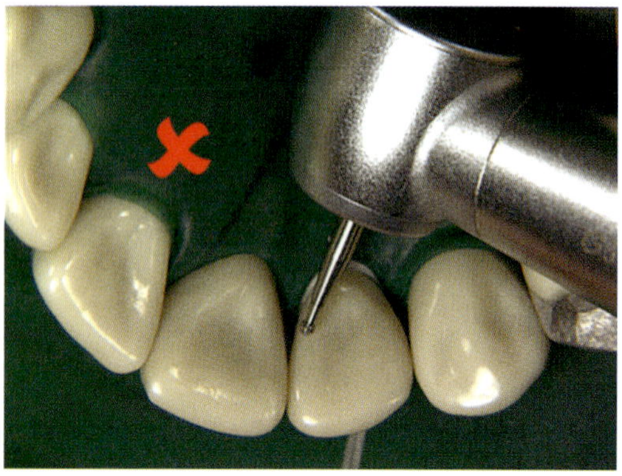

When gaining access with the air turbine handpiece, the angle of approach is important.
A 520 small round diamond coated bur is used that is 1 mm in diameter.
If the angle of approach is taken at right angles to the palatal surface (or from a distal inclination), unnecessary removal of enamel from the marginal ridge will result.
Sufficient access must be achieved, however, to allow complete caries removal.

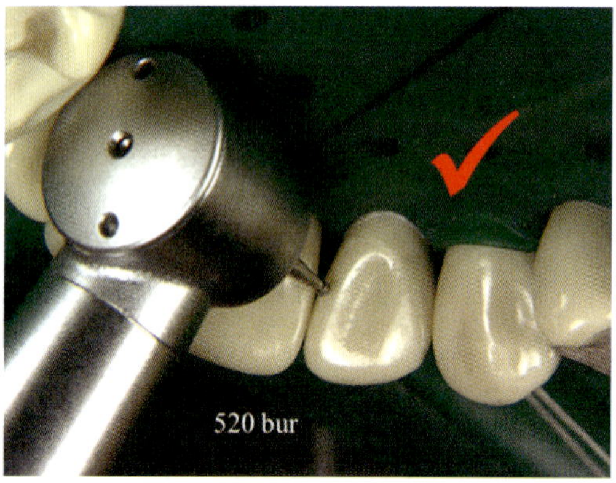

An approach from a mesial direction will limit the amount of enamel removed from the marginal ridge.
It should be remembered that the incisal edges of the mandibular incisors make contact with the opposing marginal ridge areas of the maxillary teeth. If composite restorations are placed in areas of contact, wear may result.

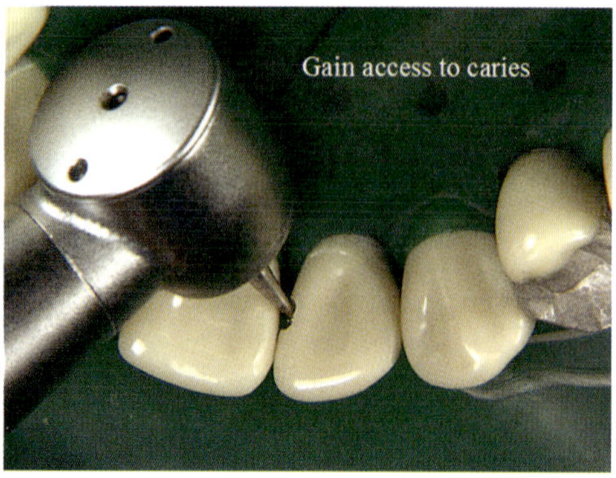

Video 7.1

In this view, access to the caries lesion has been gained. Note that the bur must penetrate right round onto the mesialsurface of the tooth to reach the facial (or labial) aspect of the lesion. Less than half of the width of the marginal ridge has been removed.
Labial enamel should be preserved where possible because the appearance of natural enamel is always better than that of composite resin.
The latter will tend to stain and may yellow with age.

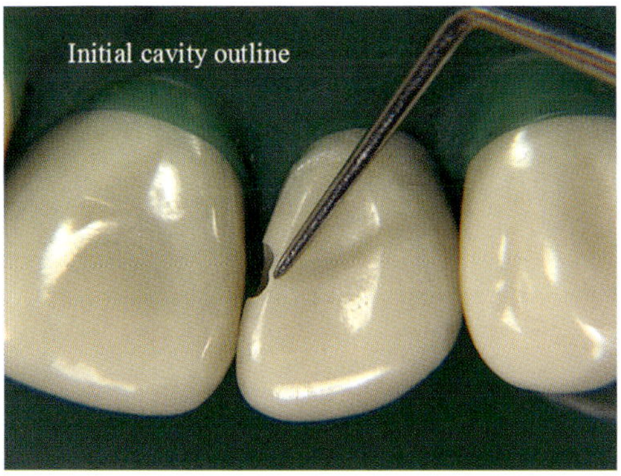

In this view, access has been gained, and the probe is highlighting the palatal margin of the cavity that lies on the marginal ridge area.

The gingival papilla has been retracted away from the gingival margin of the cavity. In healthy conditions, the interproximal space is filled with the gingival papilla.

Note that the labial margin extends to the junction of the middle and labial third of the mesial tooth surface.

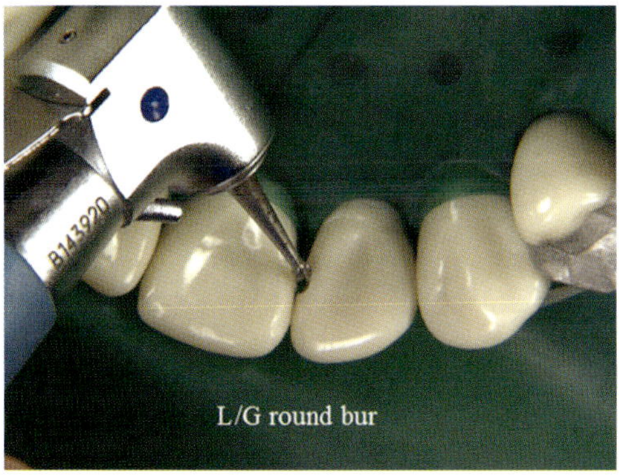

The air turbine handpiece can now be set aside. A number 3 round latch grip bur can be used at conventional speed to remove the caries from around the periphery of the cavity.
Current clinical practice dictates that all stained and softened dentine should be removed from the EDJ to prevent re-activation of altered dentine if leakage should occur.
Dentine bonding would also be affected if altered dentine were left in this situation.

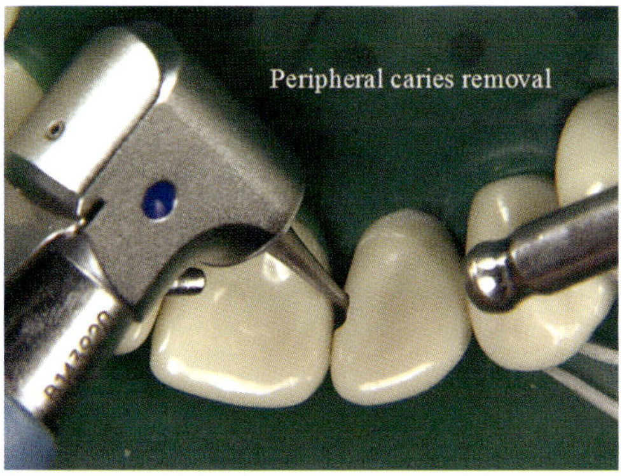

Caries is removed from around the periphery of the cavity.
In this view, the bur is being used to remove the caries from the labial wall of the cavity.

Video 7.2

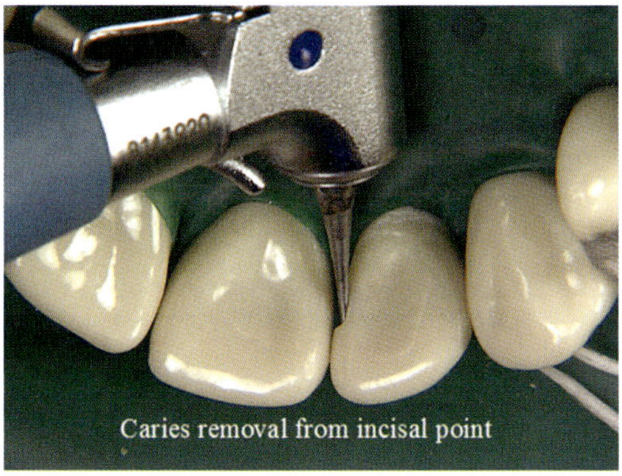

Caries removal is then extended to the EDJ junction nearer the incisal edge...and onwards to the palatal wall and then along the gingival floor.

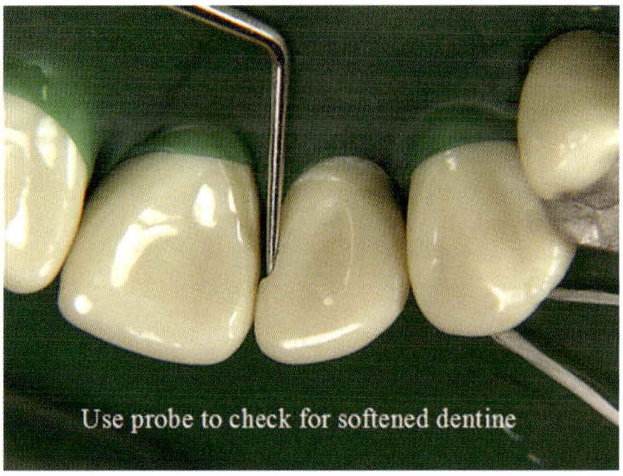

A probe can then be used to explore around the periphery of the cavity to ensure that it is firm and free from softening.
A visual check should be made also to ensure that staining is absent from the EDJ area.

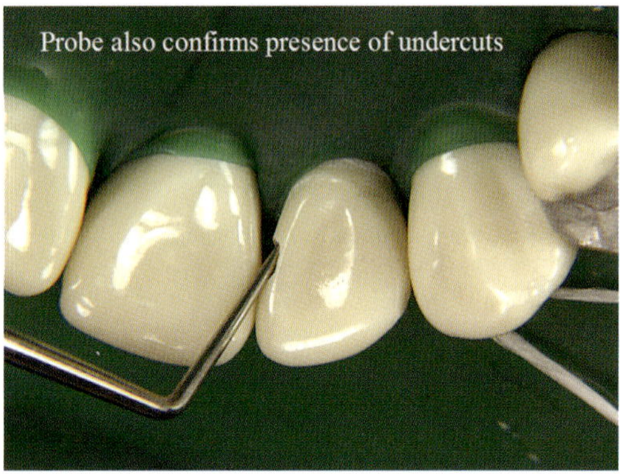

It can be seen that caries removal will often prepare a cavity with an internal aspect that is larger than the access cavity. In other words the cavity will be naturally undercut.
An undercut is present here on the gingival aspect of the cavity.

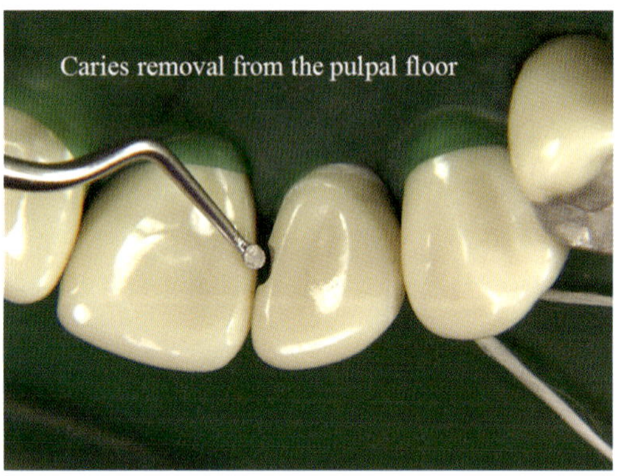

Caries removal from the central area can be accomplished by either using a round bur or an handheld excavator. Excavators are recommended where cavity depth is deep and approaching the pulp.

Work from the central area of the pulpal floor in an outwards direction.

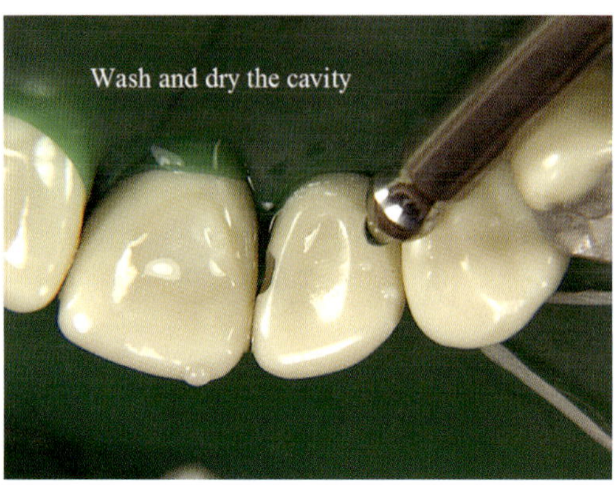

The cavity is then washed and dried using the triple dental syringe.

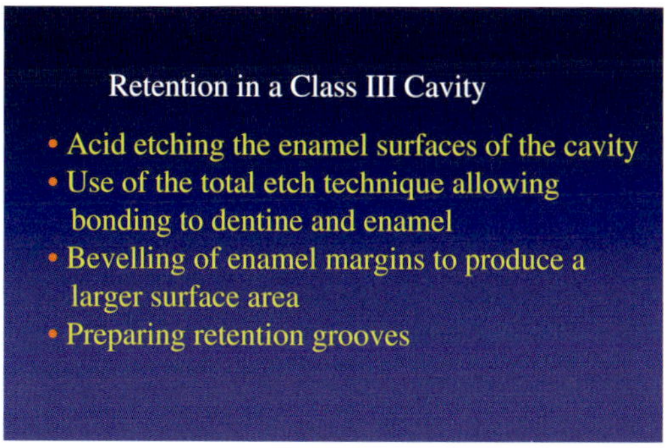

Retention must now be considered.
Most small to medium sized cavities will be naturally retentive as they will have been rendered undercut during caries removal.
Bonding to tooth structures is now commonplace in adhesive aesthetic dentistry.
Only consider preparing retention grooves in exceptional circumstances for larger cavity sizes.

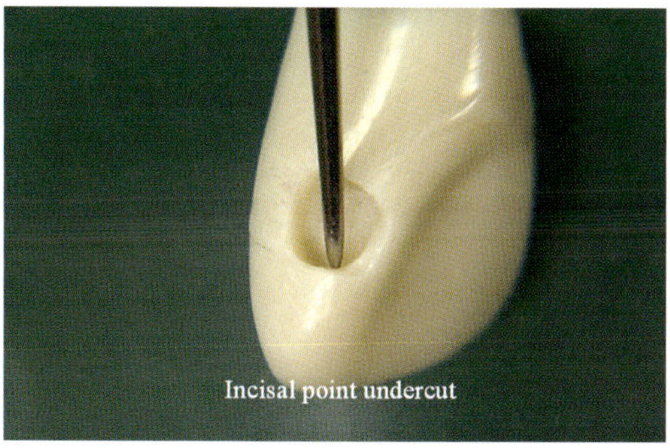

The probe can be used to check for the presence of undercut areas in the point angle incisally and along the gingival floor.
This is usually created naturally when the caries is removed from the EDJ of the cavity.

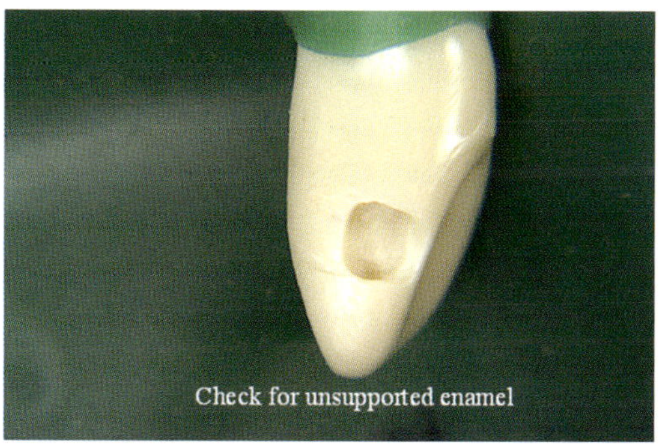

The labial margin can have enamel that is left slightly unsupported because this area of the cavity will not be subject to forces.
The enamel on the palatal side must be supported because the lower incisal edges contact this area and would fracture any unsupported enamel.
Consideration should be paid to use of bevels on enamel margins.

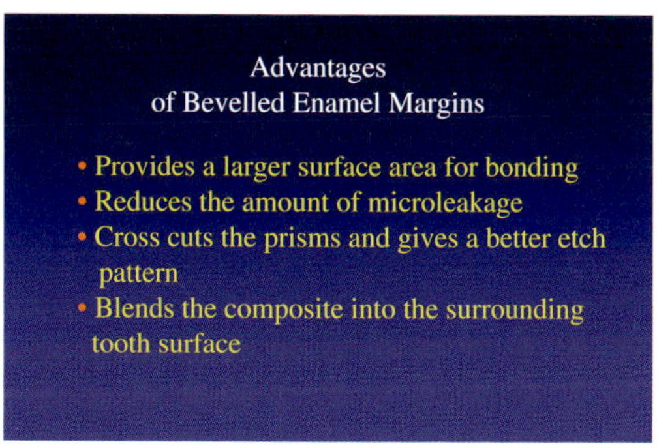

Bevelling enamel margins can be beneficial to the cavity by increasing the surface area of enamel present for bonding and providing an improved etch pattern. It has also been reported to reduce the amount of microleakage that is likely to occur.
From a purely aesthetic point of view, the composite resin is blended into the tooth surface rather than having a distinct finish line.

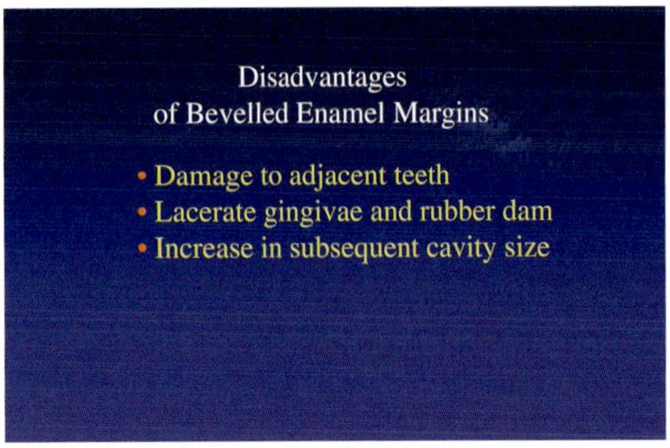

Damage to the adjacent teeth is a distinct possibility when bevelling in confined spaces.
If ginigival bleeding is initiated, the restorative material will be contaminated and detract from the final result.

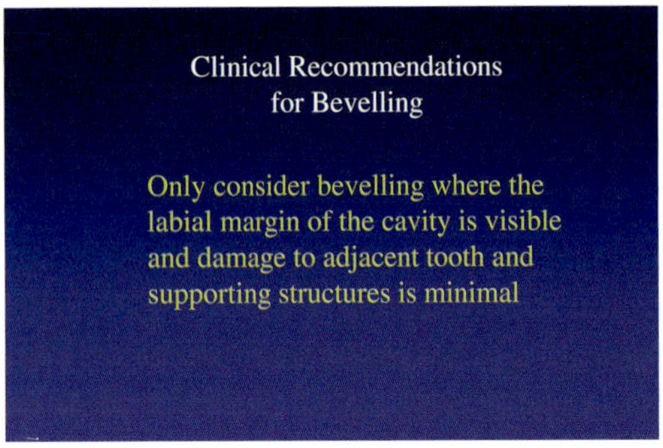

A balanced view must be taken regarding bevelling and the relative merits carefully weighed.
It is suggested that bevelling should be considered only where the labial aspect of the restoration can be clearly seen in larger class III cavities.

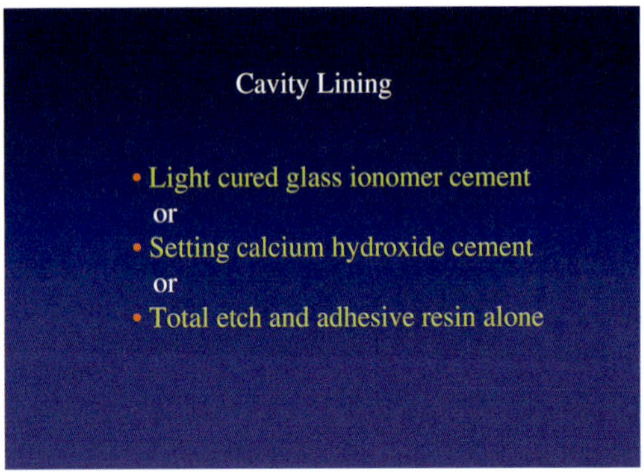

A choice of lining materials is available for lining a class III cavity. Either a setting calcium hydroxide cement could be used or a light cured glass ionomer cement that would bond to the dentine and release fluoride ions.
Many operators now believe that the dentine can be sealed or lined using the total etch technique and applying a hydrophyllic bonding resin that will infiltrate the dentinal tubules. This technique may be used in shallow to moderate depth cavities and relies on the hope that the resin will not hydrolyse with time.

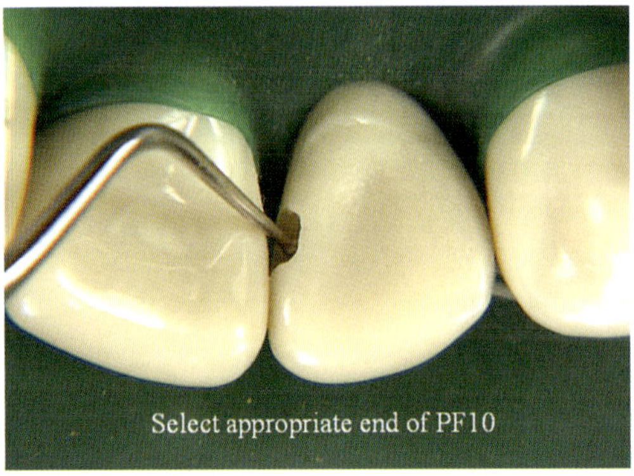

If a lining dental cement is to be used, carefully select the end of the PF10 instrument that will be used. When an inappropriately large end is used, the material will be applied to the walls of the cavity also.

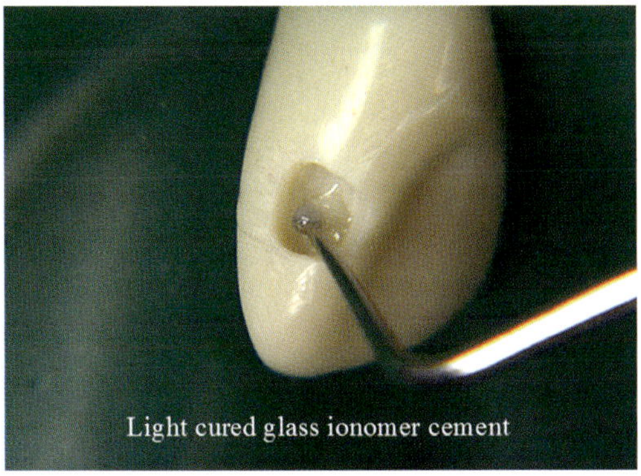

In this sequence a light cured glass ionomer cement will be inserted and spread onto the pulpal floor of the cavity using the PF10 instrument.
Undercuts should not be blocked out using this cement.

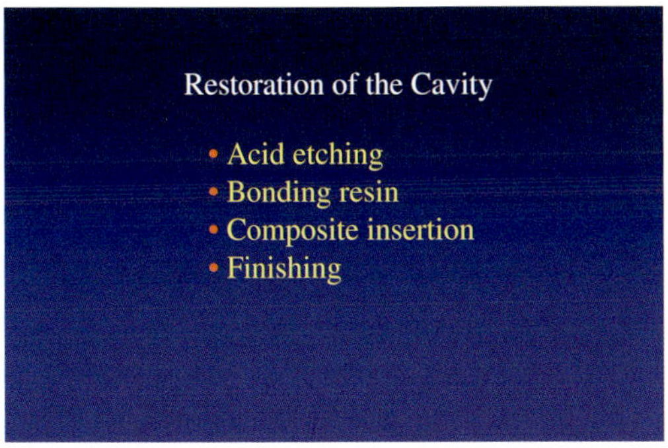

The stages of restoring the prepared cavity are outlined.
They range from etching the enamel and dentine before applying the bonding resin, through to insertion and finishing of the composite resin.

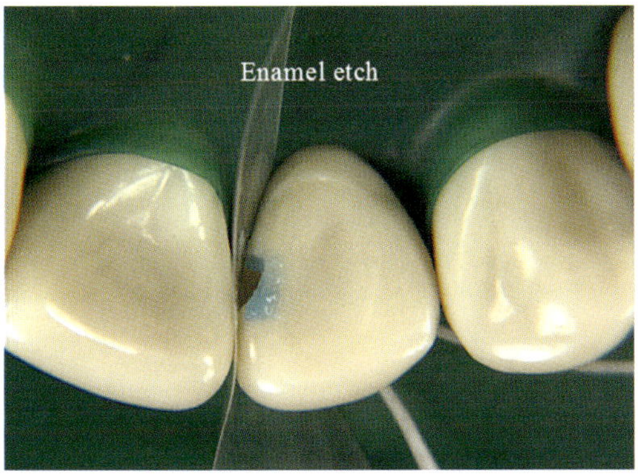

A polyester strip is inserted between the teeth to protect the adjacent tooth structure from inadvertantly etching.
The etch is applied along the enamel margins initially. This is a 36% buffered phosphoric acid gel.
The gel is applied around all of the peripheral enamel on the labial, gingival, and palatal surfaces.
It is often difficult to apply the gel onto the labial enamel margin because access to this area is hindered by the size of the access cavity.

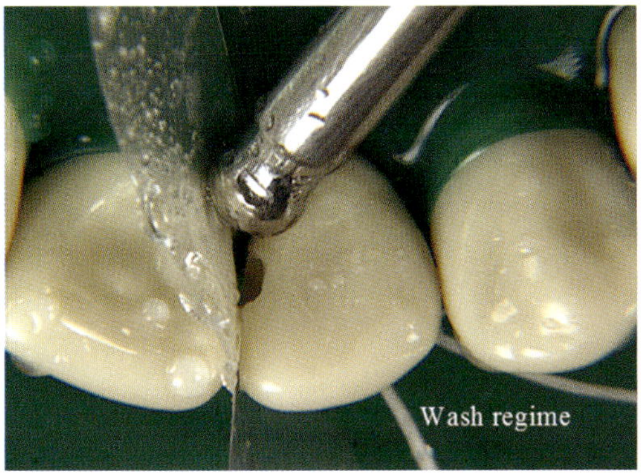

The gel is then applied to the inner aspect of the cavity so that the exposed dentine is etched to remove the smear layer and open out the tubule orifices.
In this way, enamel is etched for up to 15 seconds while the dentine receives a shorter etch time.
The cavity is then liberally washed with water from the triple dental syringe for the same length of time as the etching regime.
Air can be introduced into the water spray to improve the penetration of the wash regime into the cavity.

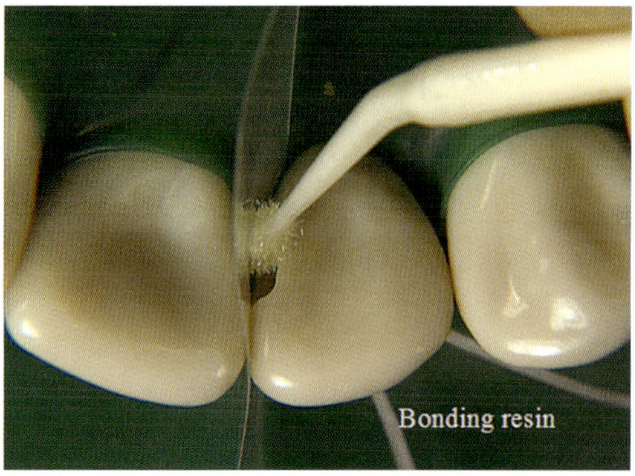

The cavity is then dried using compressed air with care taken to avoid desiccation. A drying regime should not extend, therefore, for more than 2 seconds. Many operators now only apply the aspirator nozzle to the cavity.

A layer of the bonding resin is applied to the dentine, lining material, and enamel and left for 30 seconds to allow it to penetrate into the pores of the etched enamel and the porosity of the lining material-if present. The hydrophillic resin can also penetrate the tubules and around the spaces of the collagen in the hybrid zone.

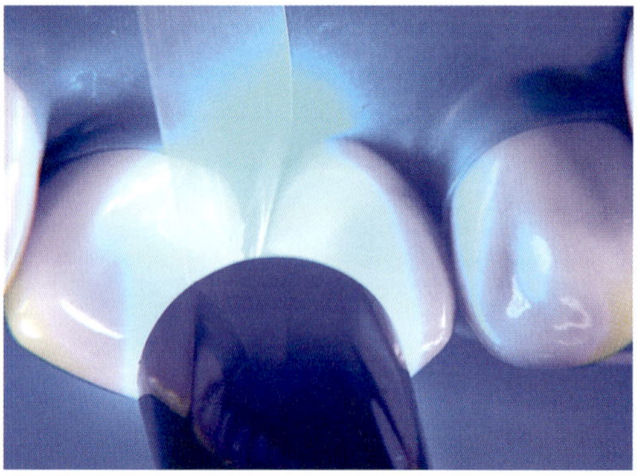

This is then light cured with visible blue light of 470 nm wavelenth. A 10 second exposure should be adequate where the light intensity of the unit being used is adequate.

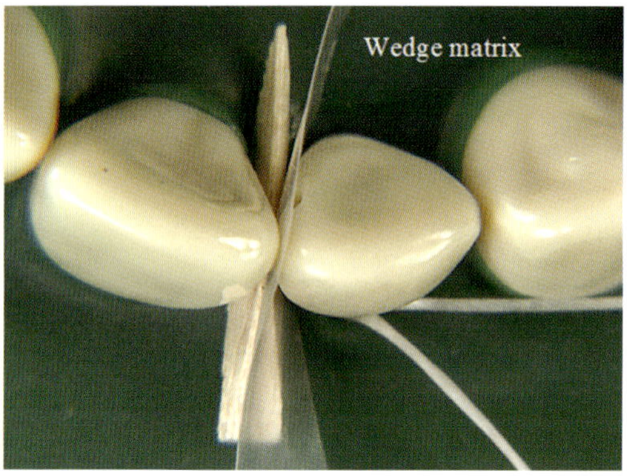

Video 7.3

A new piece of polyester strip is inserted and a wedge placed between the teeth to adapt the matrix to the gingival enamel.

This will prevent overhangs of composite resin when the restoration is polymerised.

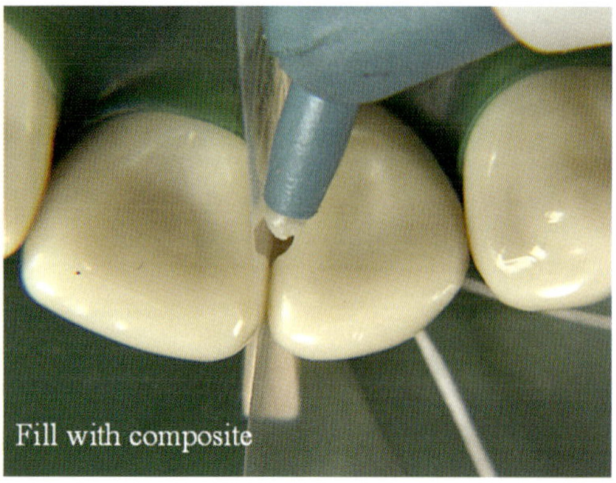

Video 7.4

A small increment of composite is inserted into the cavity from the compule of shade-matched material.

These composite tips contain sufficient material for class III and IV cavities. As they can be used on one patient only, they are an excellent way of maintaining infection control and are user-friendly to insert the composite into the cavity.

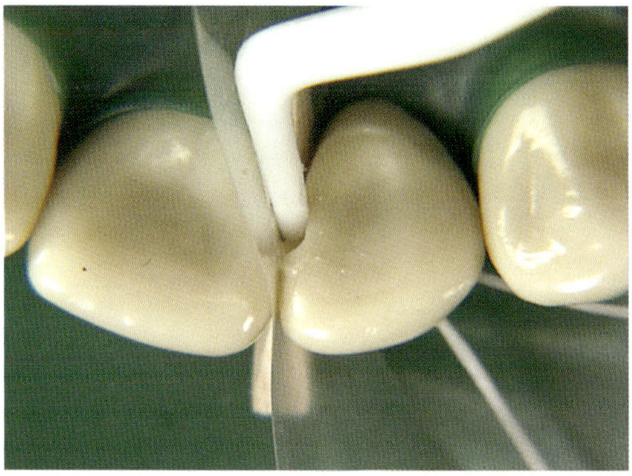

In this view, a Teflon coated instrument is being used to manipulate the composite into the mechanically retentive cavity.

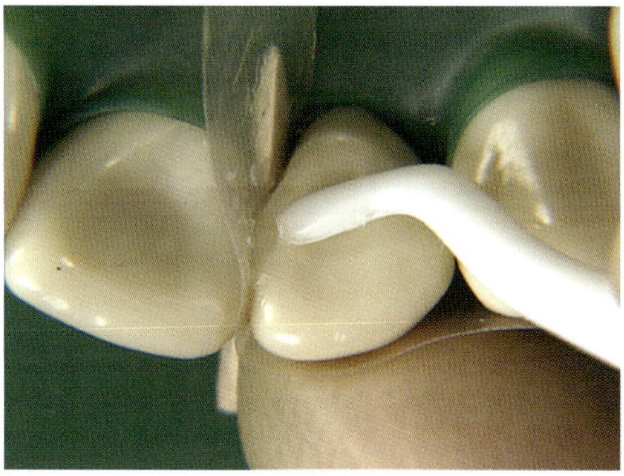

The cavity is then filled with only a slight excess of material.
The thumb of the left hand is being used to hold the matrix strip against the labial surface of the incisor.

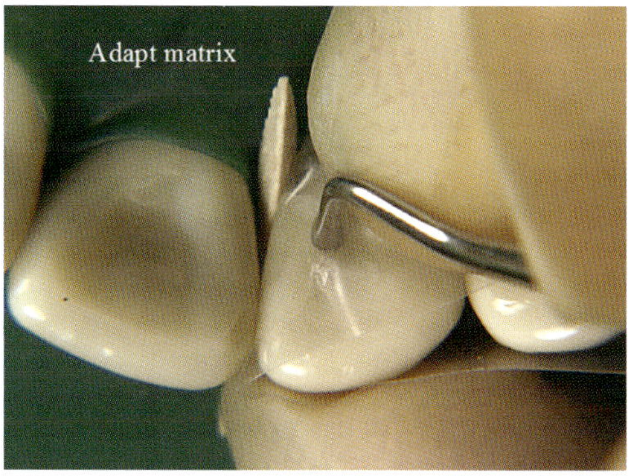

The matrix is then brought around onto the palatal surface of the tooth and held firmly with the forefinger of the left hand.
A ball ended burnisher is then used in the right hand to apply pressure to the enamel surface just beyond the cavity margins.
This ensures that excess filling material is brought into a thin layer for ease of subsequent removal.

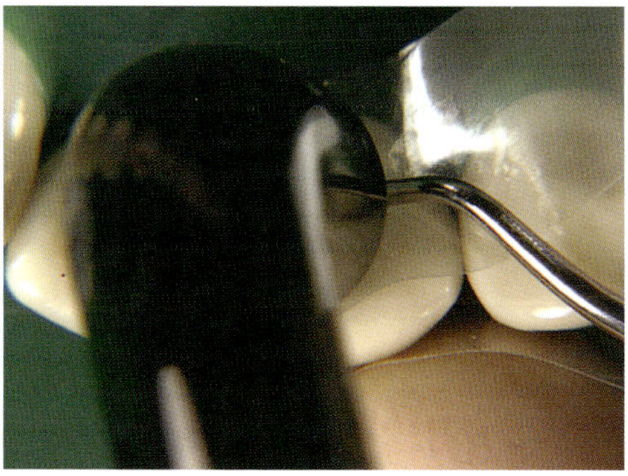

While still holding the burnisher on the surface of the matrix, the assistant can bring the curing light tip in close to the surface of the tooth and initiate curing.
In this case, the thickness of the composite is less than 2 mm and can be cured in one increment of 40 seconds.
Some operators are worried about the risk of pulpal damage by raising the temperature of the pulp during curing in excess of this time.

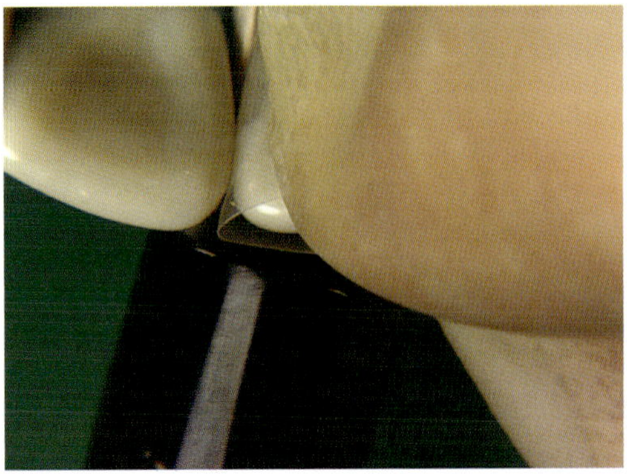

A further cure from the labial aspect will complete the curing regime.

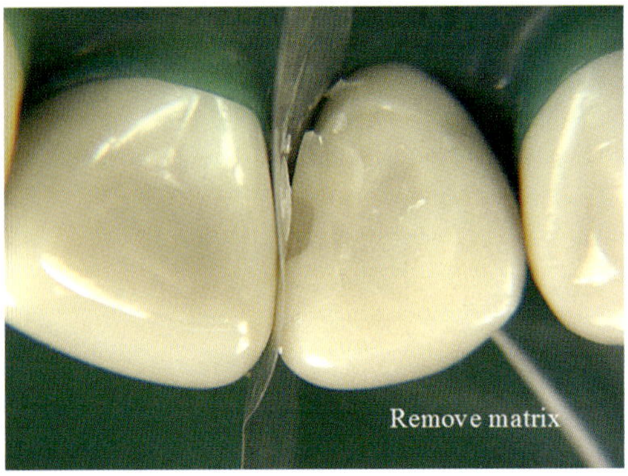

The wooden wedge is removed and the matrix loosened from around the tooth.
Small thin areas of excess composite are inevitable. These can be removed easily using sharp hand instruments.

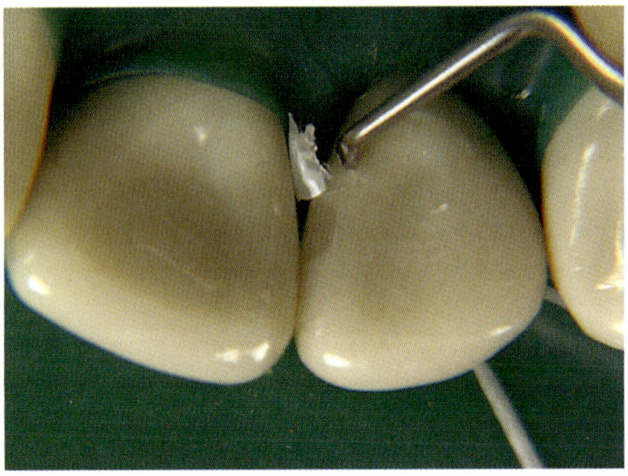

The dorsal surface of a sharp excavator may be used to prise the excess material away from the enamel surfaces beyond the cavity margin.
This slide shows how this layer will fracture back to the cavity margin when a force is correctly applied.

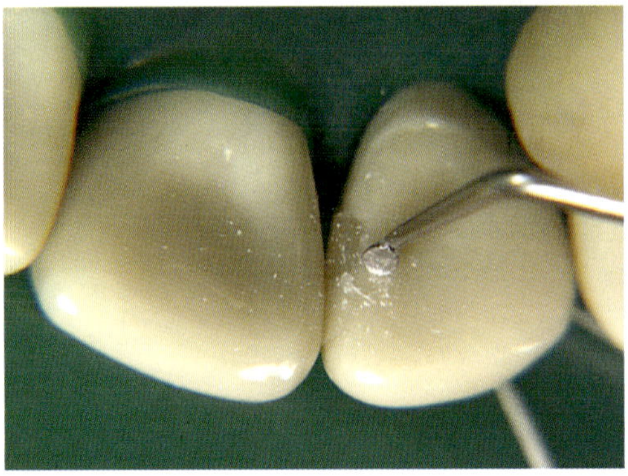

The leading sharp edge of an excavator can be used to remove further areas of excess material. As the composite is bonded strongly to the etched enamel margins of the cavity, no risk of damaging the restoration margin should be encountered.

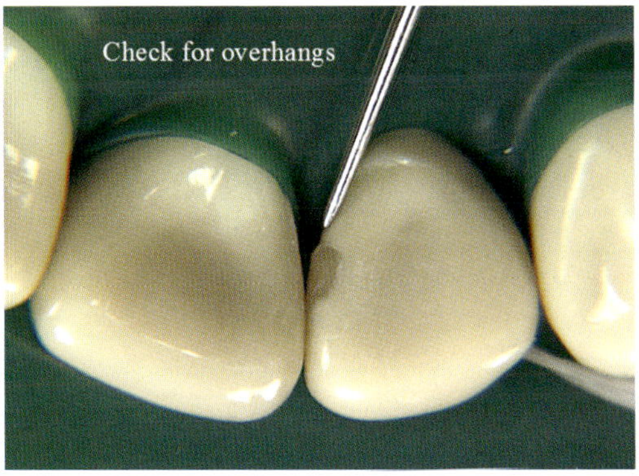

In this view the tip of the probe is high-lighting a small area of excess material at the gingival margin.

If this were left *in situ*, plaque accumulation would result with a deterioration in the local periodontal condition, and, the risk of secondary caries at this margin would be greater.

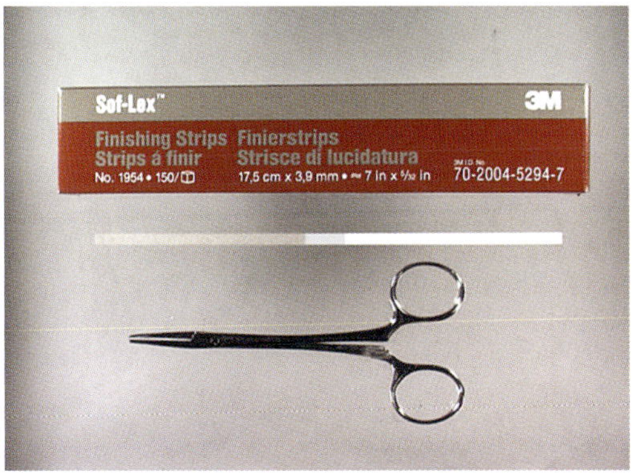

Excess composite can be removed using abrasive strips. Mosquito forceps are used to hold one end of the strip while the other hand guides the strip into position and applies a counter force on the strip to hold it firmly against the restoration and tooth surface.
The smoother end of the finishing strip should be used to produce a slightly smoother finish.

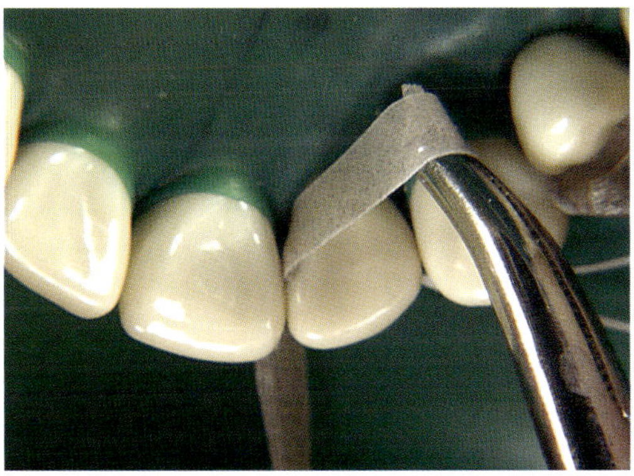

The rougher of the two ends is used initially. The forceps are inserted to the palatal aspect beacause it is difficult to insert fingers onto this surface of the upper arch.

The strip is worked in a backward and forward motion to remove the excess material.

Where no excess is present, abrasive strips are not used as they serve only to roughen the surface of the composite.

The smoothest surface finish is achieved by allowing the composite to set against the matrix strip.

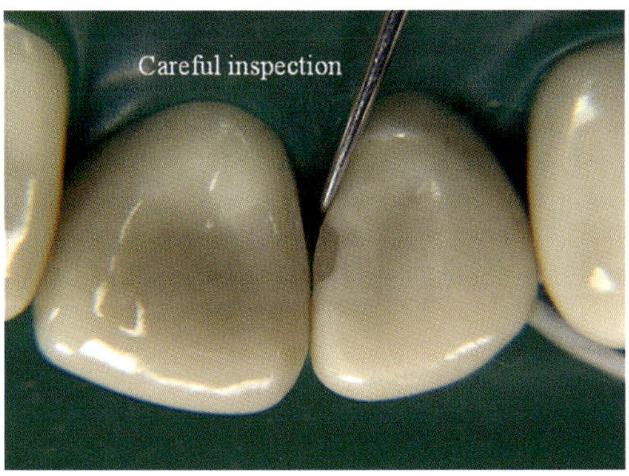

A careful inspection should then be made to ensure that excess material has been removed. Note that the surface of the palatal composite is no longer smooth and shiny as before.
It has now been roughened by the finishing strip.

Video 7.5

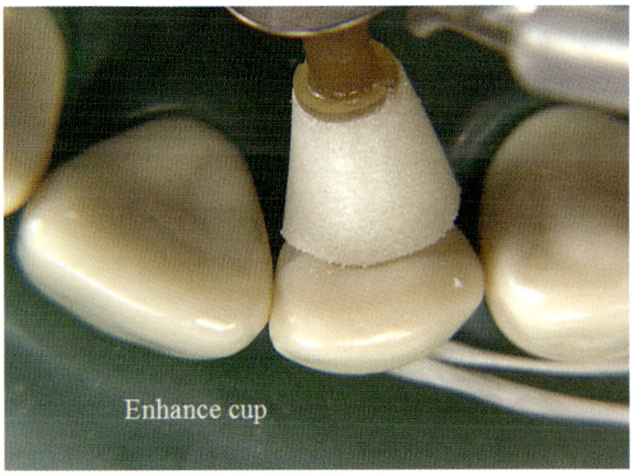

The accessible palatal surface can be smoothed and polished using impregnated polishing points and cups.

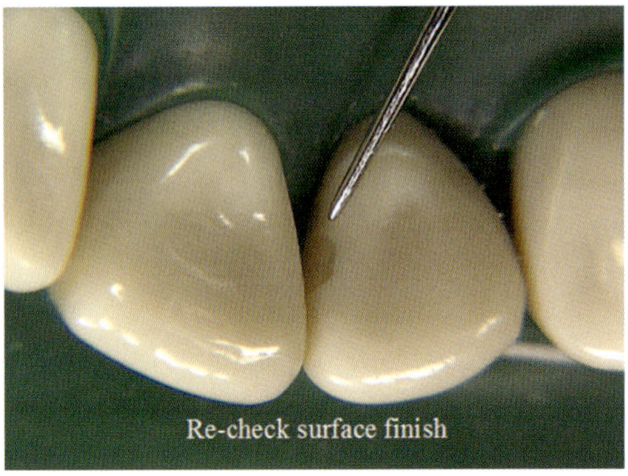

Make a final inspection of the smoothed surface using the probe.
It should not be possible to feel the interface of the restoration to tooth surface when the probe is moved from restoration to enamel surface and back again.

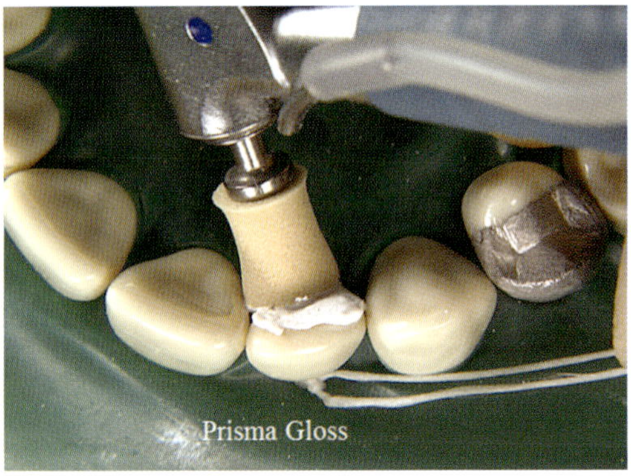

Finally, the adjusted and smoothed surfaces can be polished using a polishing paste on a felt cup.

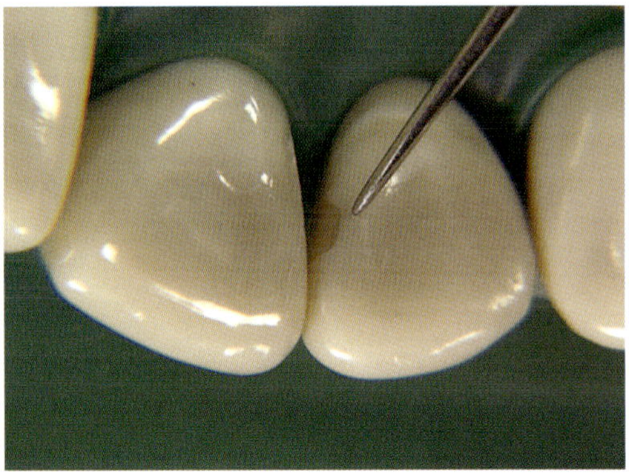

In this view, the completed restoration is being checked finally before the rubber dam is removed, the occlusion checked, and, the patient discharged.

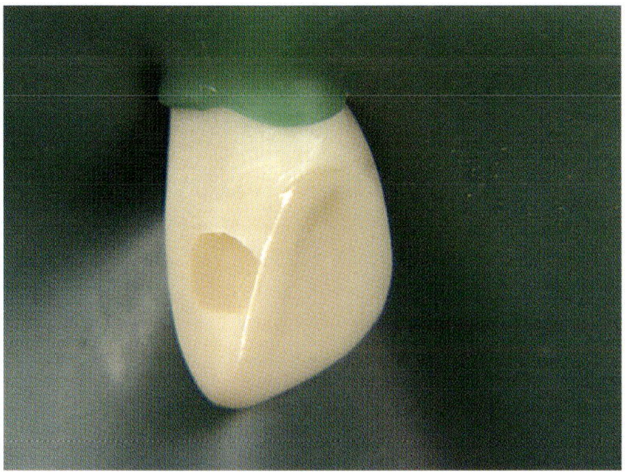

This view shows the smooth surface achieved using this system.
Smooth surfaces better resist plaque accumulation, and, the longevity of the restoration should be improved.

Restoration of a Fractured Incisor

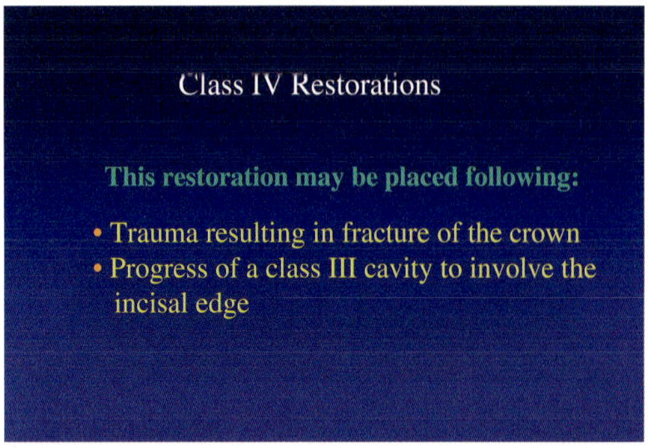

Class IV cavities may be required after trauma resulting in loss of the incisal edge. Alternatively, the progress of an interproximal cavity on incisor or canine teeth will result in weakening of the incisal edge. This may fracture, resulting, in part of the incisal edge being involved in the restoration.

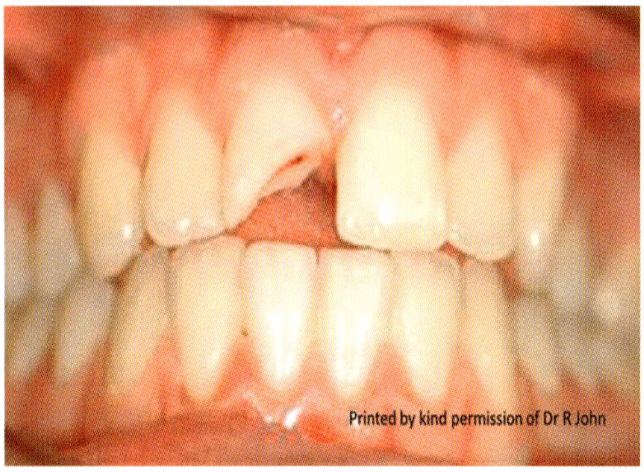

Children are the most likely group of patients to sustain trauma injuries to the teeth. This is more likely if they have prominent incisors. When traumatised they are likely to fracture at a 45° angle across the crown. This may expose dentine, or, if deeper, the pulpal tissue may be exposed. Note the oblique nature of the fracture that also runs at approximately 45° from the labial to the palatal aspectof the crown.

One of the problems following trauma is that a root fracture may also have occurred, and, the opposing and adjacent teeth must be inspected for signs of trauma.

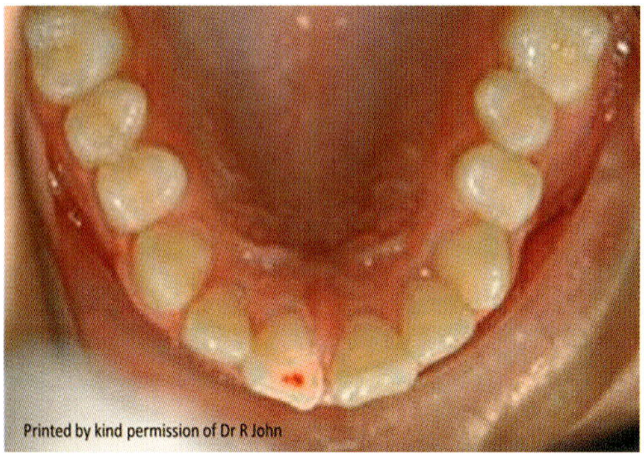

In this case of trauma, the fracture line runs obliquely from labial to palatal, but, the pulpal tissue has been exposed on the central incisor tooth.

In some cases, the palatal edge of the fracture can finish subgingivally. This makes the restoration of this tooth more problematic because isolation is difficult.

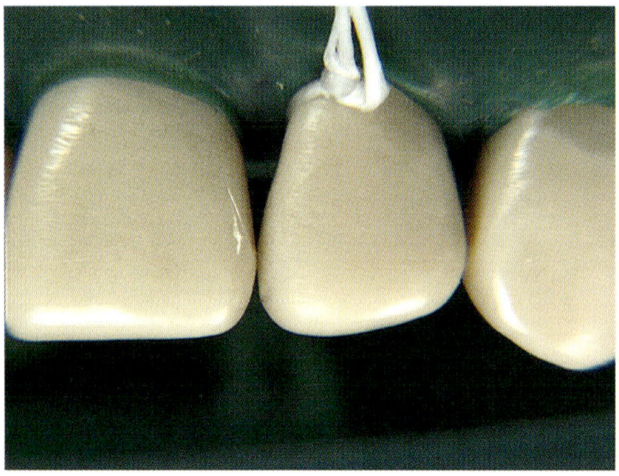

In this sequence, a simulated fracture of the maxillary lateral incisor tooth will be shown.

The stages of restoration will be demonstrated, but, readers should refer to textbooks on accidental trauma for the overall management of these cases.

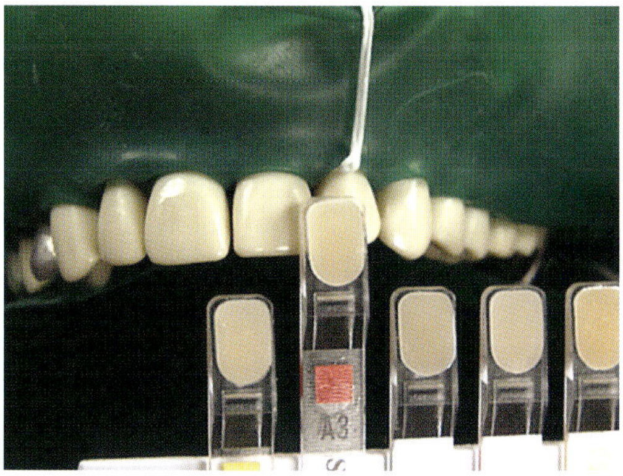

Careful shade matching of the composite resin is important when excellent aesthetics is to be obtained for the patient.

Teeth dry out and become lighter under rubber dam so the shade should be selected before the dam is applied or immediately after its application.

Ceram X Duo is an ideal material to use for anterior restorations because it is presented in a denser opaque dentine shade and a more translucent highly polishable enamel shade. The operator simply matches the final shade and reads off the shade of dentine and enamel compules that should be used.

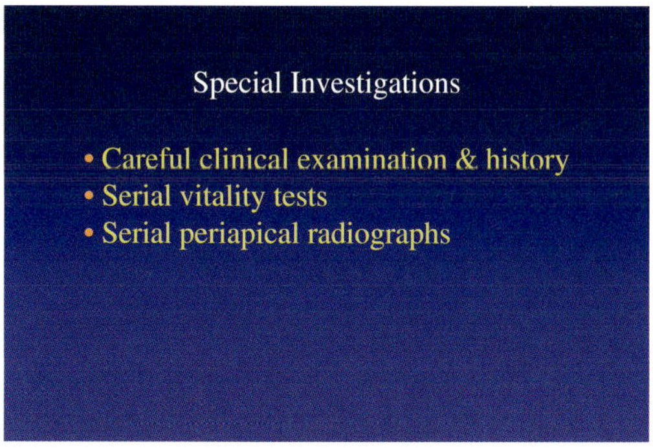

Clinical exam:
Look for discolouration of crown, mobility of tooth, position of tooth in occlusion.

Vitality:
Test vitality with at least two methods.
Need to have a series of pulp tests to eliminate concussion:

Radiographs.
Two different view are required with differing angulations to identify fracture lines.

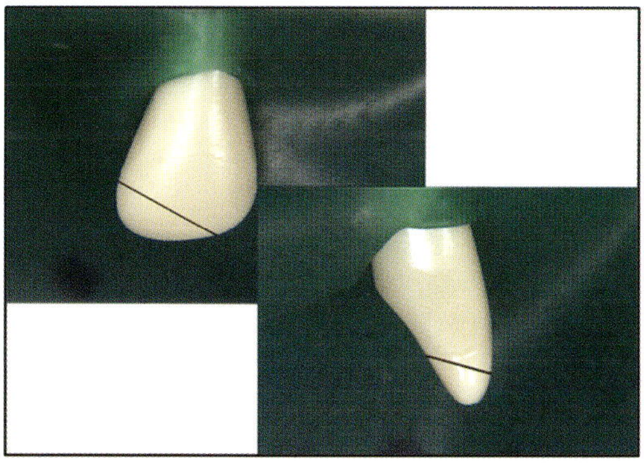

A line has been drawn across this lateral incisor tooth to simulate where the extent of the fracture is to be made. Note the mesio-incisal direction of the fracture at a 45° angle.

When trauma is applied to the labial aspect of the incisor, the fracture line is likely to run at an angle towards the palatal surface of the tooth.

From simple mechanical principles, it is likely that a fracture could occur also in the root of this tooth. If this were so, the angle of the root fracture is likely to mimic that seen in the crown.

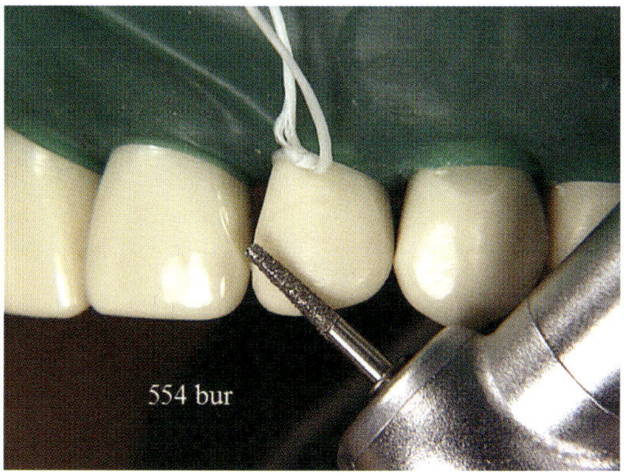

A simulated fracture is prepared using a long tapered fissure bur. With the correct angulation of the bur, the mesio-incisal corner of the tooth can be removed to show enamel and dentine without any pulpal exposure.

Alternatively, the tooth may be prepared on a dental lathe as this is not a cavity preparation that would normally be done.

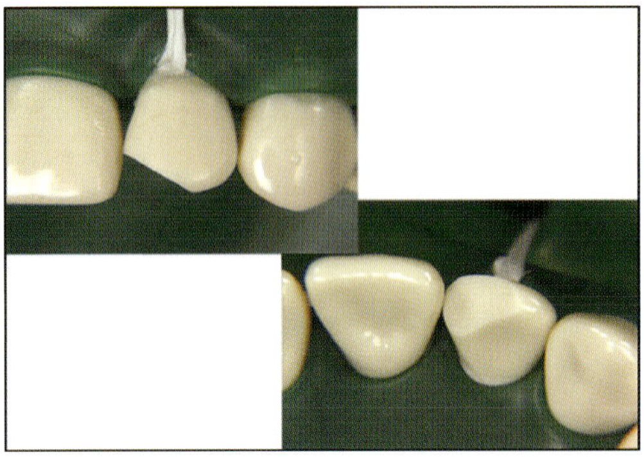

This would be the likely view of the fractured tooth from the labial and incisal aspects.

This regular enamel fracture may not be seen in reality. A previous slide indicated the rough and irregular fracture edge that is more likely to occur.

When the fracture is viewed from the incisal, the cut surface should be sloped towards the palatal surface of the tooth. The palatal edge of the fracture should be at a level closer to the gingival margin than the corresponding labial margin.

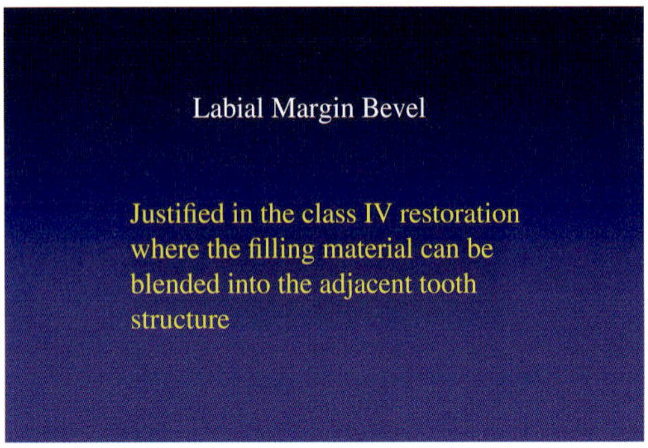

At this stage a decision has to be reached on whether to bevel the margins of the cavity.

The relative merits have been discussed for the class III restoration.

Sufficient area exists for bonding in the class IV restoration, but, the main advantage of bevelling would be to blend the filling material into the labial surface.

For this reason it is recommended that a compromise situation should exist where only the labial margin is bevelled.

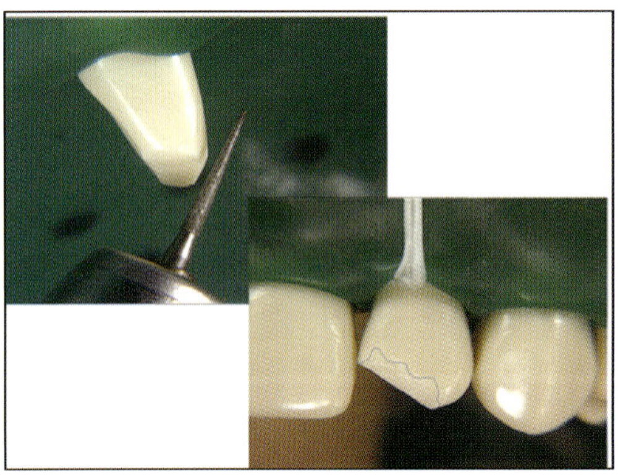

The long and slender separating bur can be used to place a bevel along the labial margin of the fracture. The main advantage of this is to blend the aesthetics of the composite into that of the enamel present on this aspect of the tooth structure. A short bevel of only about 1 mm in width should be placed all along the enamel edge. This may be achieved by holding the bur at a 45° or greater angle to the long axis of the tooth. Note the outline is somewhat jagged so that the blended composite will not form a uniform finish area but the light will be diffused and blend into the surrounding tooth structure.

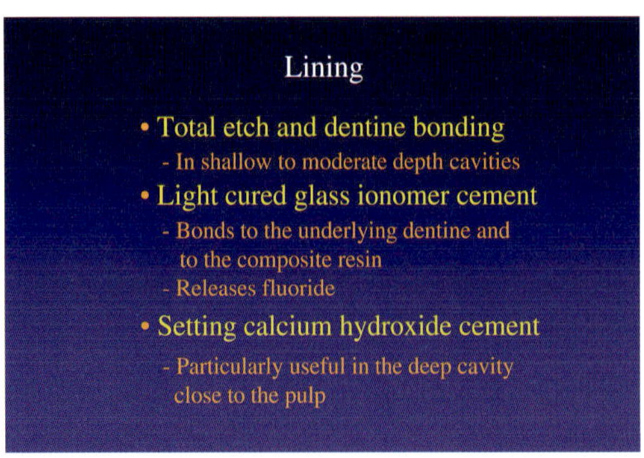

A range of lining materials are available for use in this situation.

Where the cavity is shallow some operators do not place a lining material because they believe that the dentine bonding system will seal the dentinal tubules. If the other part of the fractured tooth is available, this, may be bonded back into place using this means of attachment.

AL/C glass ionomer cement will be shown in this case.

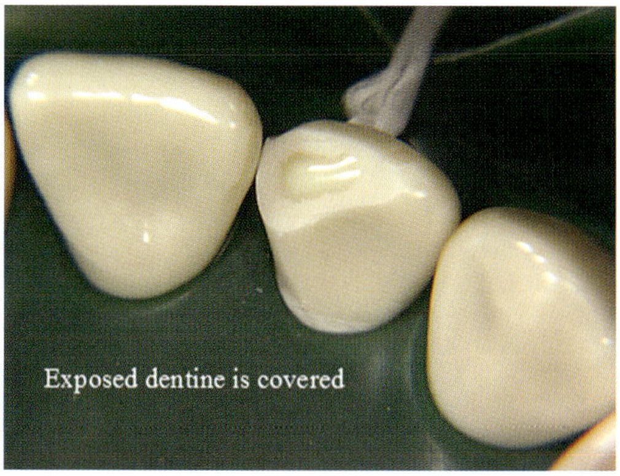

In this simulated clinical example a L/C glass ionomer cement (GIC) has been transferred to the dentine surface using a PF10 instrument. The polyalkenoate cement will bond to the underlying dentine, release fluoride and be cariostatic, and have a thermal expansion coefficient similar to that of the lost dentine. The material is light cured for 30 seconds.
In this view note the amount and situation of the centrally placed GIC, which is covering up the dentine exposed by the fracture.

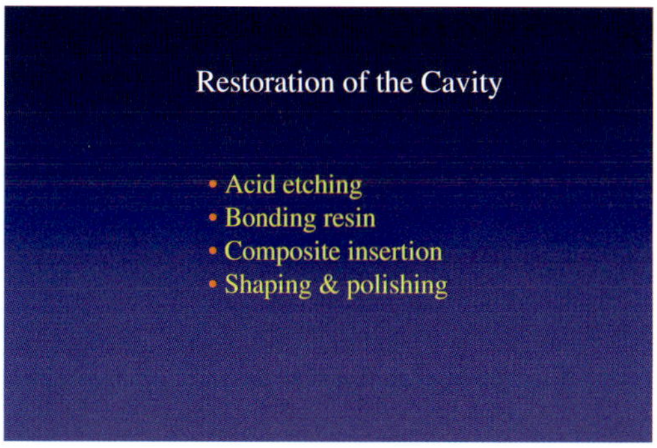

Once the cavity margins have been bevelled and a lining placed, the next stages of the restoration of the fractured incisor can be approached.

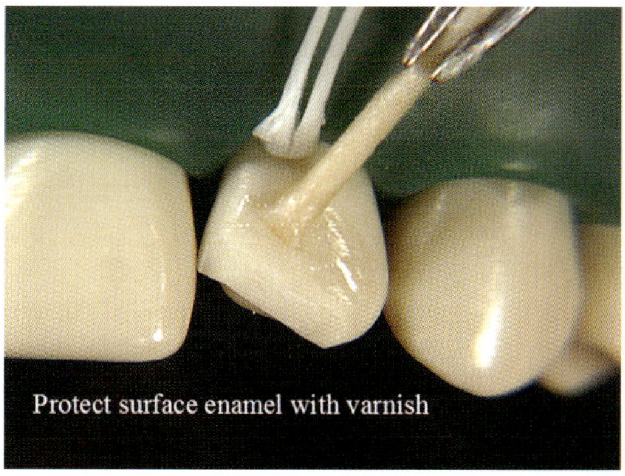

It is a good idea to place a protective layer of material over the enamel surface to prevent overextended composite from bonding to this surface. Removal of excess composite is time consuming, and it is difficult-but not impossible -to re-establish a really smooth surface finish with rotary instruments.
Copal ether varnish can be applied to the adjacent enamel surfaces beyond the bevel as a separating medium. The operator must ensure that the varnish is not applied to the cavity margins.

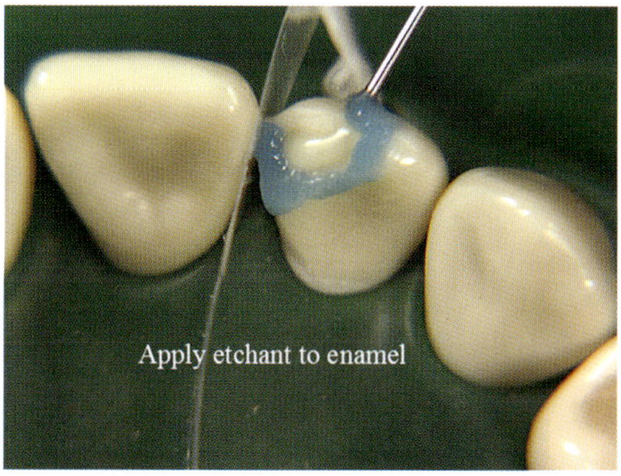

The etching and bonding procedure is performed in the same manner as used in previous restorations. Enamel etching always commences on the enamel margins of the cavity first so that the inner aspects of the cavity, consisting of dentine, are etched for a lesser time. It is important not to exceed the recommended etching times.
Contemporary bonding procedures may also use the aspirator only to evaporate the alcohol solvent in the bonding material.

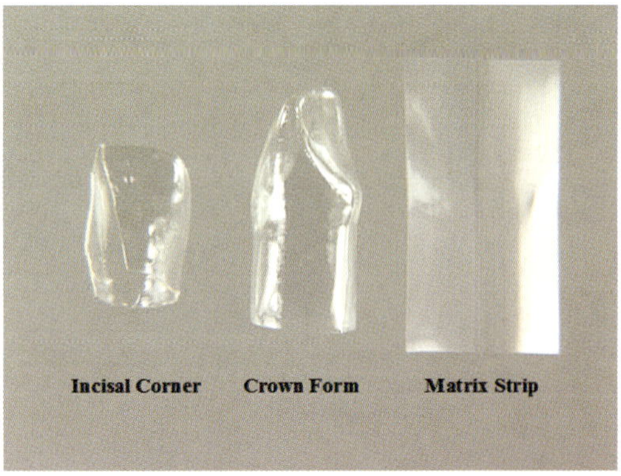

A variety of matrix systems can be used to contain and help shape the composite resin restoration.
Incisal corners are available for both mesial and distal application to incisor teeth. These are made from a thin polyester material that is easily trimmed to shape.
Crown forms may also be used but are thicker than the incisal corners. These require more trimming to fit onto the fractured tooth.
Many operators use matrix strips similar to those used for class III restorations.

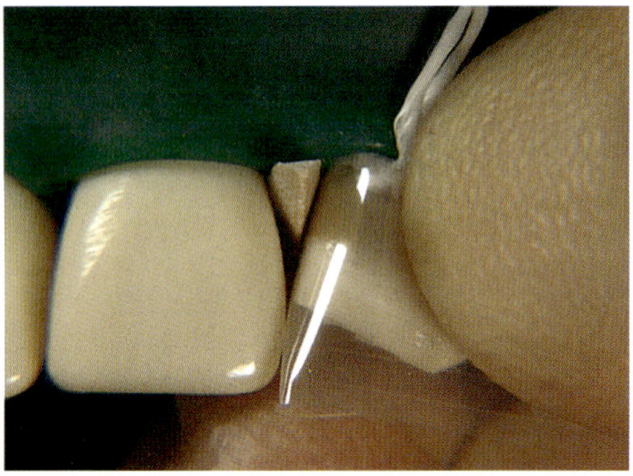

In this view, a matrix strip has been placed around the lateral incisor and wooden wedge inserted between the teeth. This locates the strip positively and adapts it to the enamel.
The operator should ensure that the strip can be brought out to form a contact with the adjacent tooth.
Using this matrix system the operator will not be able to initially contour the composite to conform with the natural incisal edge.

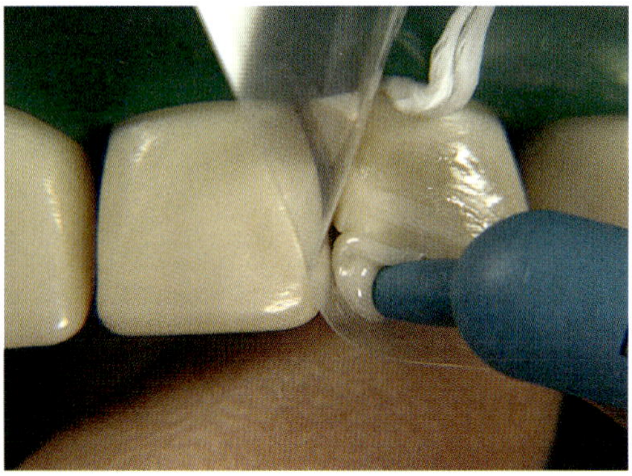

The palatal part of the restoration should be built up using an opaque dentine shade of composite to prevent too translucent an appearance from being produced.
Ensure that an opaque dentine shade is selected for this stage.

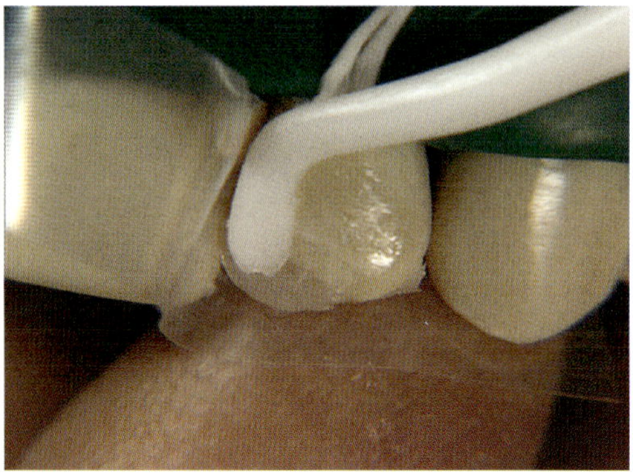

The matrix is supported with a finger from the left hand while the composite is moulded against the matrix.
Ensure that the composite does not extend to the labial surface at this stage.

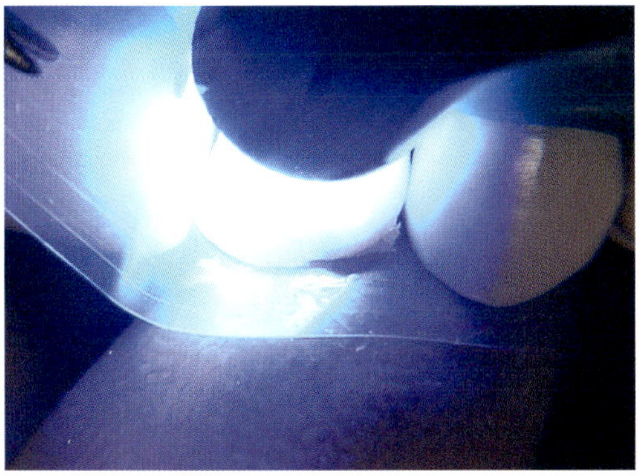

This is then polymerised for 40 seconds.
Note that the matrix has not been placed over the labial aspect of the composite at this stage so that the surface layer will not fully polymerise due to the oxygen inhibited layer.
This means that further layers of composite will bond with maximum strength to this layer if they remain uncontaminated.

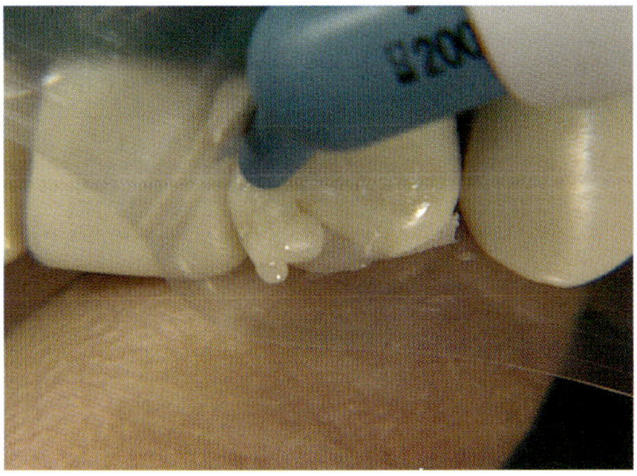

A suitable enamel shade of composite is then selected and applied to the surface of the dentine layer.
This composite will be more translucent and have a better and more natural appearance.

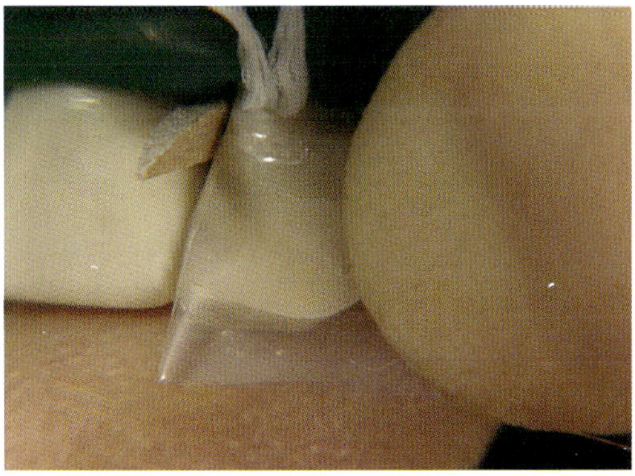

When sufficient has been applied the matrix is brought around the tooth and held firmly in place.
Ensure that the matrix does not form a concavity in its surface.
Small amounts of excess material should be present only along the incisal edge. In this position it is easy to remove at a later stage.

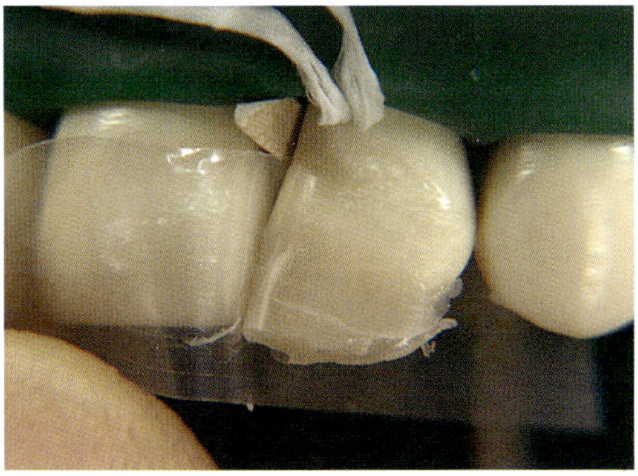

The matrix and wedge are removed after polymerising.
Only small amounts of excess should be present on the labial enamel surface of the tooth.
The bulk of the excess material is present in the incisal region. The clinical height of this tooth is now obviously too great, and, it now requires reducing to conform to the original anatomy.

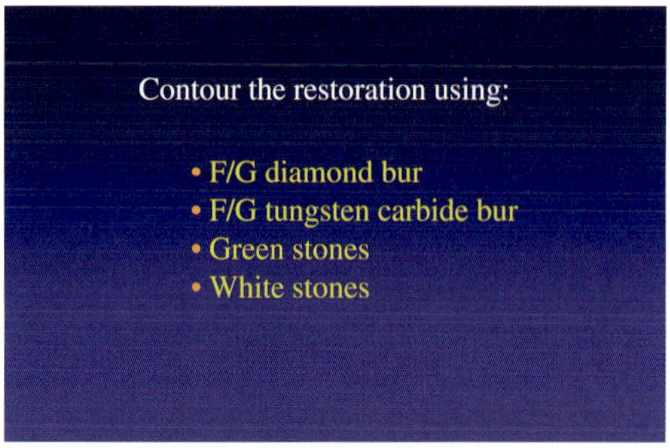

The labial surface of the restoration should have been contoured with the matrix strip and requires no or minimal finishing, but, the incisal edge can be contoured using a variety of rotary instruments. These range from stones to tunsten carbide or diamond coated burs.

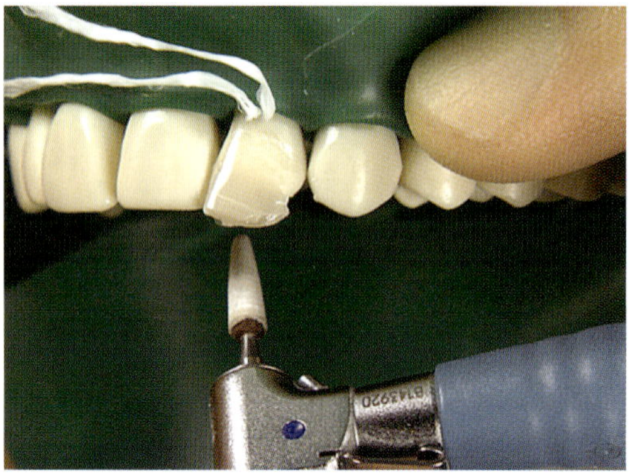

This slide indicates the use of a white stone held at an angle to the incisal edge.
Most patients prefer the use of a diamond coated bur in the air turbine handpiece because this produces minimal vibration and aids patient comfort.

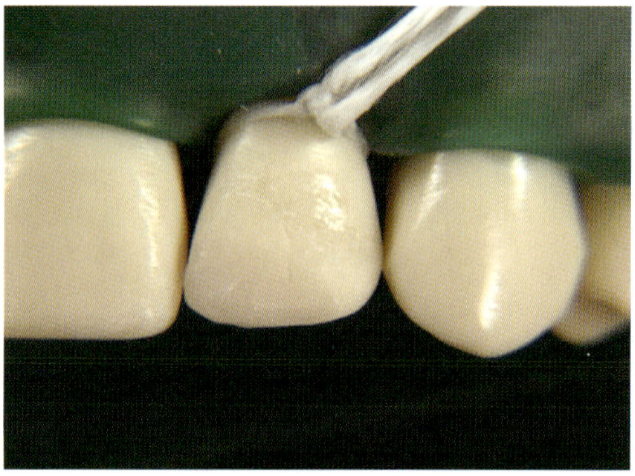

The incisal edge of the lateral incisor has been contoured with a diamond bur at this stage.
The shape of the incisal edge can be copied from the contra-lateral tooth to blend in with the overall natural appearance.

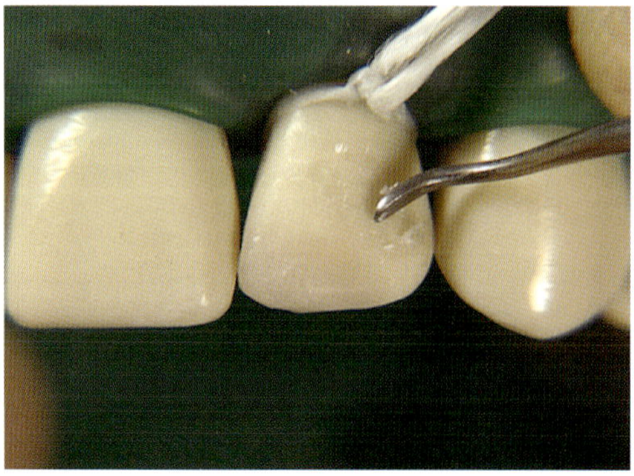

Thin flash of composite may overlie the enamel surface of the tooth. As this surface was coated with a varnish before etching, excess should be easy to remove using a sharp excavator.
If the varnish is not applied, inadvertent etching may occur, and, this surface will be overlaid with a thin layer of tenaciously bonded composite.

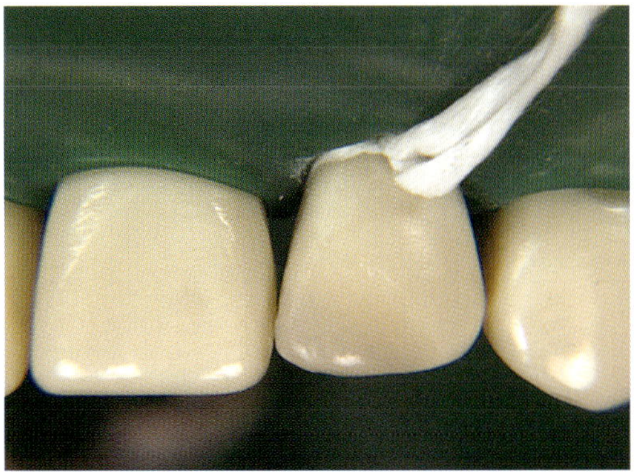

The shaped surfaces of the restoration can then be polished using an impregnated rubber polishing kit consisting of discs, cups, and, points. A final lustrous finish can be achieved by using the polishing pastes on the felt cup.

Remember that the first pastes must be washed from the tooth before the second is applied – otherwise, the larger particles will prevent a lustrousshine.

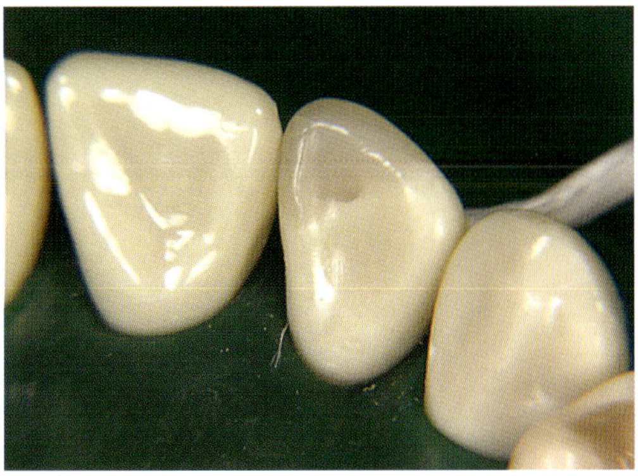

The palatal surface should also be returned to its original shape.

In this view, it can be seen that the marginal ridge has been re-established in the composite.

A Clinical Case

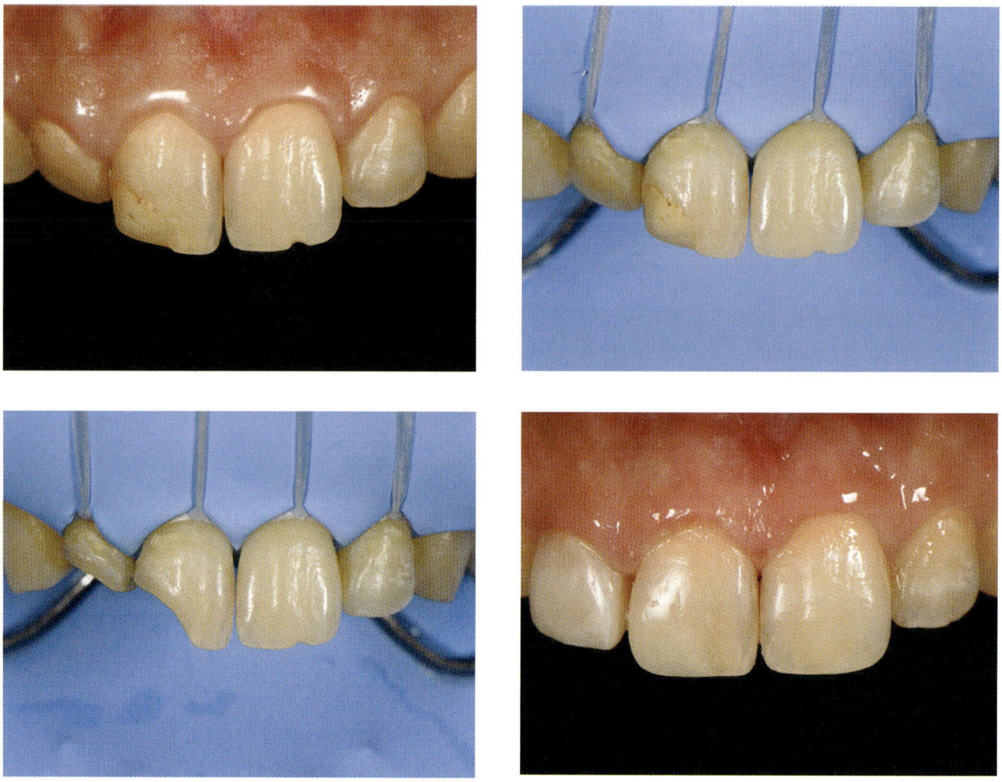

This sequence shows the re-restoration of a stained and worn disto-incisal restoration on maxillary right central incisor tooth. Modern composite resin materials can achieve a much better appearance.
Source: Printed by permission of Dr Osama Alkhatib.

Further Reading

Andreasen, J.O., Andreasen, F.M., and Andersson, L. (2018). *Textbook and Color Atlas of Traumatic Injuries to the Teeth*, 5e.

Demarco, F.F., Collares, K., Coelho-de-Souza, F.H. et al. (2015). Anterior composite restorations: a systematic review on long-term survival and reasons for failure. *Dental Materials* 3 (1): 1214–1224.

Heintze, S.D., Rousson, V., and Hickel, R. (2015). Clinical effectiveness of direct anterior restorations – a meta-analysis. *Dental Materials* 31: 481–495.

Kirilova, J., Kirov, D., and Topalova-Pirinska, S. (2014). Stratification technique in maxillary anterior incisors restoration. *Journal of IMAB – Annual Proceeding (Scientific Papers)* 20 (3): 550–553.

Romero, M.F. (2015). Esthetic anterior composite resin restorations using a single shade: step-by-step technique. *Journal of Prosthetic Dentistry* 114: 9–12.

DentalTrauma Guide. (2020). http://www.dentaltraumaguide.org/dtg-members-frontpage

8

Restoration of Lesions in Cervical Third

In the early 1900s, Black classified carious lesions occurring in the cervical third of anterior and posterior teeth as class V lesions. These lesions may occur on the buccal or lingual surfaces. In contemporary practice, lesions in the cervical third may be a result of an aetiology other than caries but are still known as class V lesions. Abrasion, erosion, and abfraction can all result in cavitation that may require restoration in this site. In the classification by Mount and Hume (1998), a lesion in the cervical third of the tooth crown is known as a site 3 lesion. Following gingival recession, a site 3 lesion could occur on the exposed root surface.

Aetiology

Caries: When caries develop in the other classes of restoration, they are related to such stagnation areas as pits and fissures or contact points. However, in the class V carious lesion, the caries commences below accumulations of dental plaque. Pit and fissure caries can develop even when patients exhibit good toothbrushing habits, but cervical caries will only develop when toothbrushing technique is poor and does not remove accumulated plaque.

Abrasion: Abrasion is the loss of tooth substance from factors other than tooth contact (attrition). A frequent cause of abrasion at the cervical margin of teeth is due to overzealous horizontal toothbrushing or scrubbing.

Erosion: Erosion is the loss of dental hard tissues by chemical action not involving bacteria. This process can be further classified according to the source of the acid with a description of both intrinsic or extrinsic types. Intrinsic sources of acids originate in the stomach and are associated with eating disorders – such as anorexia and bulimia nervosa – or with acid reflux and regurgitation. Extrinsic sources are acids contained in dietary components, such as carbonated soft drinks and fruit or fruit juices. Workers in certain industries, such as battery manufacture or chemical industries producing acids, are also prone to tooth erosion.

Abfraction: Abfraction is a theoretical process whereby occlusal forces create stresses in enamel and dentine along the cervical area of a tooth, resulting in the fracture of the overlying enamel.

It can be difficult to identify the aetiological factor for a non-carious cervical lesion in the cervical third because each description probably does not exist alone, and these lesions are likely to be multi-factorial in nature.

A Practical Approach to Operative Dentistry, First Edition. Gordon B. Gray and Alaa H. Daud.

Companion website: www.wiley.com/go/gray/operative-dentistry

Appearance

The appearance of non-carious cervical lesions may be related to the major aetiological factors:

- ***Abrasion*** can produce lesions with sharply defined margins
- ***Erosion*** produces broad, dish shaped but shallow lesions
- ***Abfraction*** lesions are typically wedge shaped, with sharp internal and external line angles

Factors Increasing Incidence of Lesions

The use of carbonated drinks and sports drinks has had a major effect on the incidence of erosive lesions. When these are combined with a high sugar content and frequent consumption, they can result in carious class V lesions. These are more prevalent on anterior teeth. and if the patient has poor plaque control, dietary advice should be given after the teeth are restored.

Patients who are undergoing fixed orthodontics with brackets or bands on their teeth are at risk of developing cervical caries. The use of fluoride rinses is recommended in this group of patients as well as meticulous toothbrushing technique.

Patients with xerostomia are at risk of class V lesions. There are more than 400 medications that can cause dry mouth. These medications include antihypertensives, antidepressants, analgesics, tranquillisers, diuretics, and antihistamines. Patients undergoing treatment for cancer are susceptible to xerostomia. Chemotherapeutic medications affect both the flow and composition of saliva. Head and neck radiation can damage the salivary glands so that the protective ability of the saliva is adversely affected due to a decrease in the immunoglobulin in the saliva.

Other conditions can also cause a decrease in salivary flow. Patients with endocrine disorders, depression, anxiety and stress, and nutritional deficiencies may exhibit symptoms of dry mouth. Sjögren's syndrome, an autoimmune disease, can cause both dry mouth and dry eyes.

Direct Replacement Restorations

The choice of restorative options is often not an easy one to make because the aetiology of these lesions affects the durability and clinical success of the restorative materials used.

Aesthetic Zone	Non-aesthetic Zone
Glass ionomer	Amalgam
Resin modified glass ionomer	Glass ionomer
Compomer	
Composite resin	
Flowable composite	

There is no single solution for treatment planning and restoring class V lesions. A thorough evaluation of aetiology of the lesion provides a sound basis for good treatment decisions and patient counselling to avoid the recurrence of these lesions.

Lesions in the non-aesthetic zone can be treated using amalgam, but the use of this material has been lessening since the Minamata Agreement. Dental amalgam can be placed in a compromised field that might be difficult to isolate due to salivary or bleeding contamination. However, cavities for amalgam require to be undercut and to have their margins with a 90° cavo-surface angle. In many instances, this requires the removal of more tooth structure than if an adhesive material were employed.

When class V cervical lesions are associated with xerostomia, the choice of restorative materials depends upon the location of the lesions. Lesions in the aesthetic zone are best treated with glass ionomer restoratives. In some cases, if the lesions are subgingival, it may be necessary to use gingival retraction cord or a rubber dam with a retentive clamp to gain the greatest chance of isolation for clinical success.

Glass ionomers are a unique restorative material. They are self-adhesive due to bonding to the underlying tooth structure. Also, the polyalkenoate cements are referred to as 'smart' materials that release fluoride to the surrounding tooth structure and allow calcium and phosphate ions present in saliva to pass through the restorative material and combine with the fluoride to produce remineralisation of the enamel as a fluorapatite. Another unique characteristic of a glass ionomer is that it provides a high initial burst of fluoride for remineralisation as well as a prolonged fluoride release over time.

To obtain a smooth surface finish, these materials can be placed using a matrix made either from aluminium that can be burnished onto the margins of the cavity or from acetate. The latter allows the passage of light for use with resin modified glass ionomer materials. Cavities that are to be restored with glass ionomer should be conditioned using polyacrylic acid to ensure an optimal bond. The matrix is only removed once the restorative material has reached an initial set. Excess cement should be removed from the surface of the surrounding tooth without damaging the surface of the remaining restoration. Care should be exercised to ensure that cement does not desiccate and turn chalky in appearance. Finally, the restoration should be protected from losing or gaining water by the application of a layer of varnish or resin. Glass ionomer restorations can be polished once they are fully set, but this will require the patient to return for this procedure.

Cervical Glass Ionomer Cement (GIC) and Compomer Restorations

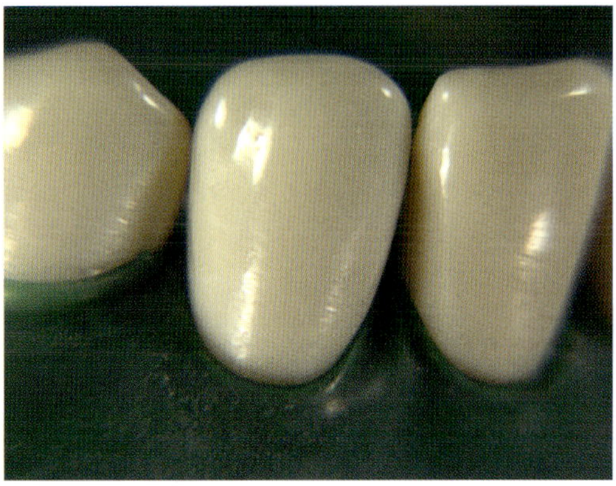

Class V cavities develop in the cervical third of all tooth types. They may be required due to the following:

- Caries due to poor plaque control
- Erosion due to intrinisic or extrinsic acids
- Abrasion due to inappropriate toothbrushing methods
- Abfracture - where occlusal stresses concentrate at the thin enamel near the enamel-cemental junction, causing fracture of the brittle enamel

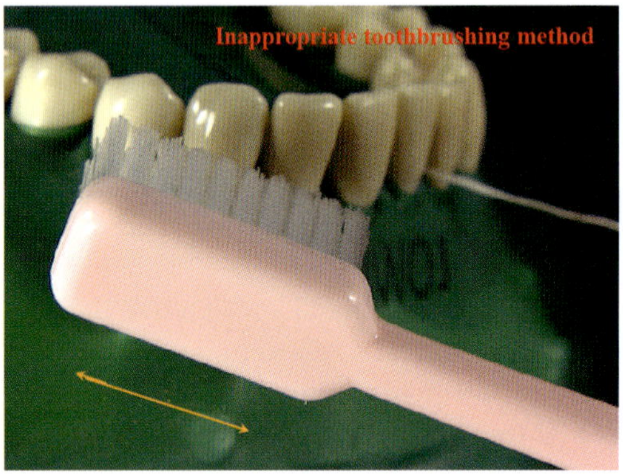

One of the most frequently seen cervical cavities is due to inappropriate toothbrushing. If the brush is used with a horizontal scrubbing action, a groove may be worn through the enamel into the softer underlying dentine.

This may be sensitive and require restoration to cover the exposed dentine.

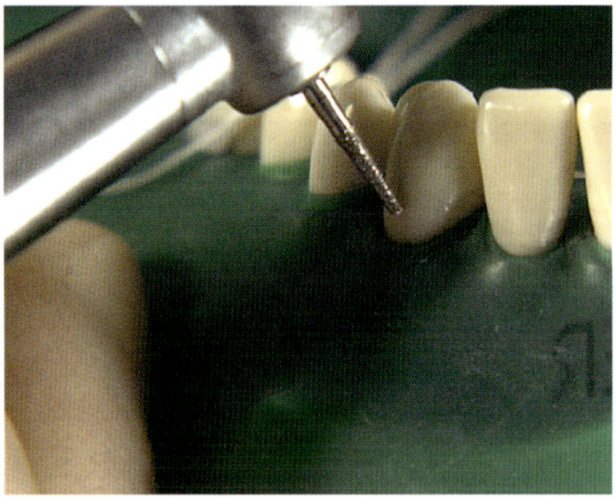

A floss ligature should be placed around the tooth to invert the rubber dam and hold it back from the cervical margin of the tooth.

A simulated abrasion cavity may be prepared to resemble a V shaped slot in the gingival third of the labial tooth surface.

This can be achieved by angling the bur at 45° above and below the horizontal plane in the gingival third.

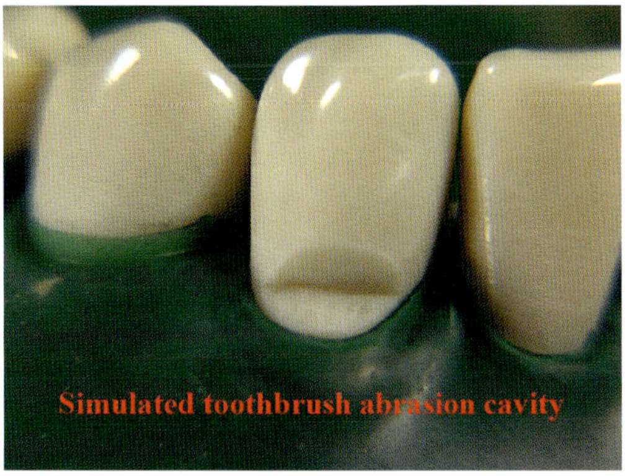

The lower surface has now been prepared with a 45° upward inclination to produce the final simulated cavity.

The depth of the lesion should be into dentine so that the cavity is at least 1.5 mm deep.

The V shaped cavity will be smooth and non-undercut as no mechanical retention is required when this cavity is restored with adhesive restorative materials.

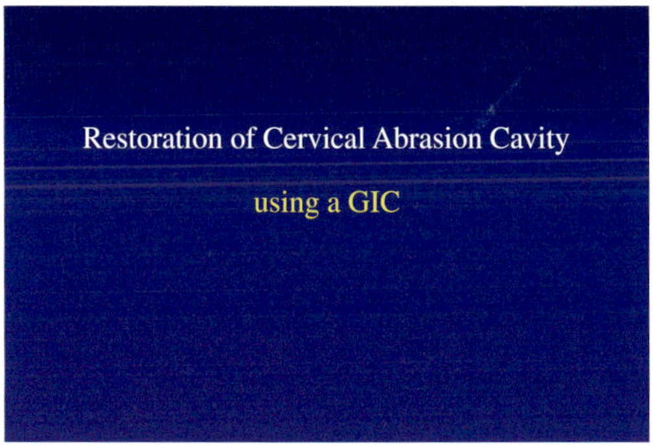

In the first of the two restorative procedures, an encapsulated chemically curing GIC will be used.

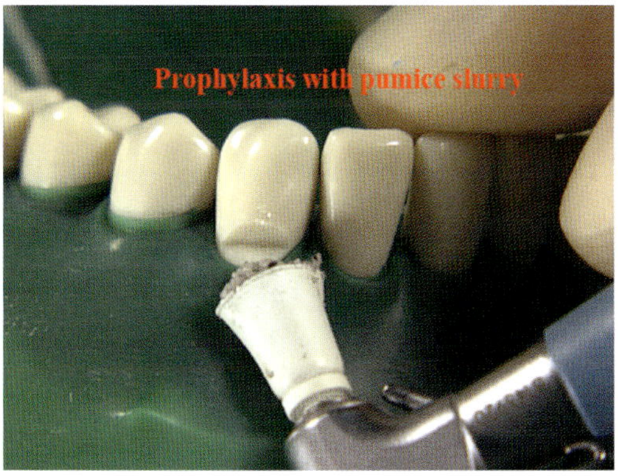

To optimise the bonding potential of the restorative material the tooth should be cleaned using an oil-and glycerine-free prophylaxis paste. It has also been reported that the paste should be free from fluoride because this may adversely affect the bonding potential of the restorative material.

A slurry of pumice can be prepared and used in a rubber polishing cup. Brushes should not be used as these may damage the rubber dam and lacerate the gingivae, resulting in bleeding. This would compromise the isolation of the cavity.

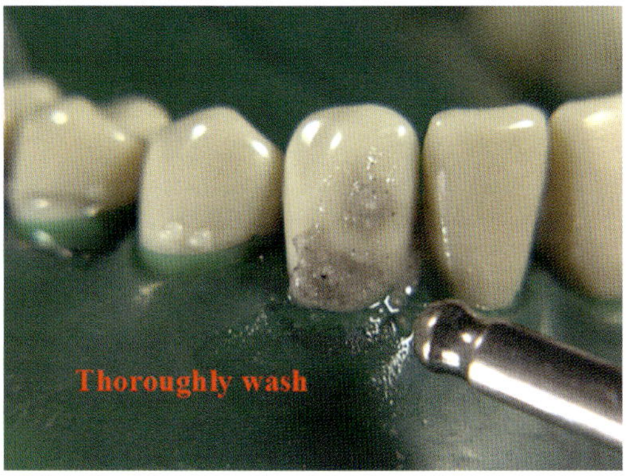

After the cleaning regime to remove surface plaque and pellicle, the area should be thoroughly washed with water...

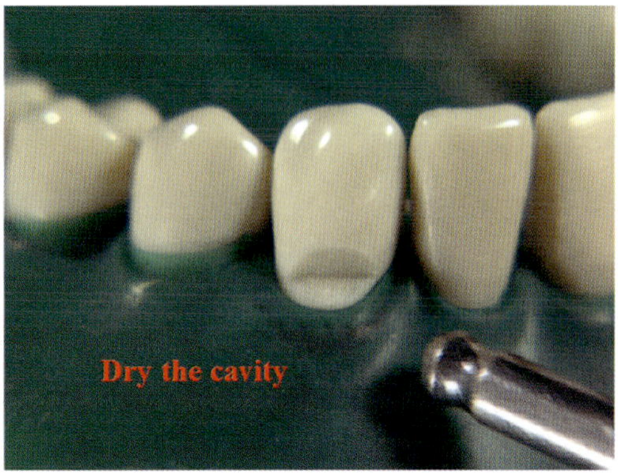

...and a gentle stream of compressed air used to dry the cavity.

It is important that the air line is not contaminated with oil from the compressor as this would have an effect on the bonding potential of the restoration.

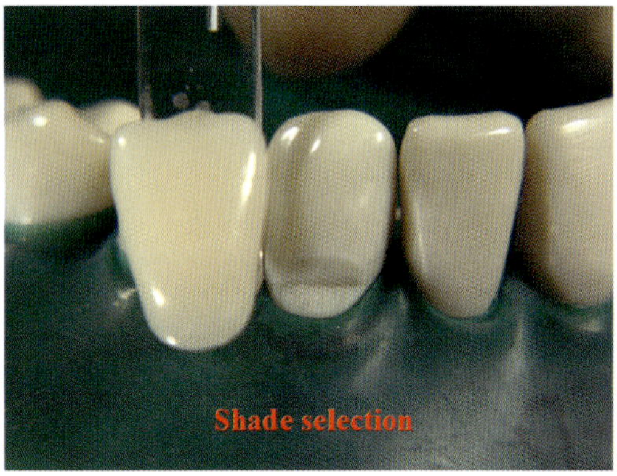

A shade may be selected for the filling material. If the tooth is not stained, the shade should be selected before the procedure commences because the shade of the tooth lightens after it is brought through the rubber dam.

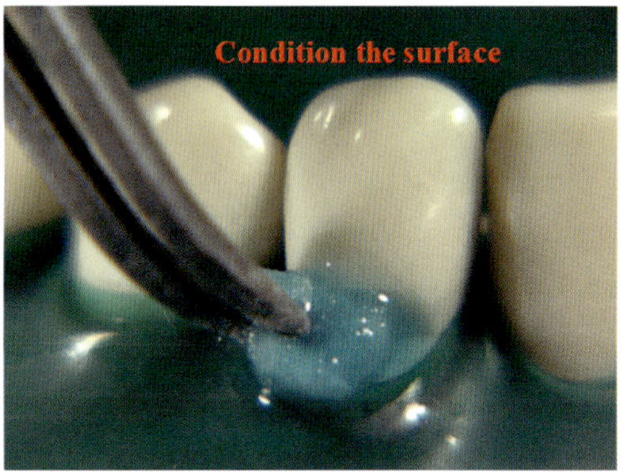

The surface of the abrasion lesion is conditioned using a solution of 25% polyacrylic acid to remove the smear layer and improve the bond strength of the GIC to the enamel and dentine surface.

This is applied with a small pledget of cotton wool and left undisturbed for 30 seconds.

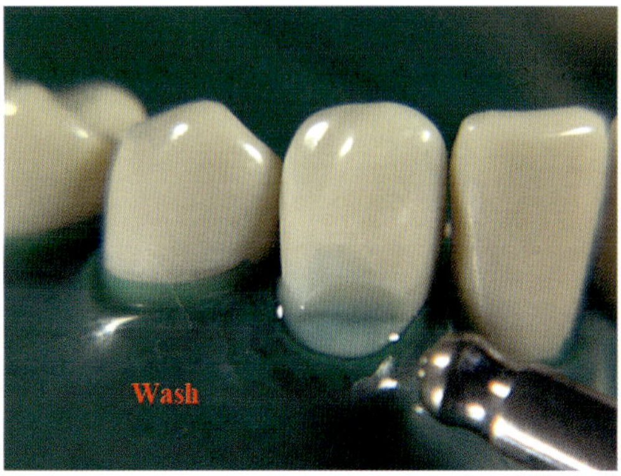

The acid should then be washed away for at least 30 seconds with a continuous stream of water from the triple dental syringe.

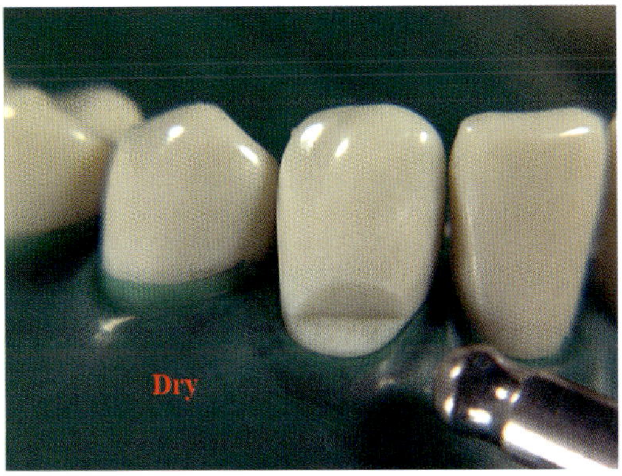

The tooth should be dried with a stream of compressed but uncontaminated air from the 3:1 syringe.

Care must be taken to avoid desiccating the dentine when this is performed, but the tooth surface must be left dry. This is dissimilar to the situation with the total etch technique for dentine bonding and composite resin.

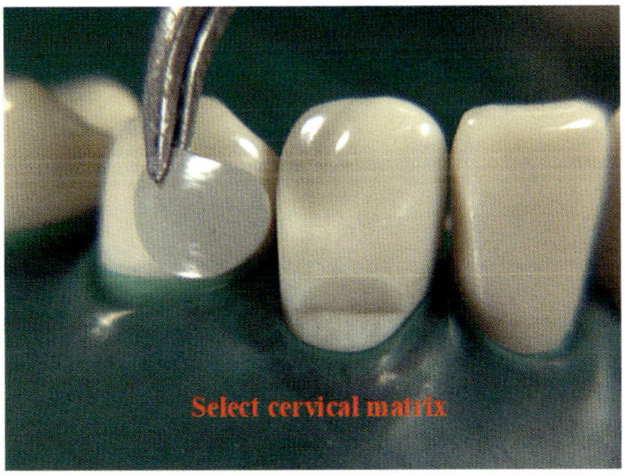

A thin, shaped foil of aluminium can be selected from the selection in the "cervical matrix" box. This will form the missing surface of the tooth and contain the filling material while it sets. In addition, it will hold the restorative material under compression while it sets and impart a smooth surface to the set filling. Care should be exercised to ensure the aluminium matrix is not indented with the serrations of the tweezers. Adhesive sticks are available to stick to the labial surface of the matrix to avoid this.

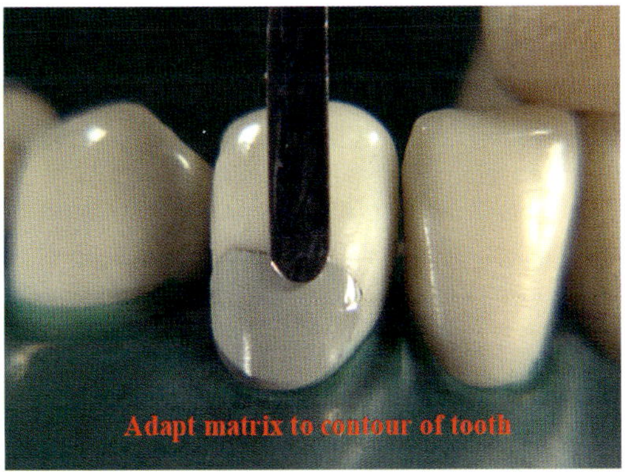

Before the filling material is mixed, the aluminium foil matrix is adapted to conform to the surface contour of the tooth.

This can be achieved by placing the matrix against the tooth and adapting the margins with a blunt plastic instrument.

If it is not well adapted, the final contour of the filling will be poor and necessitate recontouring of the GIC at an early stage.

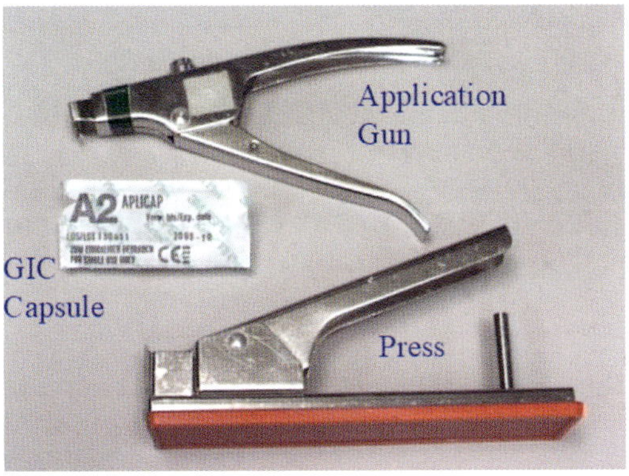

In this sequence, an encapsulated GIC will be used. This slide shows the equipment required to activate the capsule and express the mixed cement.

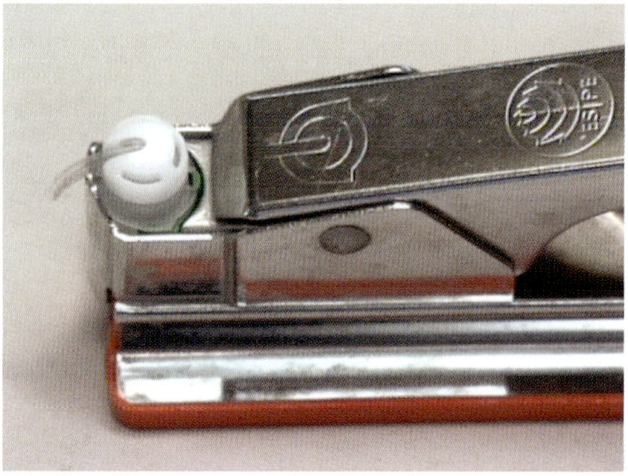

A capsule of the appropriate shade of cement is removed from its sterile package and inserted into the press. Note the nozzle faces forwards and the green plastic side of the capsule faces towards the handle of the press.

The handle of the press is pushed down and held for a full 2 seconds to rupture the internal membrane. This allows the polyalkenoic acid to come into contact with the aluminosilicate glass.

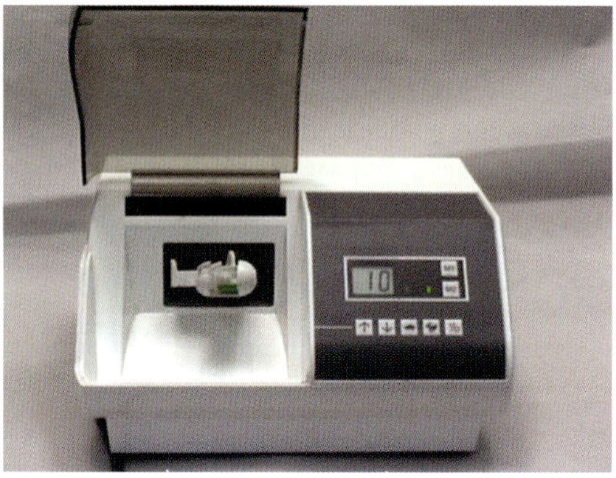

The activated capsule is placed in the cradle of the mixer with the nozzle situated to the left side in the opening. The machine is set to the faster of its two speeds and timer activated for 10 seconds.

The type of mixer shown will not operate until the protective lid is closed.

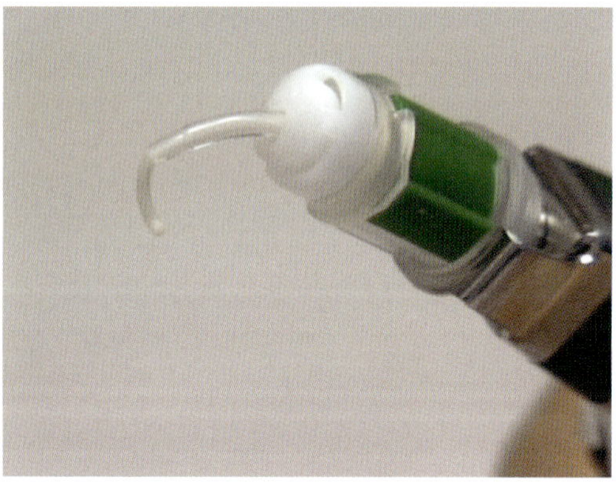

Once mixed, the capsule is removed from the cradle, and the end opposite the nozzle is inserted into the applicator gun. The curved nozzle is then pulled outwards and the handle of the gun is depressed a few times to push the internal plunger into the capsule and express the mixed cement.

The main advantage of the encapsulated cement is that a viscosity and quality of mix is obtained that is reproducible. In addition, the material can be injected directly into the cavity.

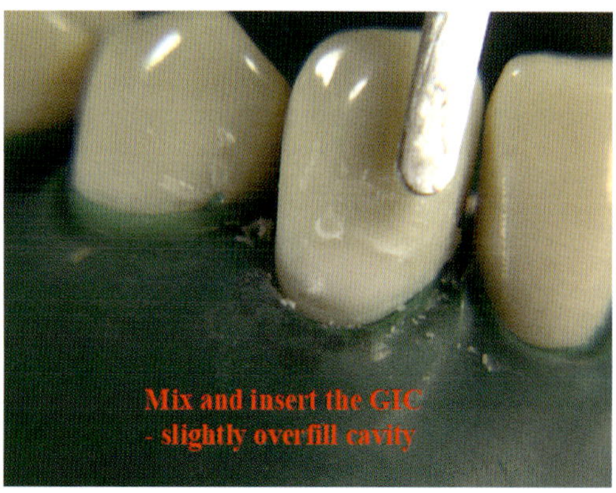

Alternatively, for a powder liquid system, the correct ratio of powder to liquid (2:2) is mixed on a paper pad with a stainless steel spatula. Mixing time should not exceed 25 seconds.

It is then transferred to the cavity using a plastic instrument.

Sufficient of the mixed material should be transferred to slightly overfill the cavity. When placed, the plastic instrument can be used to roughly achieve the correct convex contour of the filling.

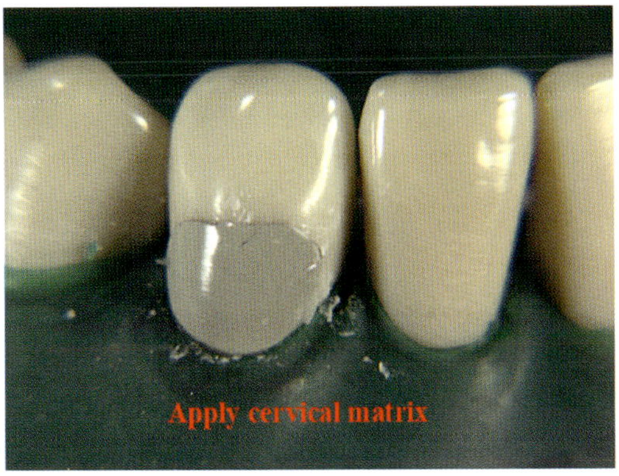

The pre-contoured and adapted cervical matrix is placed over the surface of the recently placed GIC and firmly adapted onto the surrounding enamel surface.

It should be left undisturbed for 5 minutes to ensure that the chemically curing filling material has reached its initial set.

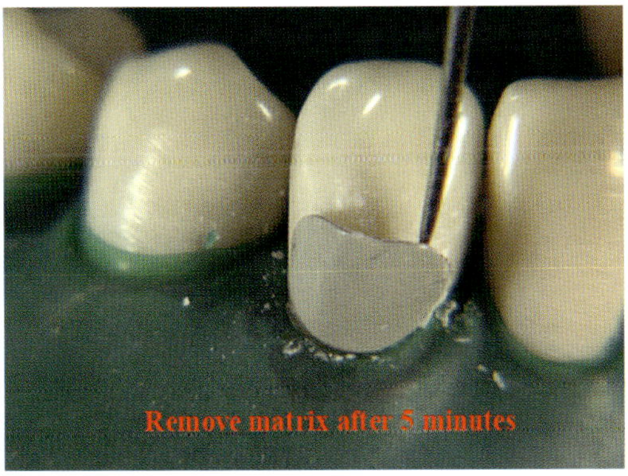

Once set, the matrix can be removed using a sharp probe to lift one of the margins.

It is important to ensure that the restorative material has reached its initial set. Some excess material left on the paper mixing pad should be tested for surface hardness using a plastic instrument.

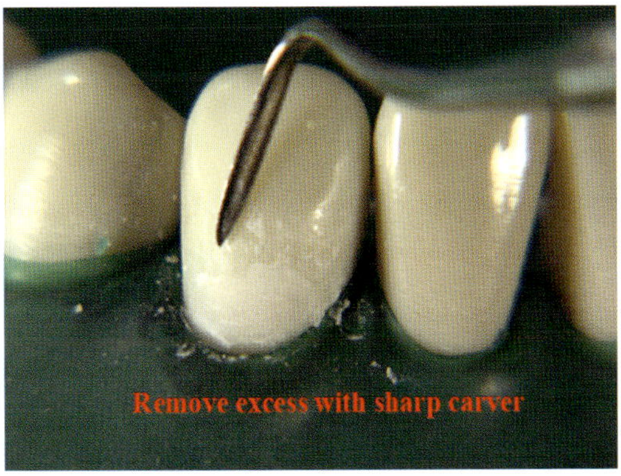

Excess filling material should be in a thin layer and will have adhered to the surface of the enamel adjacent to the cavity margins.

Where possible, finishing should be delayed for 24 hours unless such gross excess is present. A sharp half-Hollenbach carver can be used to remove the thin excess overlying the adjacent enamel tooth surface.

Note the smooth surface of the filling where it has set against the matrix.

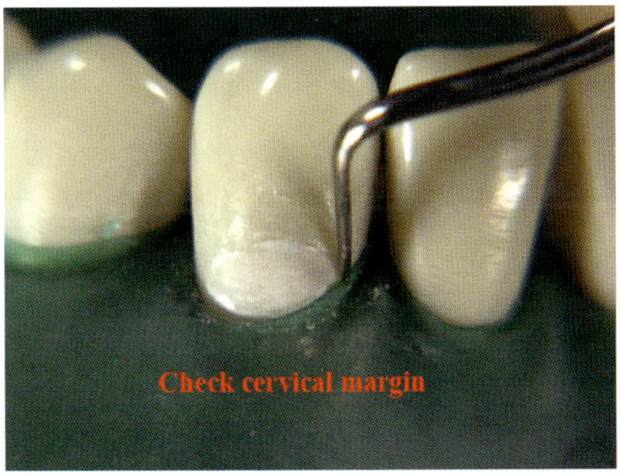

Run the carver along the cervical margin of the restoration to remove excess that otherwise may attract plaque accumulations.

Note that the majority of the surface of the filling has not been touched during this initial carving stage.

The chalky appearance demonstrates how this restorative material can dry out quickly.

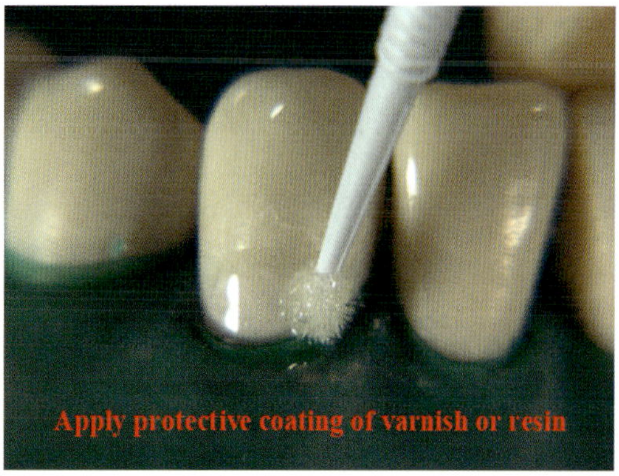

GIC must be protected during the first 24 hours because it could either take up or lose water. This would adversely affect the longevity of the filling because the matrix of the cement would be weakened.

Movement of water across the surface may be prevented by placing a preventive coat of either varnish or light-cured a bisGMA resin.

The resin has been reported as being more effective in the protection it provides.

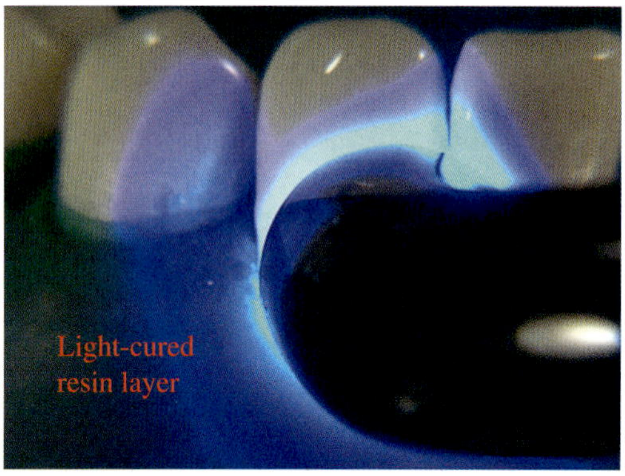

The resin should be left undisturbed for 30 seconds to allow it to penetrate into the porosity within the material. This will provide sufficient mechanical retention.

The resin layer must be light cured for 20 seconds with a visible blue light source with a wavelength of 470 nm.

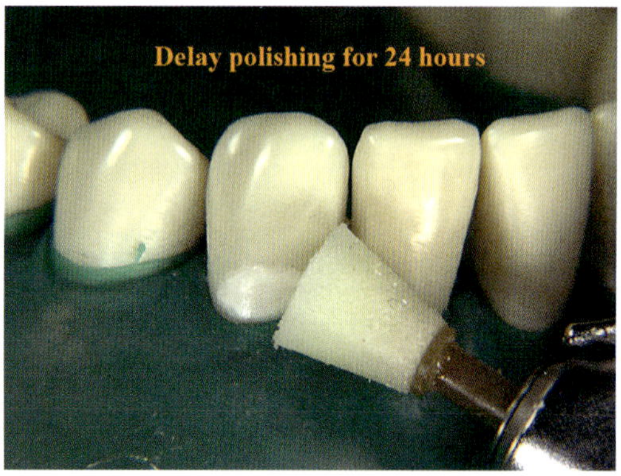

For the carefully inserted restoration this may be all that is required. Where the contour is incorrect, adjustment to shape and form can be made with impregnated rubber points, cups, and discs.

Recontouring should not be attempted until the material has matured and the second ion exchange has taken place.

This involves the mobilisation of the aluminium ions from the aluminosilicate glass and is not complete until 24 hours have elapsed from time of placement.

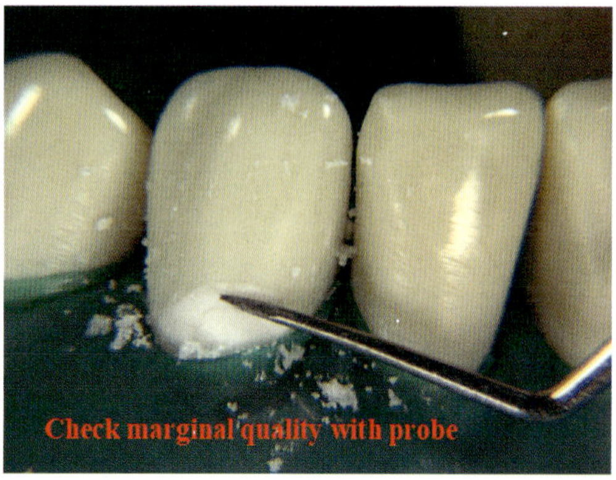

When the polishing points and cups have been used, the marginal integrity of the restoration should be checked using a probe. This is accomplished by moving the probe back and forward across the margins.
Marginal excess may be missed if the probe is used in one direction only.

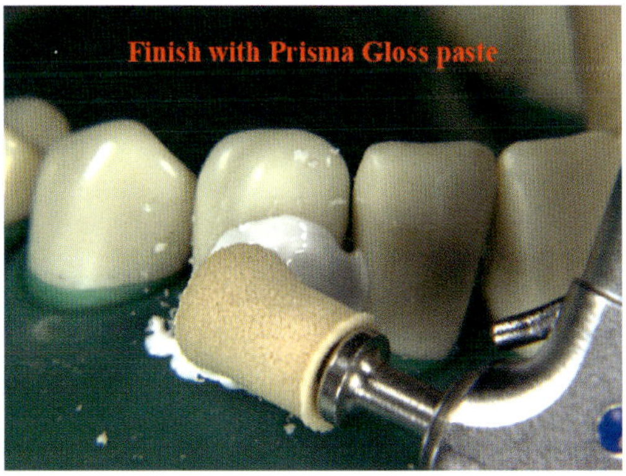

When recontouring and smoothing has been completed the surface of the filling can be finished using polishing pastes.

It is important that this material is used on the appropriate *felt* polishing cup supplied with a separate mandrel. It should *not* be applied to the impregnated rubber cups.

Ensure that the surface is washed thoroughly between the two paste applications.

Compomer Restorations

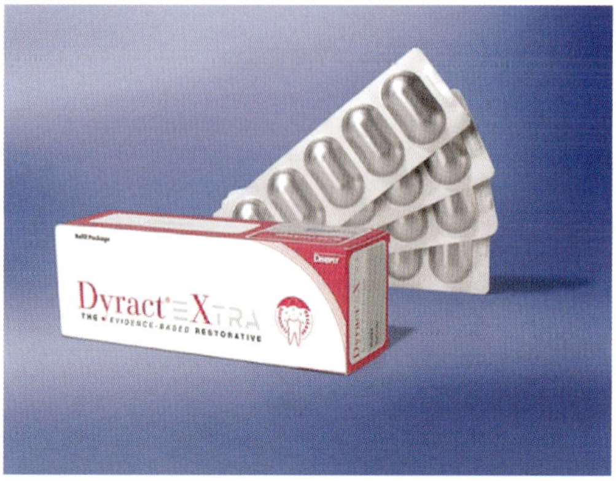

Alternatively, a compomer may be used. This filling material combines the properties of GIC with composite resins. The restorative can be made to adhere to tooth structure and may also release and absorb some fluoride ions.

The kit comprises the filling material presented in compules for use in a gun delivery system similar to that for composite resin. In addition, a bonding resin is supplied. For convenience a variety of shades are available for shade matching.
Source: Dentsply Sirona.

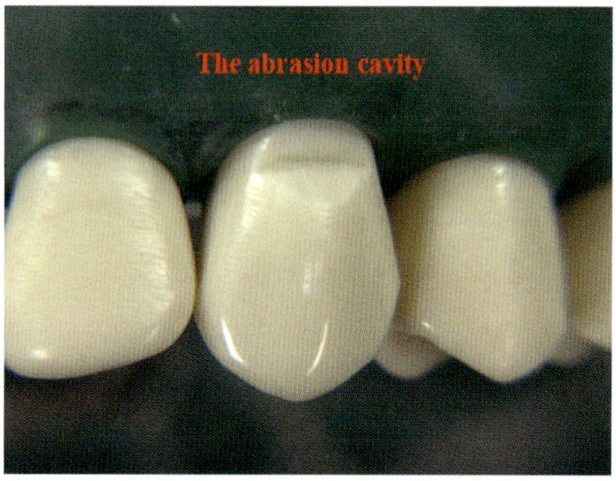

In this part of the sequence an abrasion cavity in a maxillary canine will be restored. The appearance of compomer is superior to that obtained with GIC.

For this reason, the compomer is frequently chosen where appearance is important.

The compomer comprises an aluminosilicate glass and an acid polymerisable resin (TCB) that allows methacrylate groups to polymerise into long chains while the pendant acid groups react with the glass filler surface.

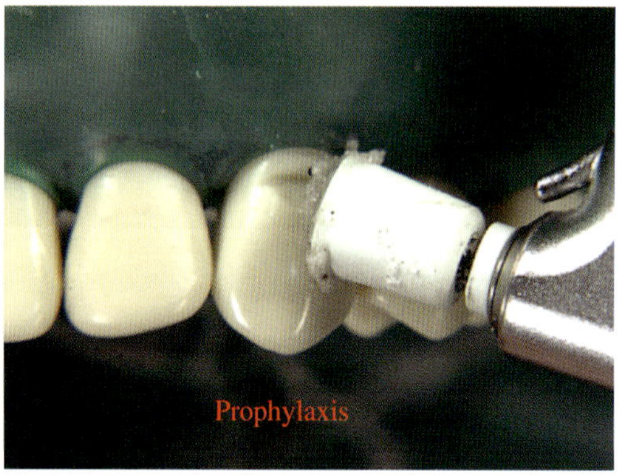

The initial stages of the procedure are similar. The surface is cleaned of accumulations of plaque using a slurry of pummice. Surface stain will also be removed at this time, allowing a more accurate shade match.

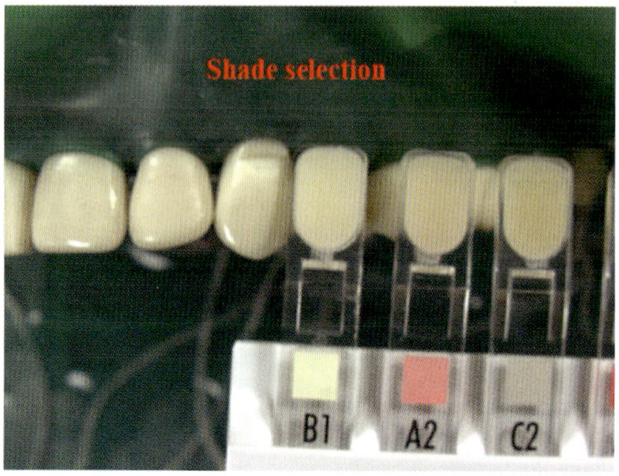

The shade must be chosen carefully for best results. Ensure that no undue delay occurs between isolating the cavity and choosing the shade. Alternatively, select the shade before isolation.

Note the colour of the square on the shade tab as this matches the cap on the compomer compule.

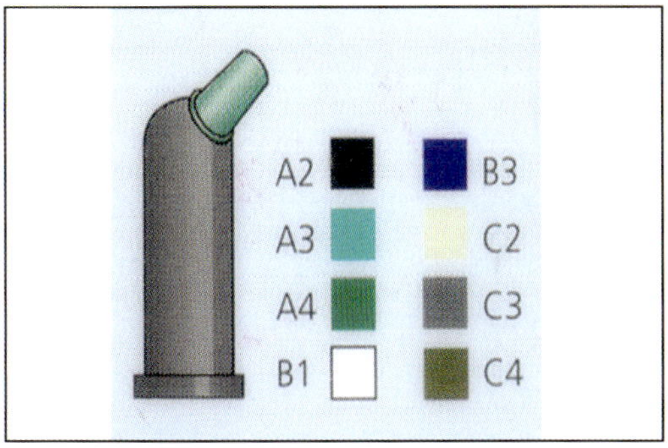

In the system demonstrated here, the coloured squares correspond to the various shades of compomer.

The cap on the compule is co-ordinated with the coloured square on the shade guide.

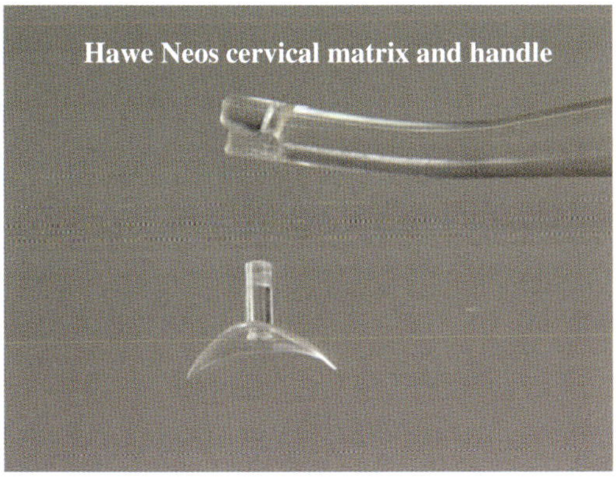

A cervical matrix should be selected that can conform to the external anatomy of the tooth.

This stage should be completed before the bonding procedure commences.

A transparent matrix is necessary when a light-cured material is used. The Hawe Neos cervical matrices are made of an acetate material and have an instrument to help with locating and holding the matrix against the tooth.

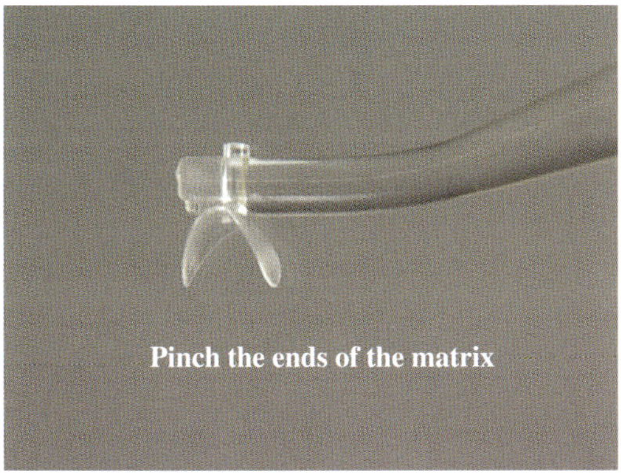

The projecting peg is inserted into the holder where it will be retained during the procedure.

To enable the matrix to be adapted to the surface of the tooth, the ends must be over-contoured by pinching them together...

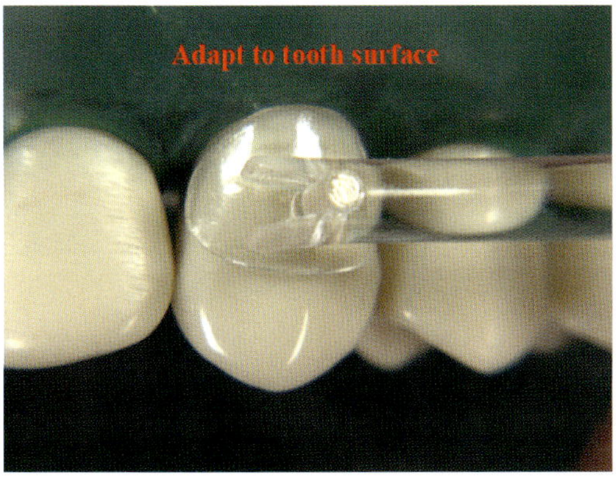

...and firmly placing onto the tooth surface. This allows the matrix to take up the correct shape.

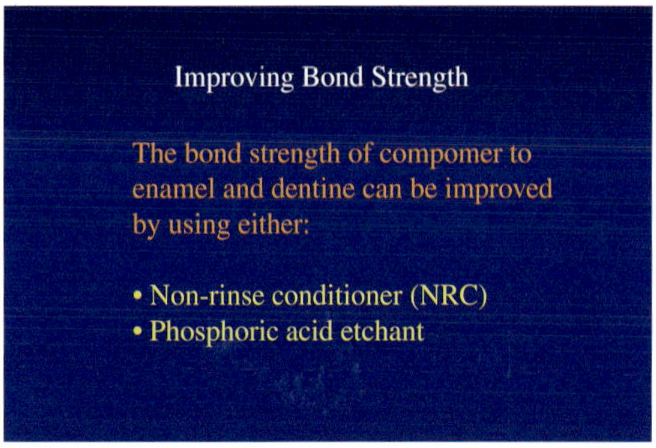

The bond strength of compomer to tooth structure is quite weak when only the bonding resin is applied to the surface of unetched enamel and dentine.

The manufacturer recommends that the enamel and dentine should be etched using either:

- NRC – a mixture of maleic and polyacrylic acids that is applied, left undisturbed for 20 seconds and then air dried
- Phosphoric acid etchant used in the same manner as for composite resin

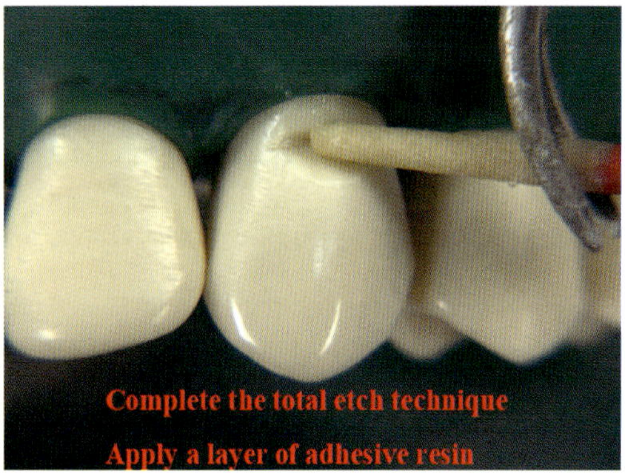

The bonding resin should be left undisturbed on the cavity surfaces for 30 seconds.

Prime and bond contains elastomeric resins and PENTA. The latter is a phosphate ester of methacrylate and is polar. It will wet the surface readily and will form ionic bonds with the apatite crystals.

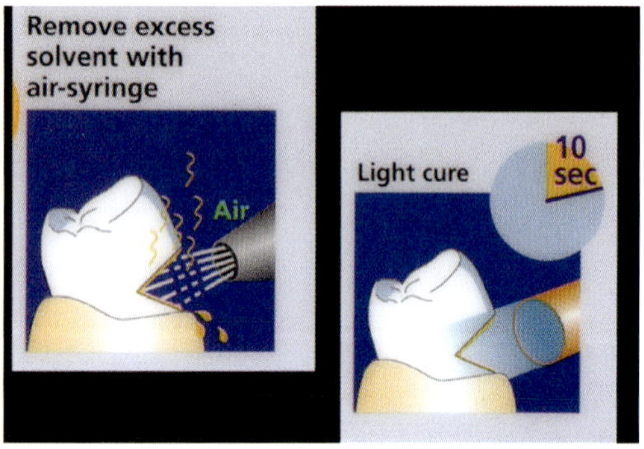

The butanol solvent can be removed by using a gentle stream of uncontaminated compressed air.

The bonding resin should then be light cured for 10 seconds.

Source: images produced by kind permission of Dentsply

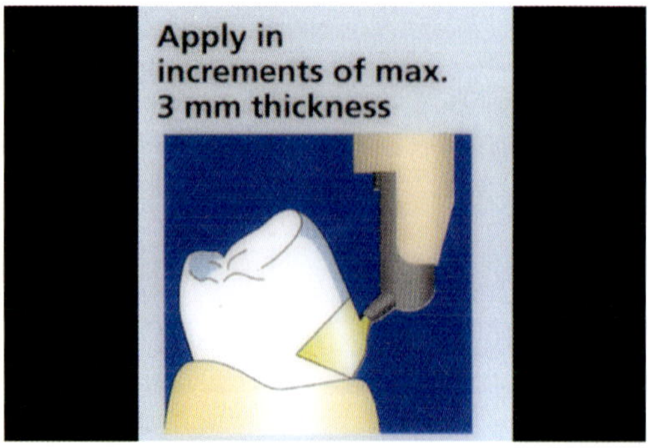

Compomer may be cured readily to a depth of 3 mm.

Most abrasion cavities would not be deeper than this dimension.

Source: image produced by kind permission of Dentsply

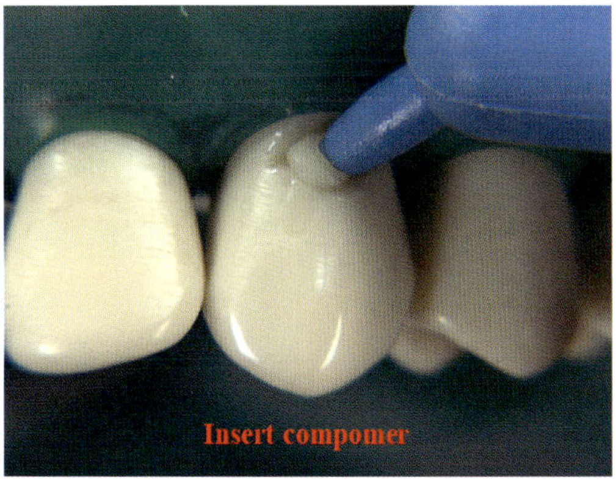

The compule is loaded into the delivery gun and the material expressed directly into the cavity.

This is easier than transferring the filling material from a paper pad on a plastic instrument.

A compule delivery system is more expensive than large syringes of filling material, but the convenience it gives far outweighs the higher cost of the material, and it is good in infection control situations.

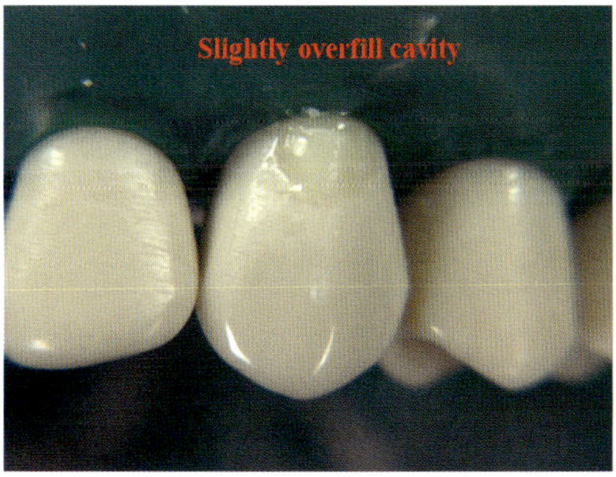

A slight excess of the material is placed into the cavity and shaped to approximately conform with the surface anatomy of the tooth.

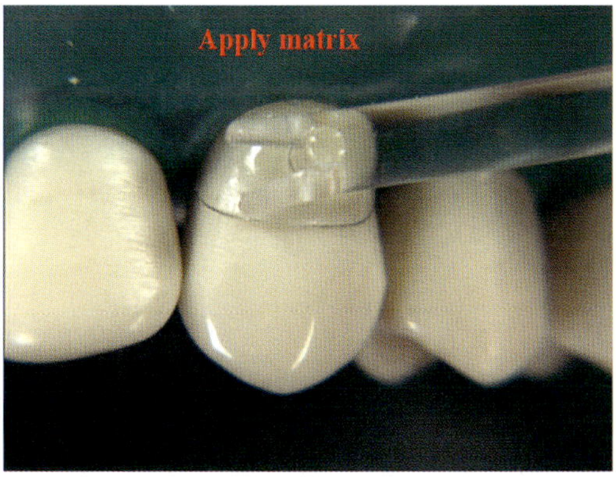

The pre-contoured Hawe Neos cervical matrix is applied over the filling material and held firmly in position to ensure that any excess material is in thin section only.

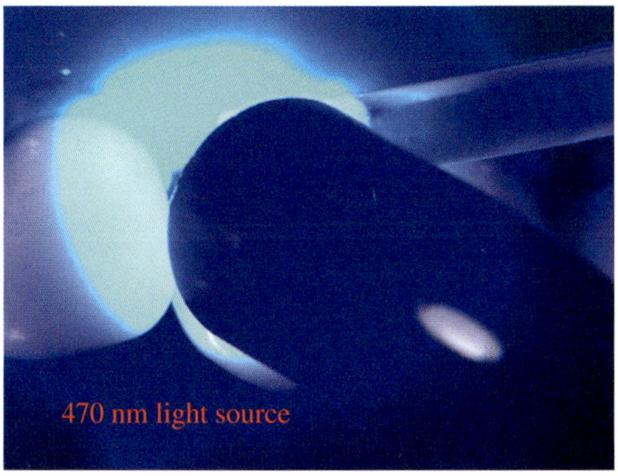

A curing time of 40 seconds is recommended by the manufacturer for compomer increments up to 3 mm in depth.

The curing gun should be held as close as possible to the tooth surface while the matrix is still held firmly in position.

Very little of the light intensity is lost as it passes through the acetate matrix system.

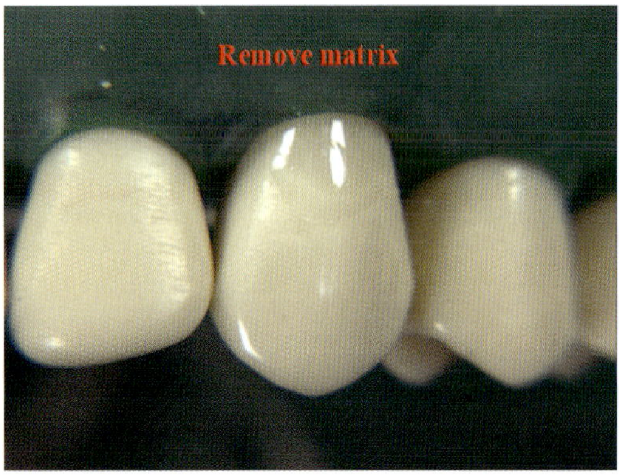

When the matrix is removed the smooth surface of the underlying compomer can be inspected for surface blows.

Only a thin layer of excess should be present over the adjacent tooth structure.

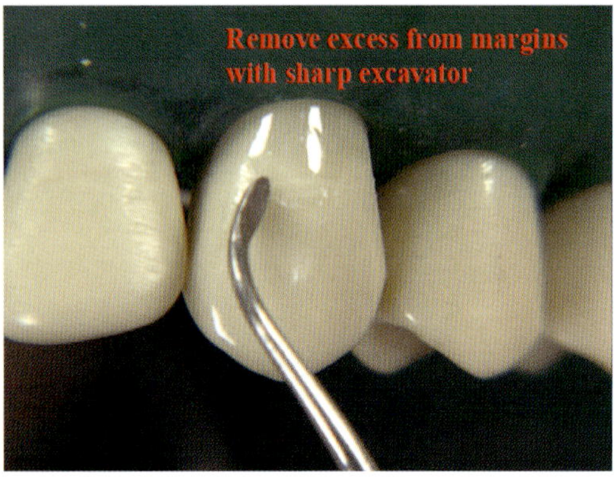

Excess filling material can be removed using a sharp excavator.

If care has been exercised when placing the bonding resin, this excess will come away cleanly and easily from the tooth surface.

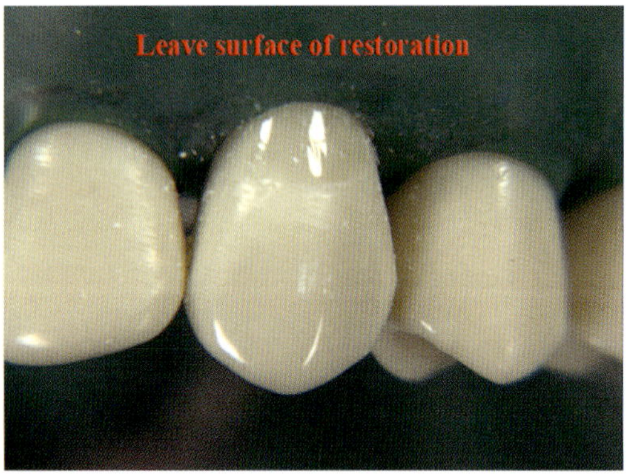

With a careful placement technique, it should be possible to leave the surface of the smooth compomer at this stage.

Check the margins with a probe and adjust, if necessary, with rotary finishing instruments.

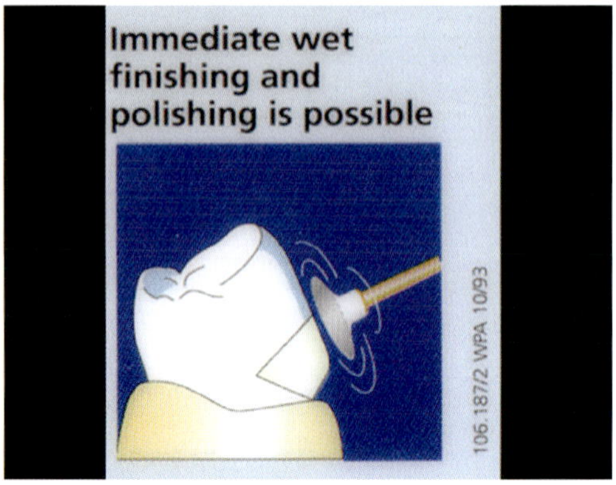
Immediate wet
finishing and
polishing is possible
106.187/2 WPA 10/93

Compomer can be finished immediately unlike the chemically cured GICs.

The "Enhance" system is ideal for finishing and polishing as most surfaces are accessible to the discs, points, and cups.

Source: image produced by kind permission of Dentsply

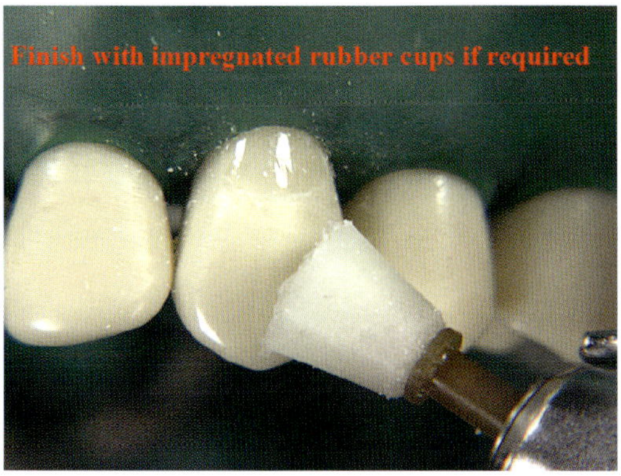

The impregnated rubber cups will be used only on the margins of the restoration, and care should be exercised, where possible, to avoid the contoured and smooth surface.

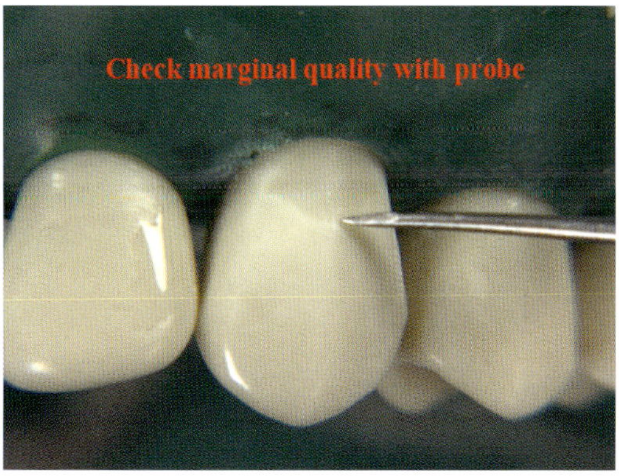

The marginal quality should be re-checked at this stage using a sharp dental probe.
This should be used to explore across the margins in two directions.

The junction between tooth and restoration should be imperceptible.

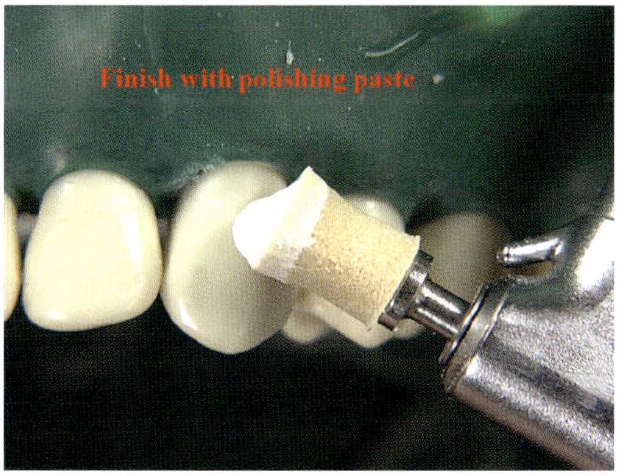

The surface can then be finished using the polishing pastes. This is used on the felt cup and stainless steel mandrel - do *not* use the impregnated rubber point or cup.

Please remember to wash the first paste before applying the extra-fine material.

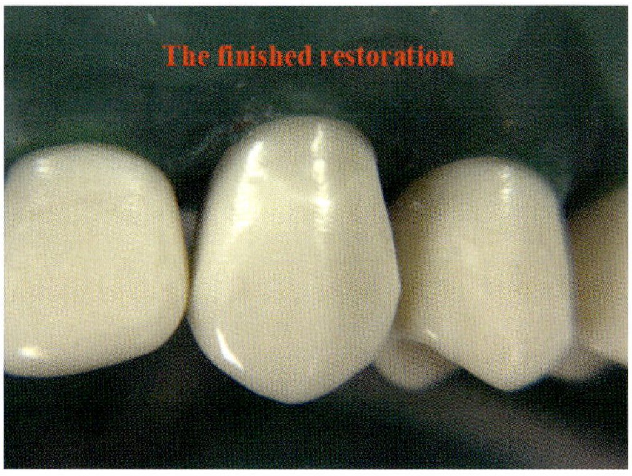

A restoration with a high quality surface can be achieved readily.

Once this restoration has absorbed water, the glass ionomer reaction may proceed via the ionised pendant groups of carboxyllic.
These will react with the filler particles of alumina silicate glass.

The latter reaction allows some ionic interchange with the tooth surface for bonding and also to release fluoride ions, which may have some cariostatic properties.

Further Reading

Brennan, D.S., Balasubramanian, M., and Spencer, A.J. (2016). Restorative treatment for initial, cavitated and gross coronal carious lesions. *Australian Dental Journal* 61: 350–356.

Canali, G.D., Ignácio, S.A., Rached, R.N., and Souza, E.M. (2019). One-year clinical evaluation of bulk-fill flowable vs. regular nanofilled composite in non-carious cervical lesions. *Clinical Oral Investigations* 23: 889–897.

Michael, J.A., Kaidonis, J.A., and Townsend, G.C. (2010). Non-carious cervical lesions on permanent anterior teeth: a new morphological classification. *Australian Dental Journal* 55: 134–137.

Sawlani, K., Lawson, N.C., Burgess, J.O. et al. Factors influencing the progression of noncarious cervical lesions: a 5-year prospective clinical evaluation. *Journal of Prosthetic Dentistry* 115: 5.

Teixeiraa, D.N.R., Zeolaa, L.F., Machadoa, A.C. et al. (2018). Relationship between noncarious cervical lesions, cervical dentin hypersensitivity, gingival recession, and associated risk factors: a cross-sectional study. *Journal of Dentistry* 76: 93–97.

Section III

Indirect Restorations

9

Indirect Restorations

An indirect restoration is one that requires either a cavity or a preparation that is free from undercuts to allow a path of insertion and withdrawal for a restoration made in the dental laboratory. The restoration should be able to be inserted into or over the prepared tooth without generating stresses. These indirect restorations should ideally be able to protect and reinforce the remaining tooth structure.

Indirect restoration must be cemented or bonded into place to provide the required retention and marginal seal. When cemented into place, non-adhesive restorations depend on the surface area of opposing walls of the preparation and their degree of convergence. Restorations that are bonded using resin-based luting materials contribute majorly to the overall retention.

There are three types of Indirect restoration:

- ***Intra-coronal,*** e.g. an inlay. This fits entirely within a cavity in the crown of the tooth.
- ***Extra-coronal,*** e.g. a crown. A crown fits over a prepared tooth. These can be full or partial coverage, e.g. three-quarters or seven-eighths crowns.
- ***Combined Intra- and extra-coronal,*** e.g. an inlay/onlay. This fits partly into a cavity within the crown but has an extra-coronal part that fits over the cusps to protect them. In the treatment of tooth wear, a metal or tooth coloured onlay can be constructed that has no intra-coronal part but is bonded to the worn occlusal surfaces to replace the missing tooth structure (see Figure 9.1).

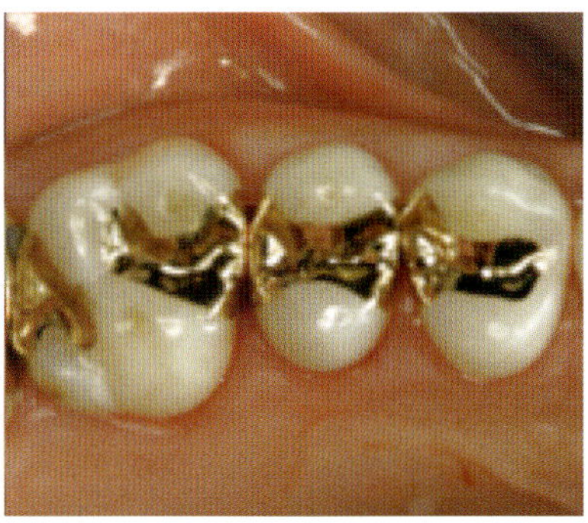

Gold inlay

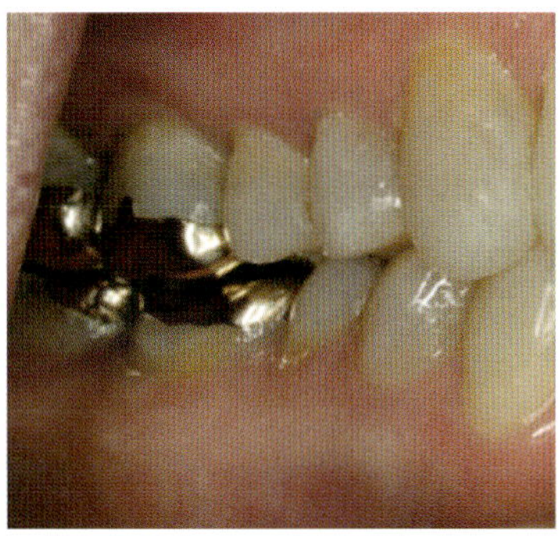

Gold onlay

Figure 9.1 The picture on the left shows some two-surface intra-coronal restorations, while the picture on the right shows multi-surface restorations where the gold has been brought over the cusps to protect them from future fracture.

A Practical Approach to Operative Dentistry, First Edition. Gordon B. Gray and Alaa H. Daud.

Companion website: www.wiley.com/go/gray/operative-dentistry

Crowns can be made from various materials. These include

- Dental alloys – precious, semi-precious, or non-precious alloys
- Porcelain
- Composite resin
- A combination of alloy and ceramic, e.g. a porcelain fused to metal (PFM) crown

A ***gold alloy*** does not have good appearance but otherwise has many advantageous properties. The hardness and wear is similar to that of enamel, so this makes it ideal for onlays and full and partial coverage crowns. The restorations are made by the lost wax technique so the wax pattern can be shaped anatomically in the dental laboratory before casting in molten alloy. The alloy can be cast in a very thin section.

A traditional ***porcelain*** is a brittle material that will fracture in clinical use unless it is at least 0.5 mm thick and is supported by tooth structure. Performance of this material is improved if it is bonded to the underlying tooth structure. Previously, these materials were used in the restoration of anterior teeth only, but nowadays, high strength ceramics are available that allow porcelain crowns to be made for posterior teeth, e.g. In-Ceram and Empress.

Composite resin for use in indirect techniques has improved strength and wear characteristics. This allows it to be used for inlay, onlay, and single unit crowns. These materials can be made to bond with the underlying dentine and enamel. The wear characteristics show these materials to be less resistant, and they will therefore not cause wear of the opposing teeth.

PFM crowns combine the good aesthetics offered by porcelain with the strength and wear resistance of gold alloy. The preparation for this style of crown requires a greater shoulder depth of 1.3–1.5 mm compared to porcelain or gold alloy alone.

Principles of Crown Preparation

The following lists cover indications for crown preparation, general principles for all restorations, and particular principles for extra-coronal restorations, which are covered in the following sections.

Indications for crown preparation:

- Badly broken down teeth
- Primary trauma
- Tooth wear
- Hypoplastic conditions
- To alter shape/size/inclination of teeth
- To alter occlusion
- As part of another restoration, e.g. a bridge
- Restoration of root filled teeth
- Appearance

General principles that apply to ALL restorations:

- Biological/mechanical, etc.
- Elimination of diseased tissue
- Preservation of tooth structure
- Restoration of form

- Occlusal stability
- Pulpal health
- Periodontal health
- Durability of tooth and restoration
- Acceptable aesthetics

Principles of particular relevance to extra-coronal restorations:

1) Preservation of tooth structure
2) Retention and resistance
3) Marginal integrity
4) Strength and structural durability
5) Occlusal stability

1) Preservation of tooth structure

   It is important to note that although destructive, the provision of an extra-coronal restoration may preserve tooth substance in the longer term – for example, posterior root filled teeth have a much higher fracture rate compared to similar teeth that have been crowned.

   There are three main considerations: the type of restoration, the materials to be used, and the amount of reduction needed.

   The type of extra-coronal restoration should be as conservative as possible whilst achieving the aims of treatment. These are principally considered by

   a) Full or partial coverage
   b) Type of material to be used

      Full or partial coverage:

      If retention can be maintained from the height and convergence angle of the preparations, intact surfaces of tooth structure should be saved and not removed for convenience or speed.

      – ***Relative merits of partial coverage:***

        These include such restorations as the MOD onlay and three-quarters or seven-eighths crowns. These restorations have a more minimal preparation and leave a surface of the tooth unprepared. This allows pulp testing or sensibility testing to be carried out in the future. The natural landmarks on the tooth are more likely to be preserved, and this may aid preparation and the subsequent laboratory construction. The margins are more likely to be supra-gingival, making the recording of an impression easier. When it comes to fitting the restoration, it is likely to be easier because the axial walls are not covered to such an extent, thus expression of excess cement is facilitated.

        The disadvantage is that the area of margin is much greater with the risk of secondary caries. In addition, the retention and resistance forms may be inferior as may the aesthetic limitations.

      Materials used:

      The material chosen will dictate the amount of tooth substance removed due to differences in characteristics.

      – ***Gold crowns:***

        Regarded by most to be the most satisfactory extra-coronal restorative material. Has a hardness similar to enamel, does not creep intraorally, can be cast accurately, and wax carving allows good detail and contour. It can be used in thin section thus allowing fine margins. Not very aesthetic, though liked by some.

- ***Porcelain crowns:***

  Traditional ***feldspathic porcelain*** crowns are the most aesthetic. They are brittle and liable to fracture, especially in thin section. Therefore, more bulk was needed than for gold crowns. These traditional porcelains were not strong enough to be used alone for posterior teeth or bridgework. Cracks could arise from micro-pores on the surface, which could then open in tension or during bending, especially if not supported, which influences margin design. Dental porcelain is harder than enamel and if unglazed may abrade tooth surface.

  Contemporary porcelain crowns are much stronger and often referred to as ***all-ceramic crowns***. These are based on ***zirconia-containing porcelains***. Zirconia-based ceramics have better mechanical properties and are named by the companies who produce these materials and techniques, e.g. Procera, Lava, In-Ceram, E-Max.
- ***PFM crowns:***

  This combination allows good strength along with good aesthetics but requires more tooth reduction than the full gold or the all-ceramic crowns. Although porcelain is frequently used for the functional surface, ideally this should be in metal.
- ***Amount of reduction:***

  Reduction of the tooth structure should be appropriate and not excessive. It needs to be sufficient to provide bulk for the restoration without necessitating over-contouring the restoration simply to achieve sufficient thickness. If too much tooth structure is removed from the tooth, it will compromise its strength.

  Reduction must be anatomical, i.e. broadly following the contours of the tooth – a flat occlusal surface may shorten an already low clinical height of preparation, giving minimal retention. In addition, it will remove more tooth substance than is necessary. Conversely, inadequate reduction in the occlusal grooves will not provide adequate space for good functional morphology.

  The amount of tooth reduction will depend also on the type of material to be used for the final restoration. Gold alloy requires 1 mm coverage occlusally with 1.5 mm over the functional cusps. It may be 0.8 mm on palatal aspect of anterior teeth. Conversely, an all-ceramic crown requires a 1.1 mm reduction on its axial surfaces, whereas a PFM crown requires 1.3 mm minimum reduction on its labial or buccal surface.

  There should be greater reduction over the functional cusp, i.e. palatal of maxillary cusps and buccal of mandibular cusps. This is achieved by means of a wide bevel. If this is not done, the wax pattern and the casting will be too thin in this area. If adequate bulk is provided by over-contouring, the occlusal contacts will be incorrect and result in them being too high or in excursive interferences during lateral movements of the mandible.

  Reduction is often overestimated. The use of depth grooves or the use of a bur tip of known diameter can be a useful aid.
- ***Protection from fracture and wear:***

  The extra-coronal restoration is able to preserve tooth structure by protecting it from fracture or wear. The restoration can control loads on the tooth by maintaining stable occlusal contacts and by protecting the remaining axial walls from stresses that may otherwise lead to fracture.

2) Retention and resistance

   It is important to know what the difference is between these two terms.

Retention form includes those features of the preparation that resist removal of the restoration along its long axis.
Resistance form includes those features of the preparation that resist dislodgement due to forces outside the path of withdrawal of the restoration.
Resistance is probably the more important of the two features, although there is a relationship between the two but not a direct one. A cement lute is strong in compression but weak in shear loads. Therefore, good resistance and retention are necessary to minimise the shear loading on the luting cement.
Retention:
Retention is primarily a surface area effect and is dependent on
- Height of preparation
- Diameter
- Taper

Theoretically, the more nearly parallel the opposing walls of a preparation, the greater the retention. To avoid production of undercuts and to allow seating of the crown, a slight taper is necessary. The taper also allows the luting cement to escape at the time of fitting. Optimal taper is 6°, which is difficult to achieve clinically. Teeth with good clinical height may need a greater taper (of up to 10°) to allow seating of the final crown. Less taper should be used for teeth with a low clinical height, where retention and resistance are poorer. The burs commonly used for crown preparation are tapered and should be held parallel to the long axis of the preparation to produce an acceptable taper.
Resistance:
In some clinical situations, even the use of additional features will not provide enough resistance. In these circumstances, surgical crown lengthening may be necessary to increase available crown height. Such additional features as grooves, slots, and boxes can improve the resistance form significantly by reducing the radius of rotation of the final crown. These features should be prepared in the long axis of the preparation and not just placed in line with the axial wall. Axial grooves should be placed, if possible, into sound tooth tissue and not into restorative core material that has been used to replace tooth structure missing due to caries or fracture. There should be a definite wall perpendicular to the direction of the force to limit the freedom of displacement and provide adequate resistance. Axial grooves effectively improve the height to diameter ratio and enhance retention as well as resistance.

3) Marginal integrity
Finishing lines should not routinely be placed subgingivally but should be placed where they may be easily finished by the dentist, cleaned by the patient, and duplicated by the impression. They should be placed on sound tooth substance rather than on restorative material of the core buildup. If possible, margins should be placed on enamel.
A subgingival margin may be inevitable where

- Caries or a crack extends subgingivally
- A restoration or a core buildup extends subgingivally
- Extra axial length is required for retention
- Appearance is of prime importance

The aim must be to produce as small a marginal gap as possible. The margin design utilised will depend on such factors as material to be used and ease of construction.

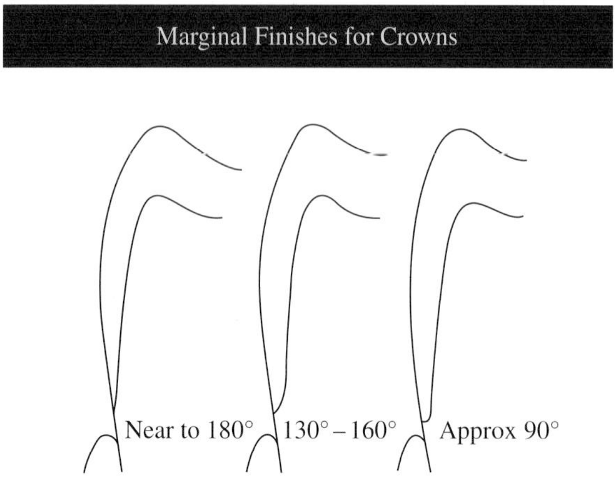

Figure 9.2 This figure demonstrates the various marginal finish lines for crowns.

Types of margin design:

See Figure 9.2 for types of margin design.

- ***Feather edge:***

  The feather edge is the closest to a 'slip-joint' that can be produced. It results in an acute angle of metal at the margin such that any failure to seat fully occlusally is not reflected totally at the margin. The feather edge margin is only applicable for a metal restoration of cast gold where the margin may be burnished easily. The disadvantages of this marginal design far outweigh this advantage because

  - This design does not provide a definitive and easily seen finish line for the dentist
  - It does not provide a definitive finishing line for the technician
  - The axial wall of the casting may lack rigidity due to the fine edge of metal
  - The restoration margin may be over-contoured as a compromise to provide definition and rigidity

- ***Shoulder:***

  A shoulder or rounded shoulder is the margin type necessary for porcelain restorations due to the latter's brittleness and liability to fracture other than in compressive loads. The margin ensures that the wide ledge provides support for the porcelain to resist occlusal forces and minimise stresses that may lead to fracture of the porcelain. Fine edges of porcelain may be rounded during firing, resulting in reduced accuracy of fit.

  The sharp, 90° internal line angle classically associated with this margin concentrates stress in the tooth, thus this angle should be rounded, and hence the term 'rounded shoulder'.

  The shoulder is generally not used for metal restorations because it will not provide the acute margin that would minimise marginal gaps and allow the margin to be burnished. This shoulder preparation is more destructive of tooth structure than other margin types.

- ***Chamfer:***

  The chamfered finishing line is the one of choice for metal restorations because it is a practical compromise between the feather and shoulder finish. It provides the acute margin that is desirable yet also will result in a restoration that has adequate axial bulk to provide rigidity without the need to over-contour and without being overly destructive of tooth substance. It also exhibits the least stress so that the underlying cement lute will have less likelihood of failure. It also has the advantages of being easily seen by the clinician and recorded on the impression and can be readily identified on the die by the technician.

4) Strength and structural durability
   The crown must be
   - ***Rigid enough*** to resist flexure. This is especially important at the margins of restorations where, if the axial portion is too thin, e.g. with an acute feather edge finishing line, the crown is at risk of deformation. This may result in fracture of the cement lute.
   - ***Thick enough*** to resist wear and fracture. A gold crown should have a 1 mm occlusal reduction and should be 1.5 mm thick over the functional cusps. In PFM crowns the thickness should be 1.75–2 mm.
   - ***Structural durability*** requires control of stresses. Chamfers concentrate stresses less than shoulders, but, where a shoulder is to be used, the junction between the base of the axial wall and the gingival margin of the preparation should be rounded to minimise stress in this area.
5) Occlusal stability
   Any crown provided for a patient must be in harmony with the existing occlusion if this is satisfactory. However, the provision of a new crown may be used to create a new occlusal relationship in those patients where the existing pattern is not harmonious.

   Pre-operative examination of the occlusion is essential, and this should be done using study models mounted with a face bow record. Note must be taken of existing relationships, such as canine guidance or group function and anterior guidance as well as the presence of excursive interferences or gross retruded contact position (RCP) to inter-cuspal position (ICP) discrepancies.

Assessment of a Patient for an Onlay or Crown

The decision to provide a tooth with an indirect restoration should not simply be a mechanical one, and factors other than the tooth in question must be addressed. If this is not carefully addressed, the restoration may fail.

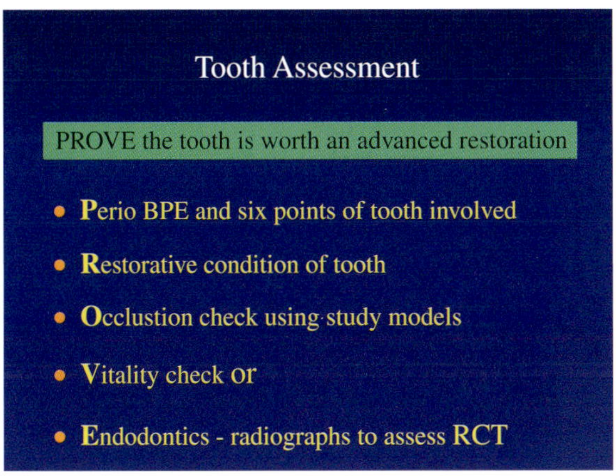

MOD Gold Onlay

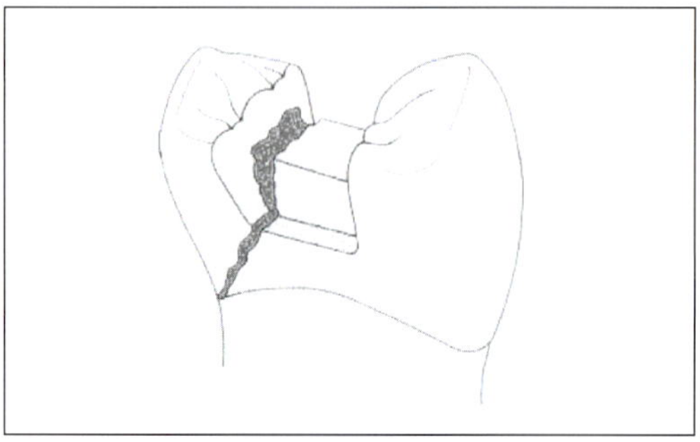

In this slide the premolar tooth shown has a wide cavity. When bisected with an MOD cavity, the premolar tooth has only 36% of its intact strength as the margin's ridges have been removed. These impart considerable strength to the tooth. The remaining strength depends, of course, on the width of the occlusal part of the cavity.

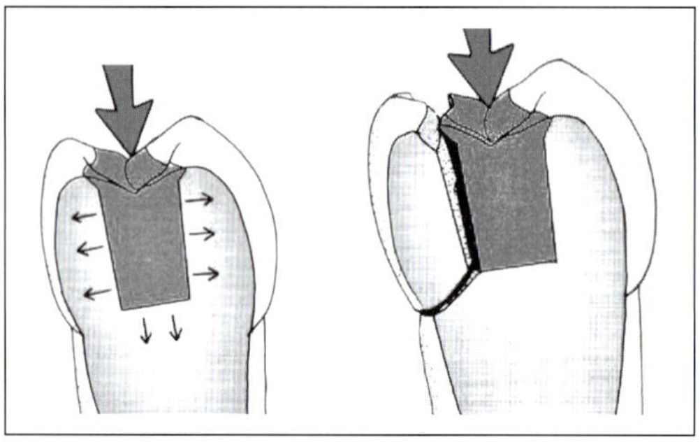

Cavities prepared for gold inlays are non-undercut and slightly divergent. It has long been recognised that this design has a tendency to wedge the cusps apart. This is even more pronounced where the isthmus of the cavity is large.

When occlusal forces are applied to an inlay, stresses are applied along the sides and base of the restoration. This results in stresses to the walls of the cavity and fracture of a cusp from the tooth. This will frequently occur at a 45° angle from the corner of the cavity.

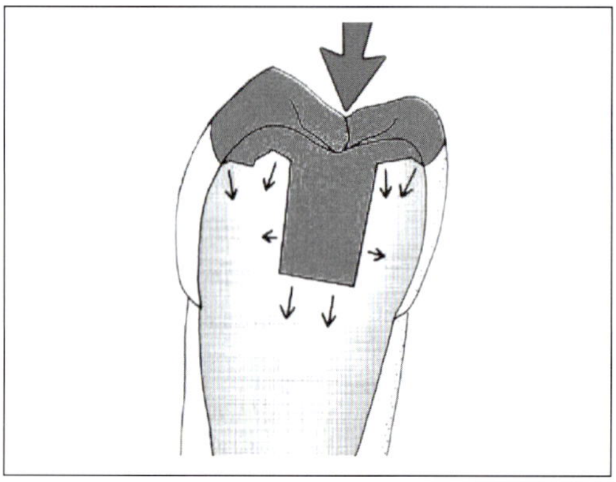

An onlay distributes the forces over a wider area, reducing the potential for fracture. In addition, the onlay covers the cusps in such a way that outward displacement is prevented when occlusal forces are applied.

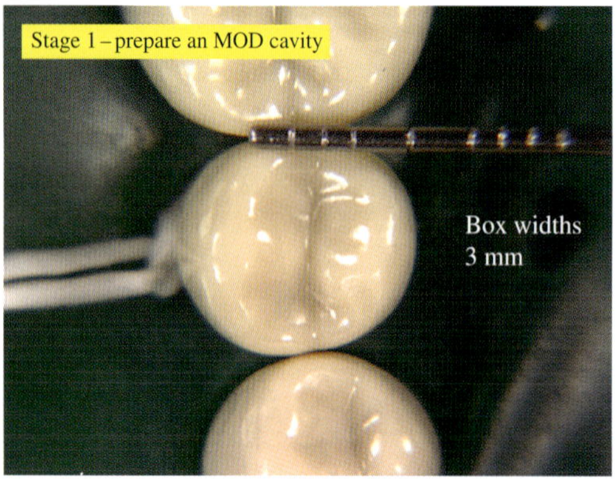

Stage 1

The first stage is to prepare an MOD cavity to eradicate caries and allow the clinician to assess the strength of the remaining cusps.

In this particular case, the caries is situated mesially and distally just below the contact points and is 3 mm in width. Substantial spread along the enamel dentine junction is also present even at the base of the occlusal fissures.

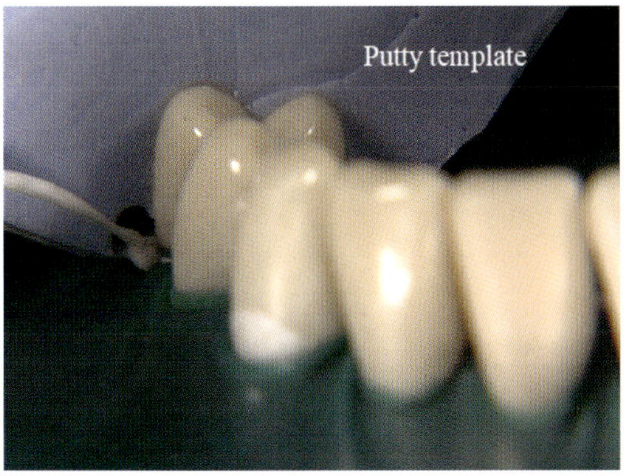

As an aid to assessing reduction of the cusps at a later stage, a putty replica has been made for visual clarity of the presentation.

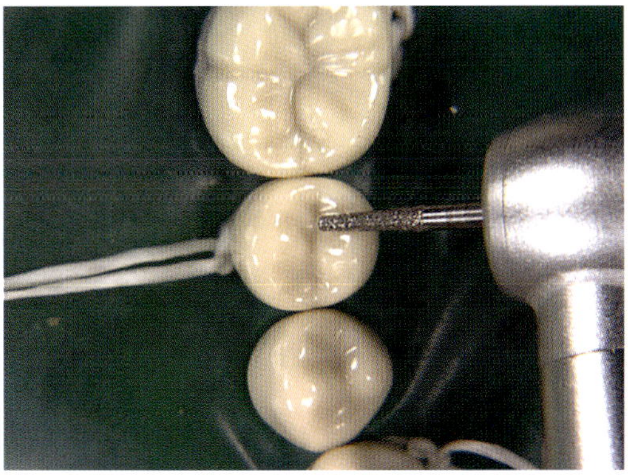

In this sequence the tapered fissure bur will be used to perform the preparation. It is a tapered F/G diamond coated bur for use in the air turbine handpiece.

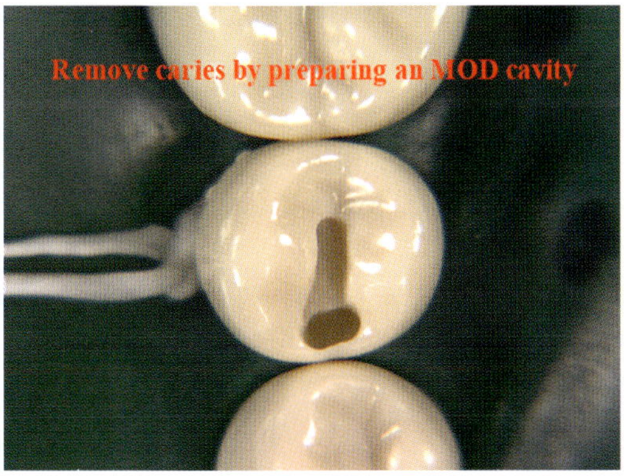

The caries has been approached mesially by entering the carious fissure first and then progressing towards the marginal ridge. The bur has fallen deeper into the caries associated with the mesial surface.

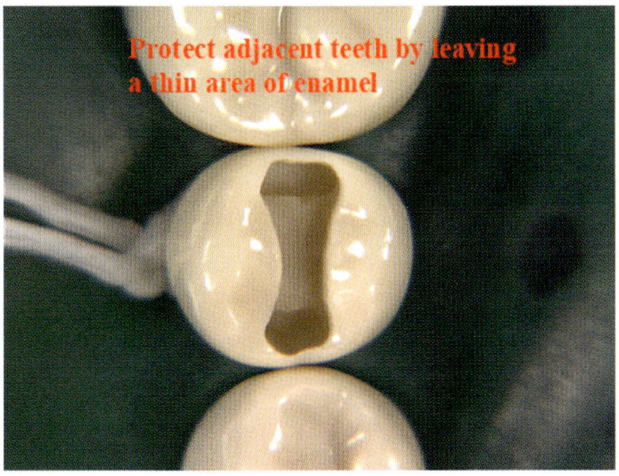

The distal aspect of the cavity is then prepared in a similar manner. The marginal enamel is maintained, where present, to help protect the adjacent teeth.

The gingival aspect of the preparation in the mesial and distal boxes should be taken sufficiently far gingivally to reach onto sound tooth structure.

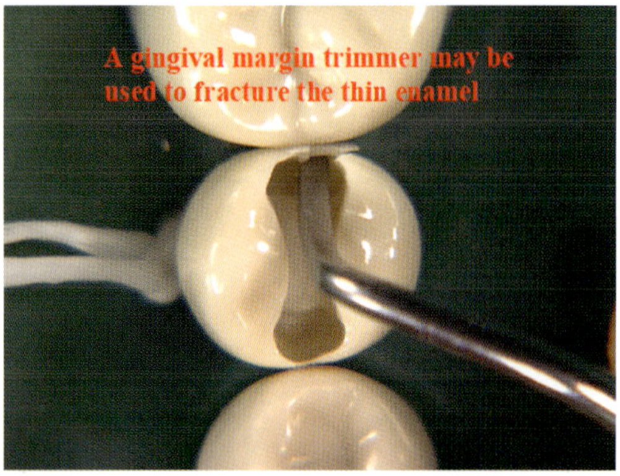

A gingival margin trimmer may be used to fracture the thin enamel at the boxes so that the adjacent teeth are not damaged during the process.

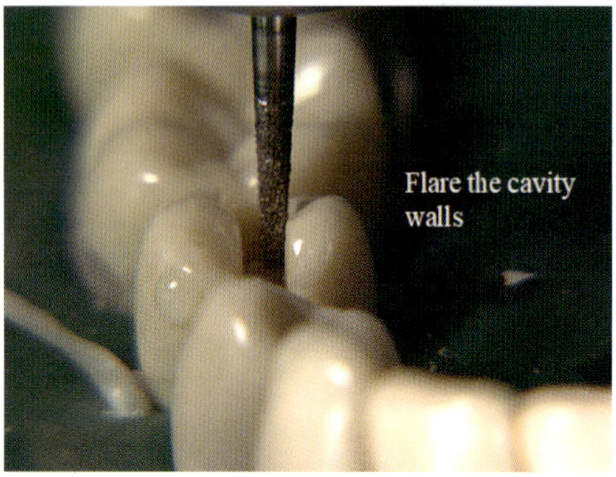

The walls of the cavity should be slightly divergent with a flare of 3°–5° only.

The taper on the fissure bur can be used to provide the correct amount of divergence. The bur should be held perpendicular to the occlusal plane of the tooth to produce the correct mount of flare.

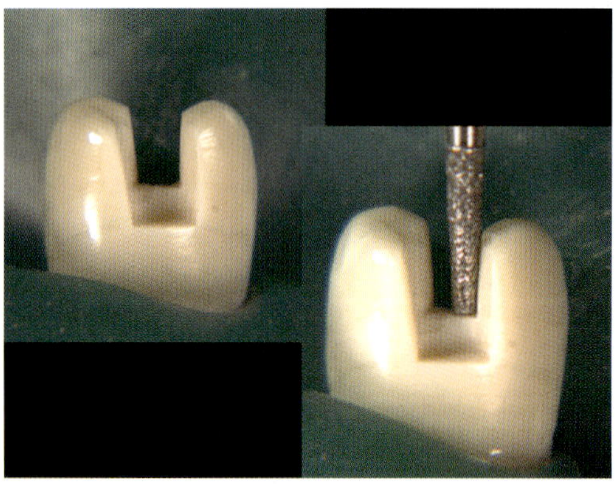

This view of the cavity shows the amount of taper that is required in both the boxes and the occlusal key-way joining up the two boxes.

Extending the taper to an amount greater than this will be detrimental to the retention of the restoration.

The degree of taper can be checked by holding the tapered bur parallel with one wall and moving it across to the cavity to the other wall...

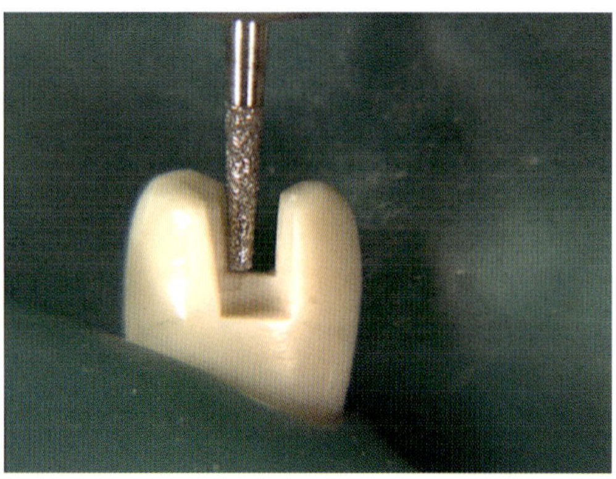

...and checking for the presence of undercut here.

If a space is present between the bur and the cavity wall, the walls are probably too tapered.

A slight space is present here.

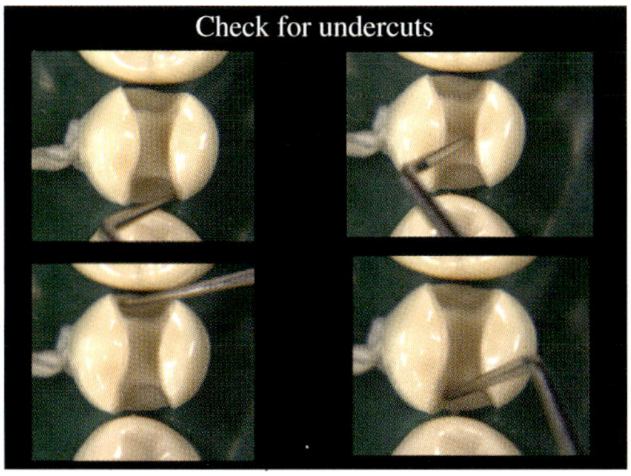

It is important that a check is made for undercuts. This can be accomplished using monocular vision.

In this view, a probe is being used to explore around the cavity while using only one eye to track its movements.

Mirror and monocular vision are important concepts in assessing cavities for the presence of undercuts.

The tip of the probe should be seen at all line angles in the cavity while using the monocular vision technique.

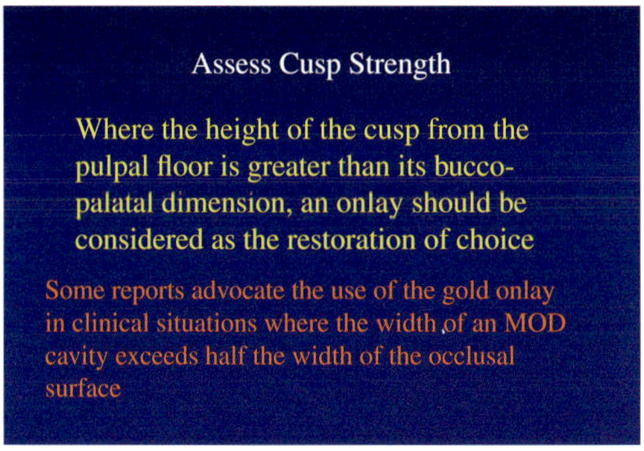

If the cusps are weak, an onlay should be considered to protect the cusps from fracture.

Many clinicians advocate the provision of cuspal coverage for all root treated teeth.

This is advocated because some think that the tooth becomes more brittle after root canal therapy, whereas others maintain that greater forces are applied to the tooth due to altered proprioception within the periodontal ligament.

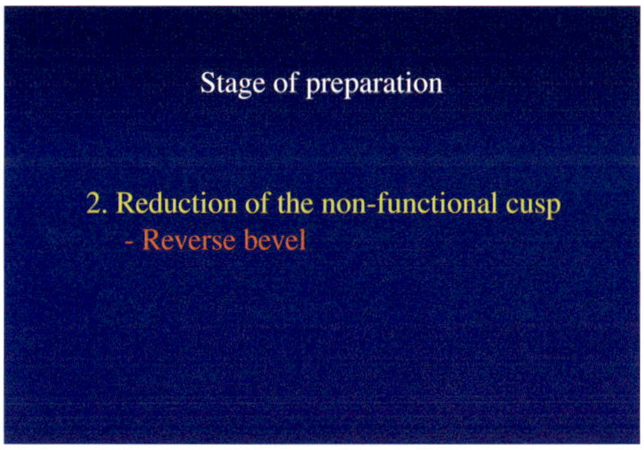

In the next stage of the preparation, the non-functional cusp is reduced by a height of about 1 mm.

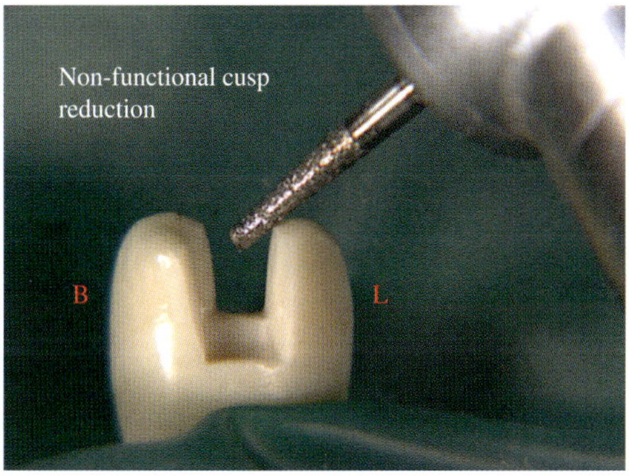

This is done in an anatomical manner by using the bur again but held at a 45° slope in towards the cavity preparation.

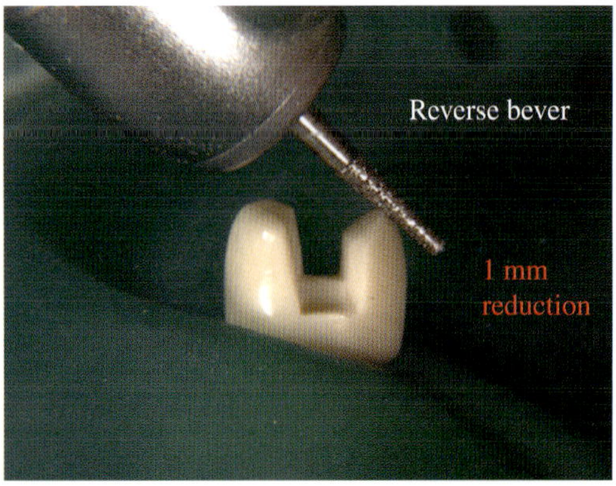

The reverse bevel is completed by preparing the outer surface of the cusp at a 45° slope.
This preparation stage should follow the individual anatomy of the cusp so that from the buccal surface, the cusp will be reduced but still have a mesial and distal slope.

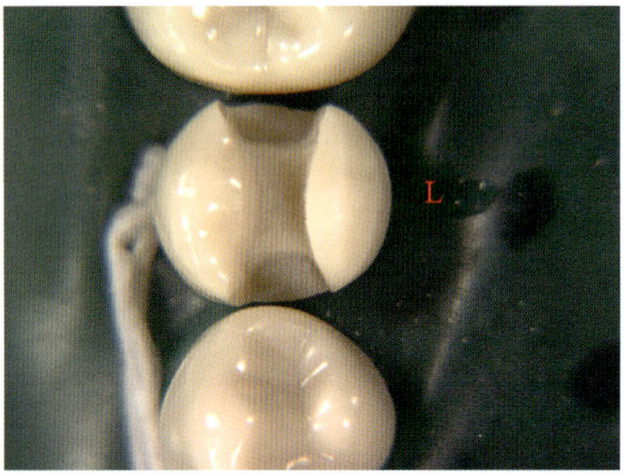

On final inspection of the non-functional cusp the cusp should resemble a roof top preparation.

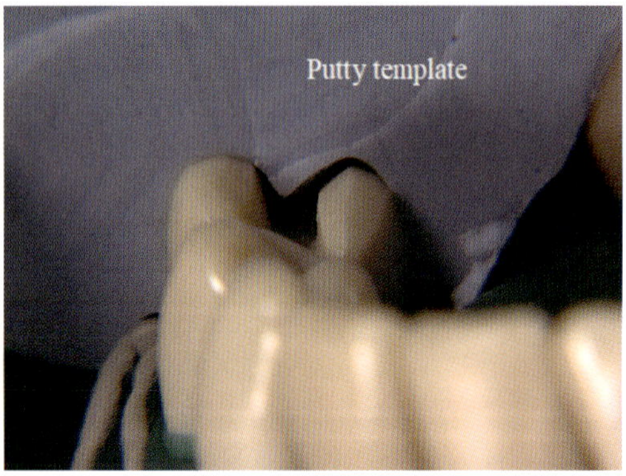

When the putty template is replaced on the tooth, the cusp should be seen to have been reduced by approximately 1 mm.

The margin of the preparation to the buccal side should be noted to have a low angle so that the gold will taper to a thin margin in this area.

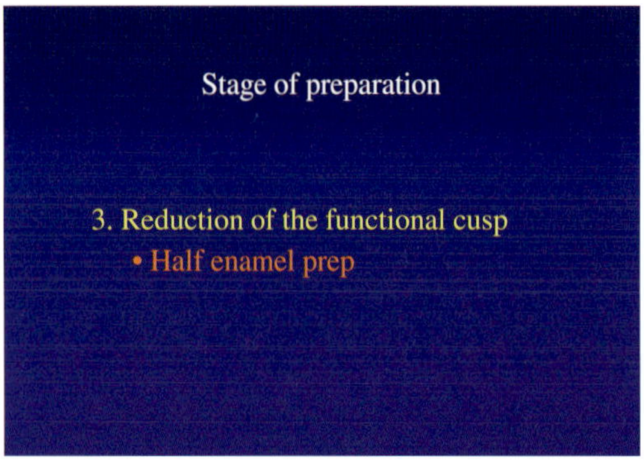

The extra demands placed on the functional cusp dictate that this should be prepared in a different manner to that just described.

This area of the preparation is known as 'the *half enamel preparation*'.

The function of it is similar to that of the reverse bevel in that it is to prevent outward displacement of the cusp under loading.

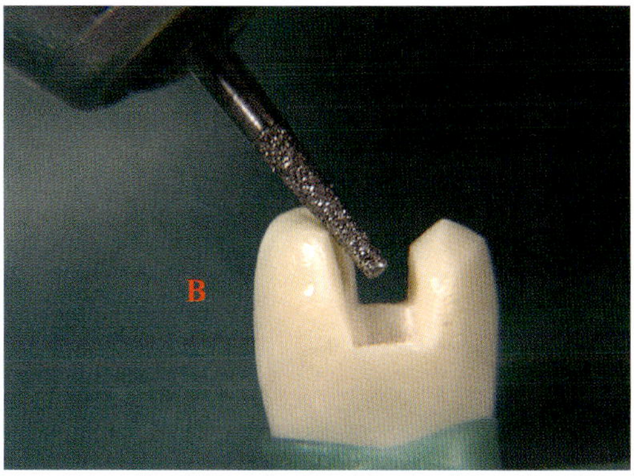

Initially, a reverse bevel is prepared but this time the reduction must be greater at 1.5 mm - this is to allow for the greater functional loads.

The inner aspect of the roof top preparation is made at 45° angle as shown here.

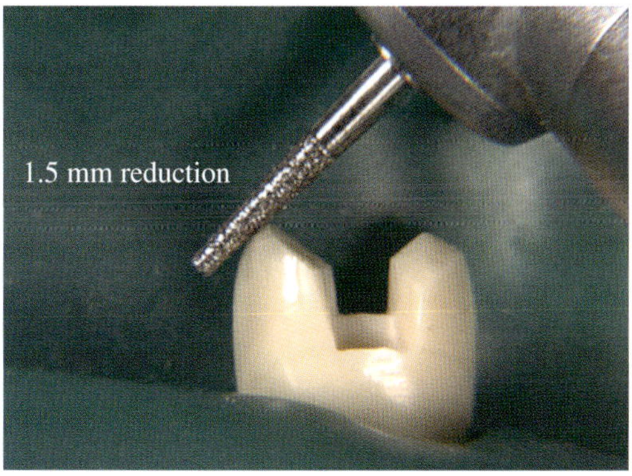

This is then followed by the preparation of the outer aspect of the roof top preparation.

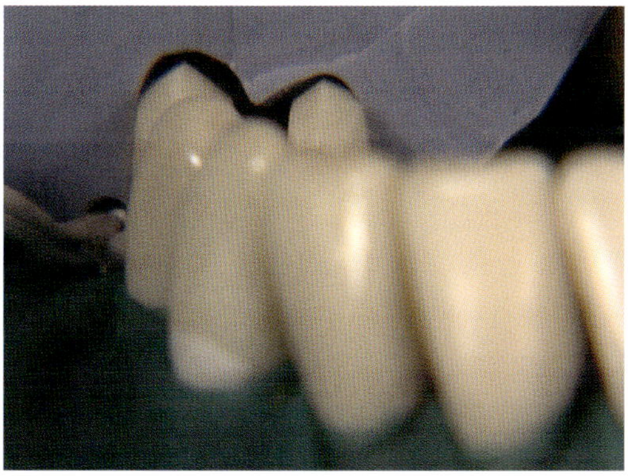

Check the reduction is 1.5 mm on the functional cusp.

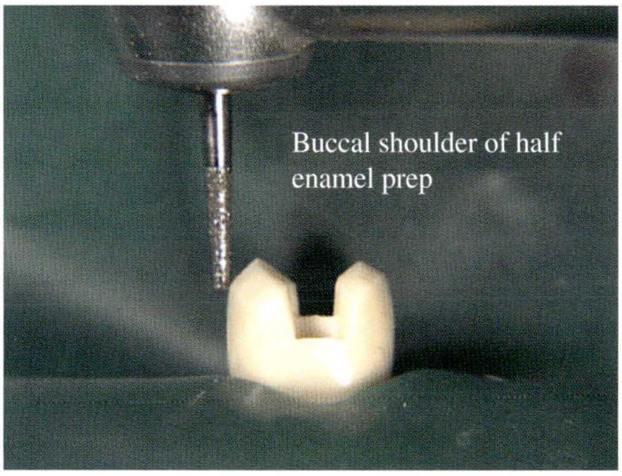

To provide greater marginal strength and improve the bracing effect of the preparation, a small shoulder should be prepared at the edge of the reverse bevel.

It is important to note that a small wall will be created while completing this stage. It must be parallel with the cavity wall and not form an undercut.

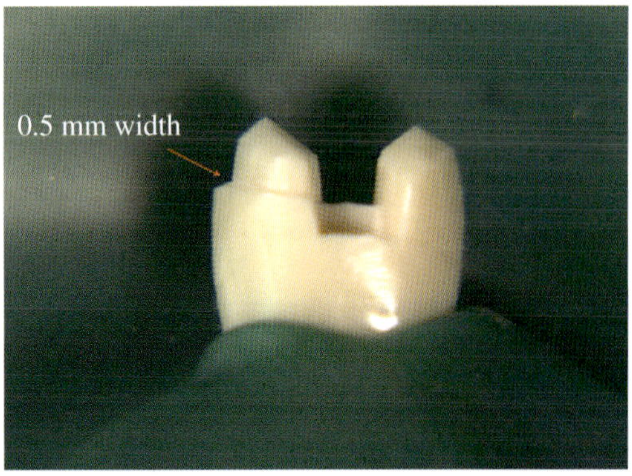

The depth of the shoulder should be 0.5 mm and should extend from one buccal wall of the intra-coronal box to the other.

When the patient is asked to occlude the teeth, the shoulder should have been positioned just gingival to the area of contact.

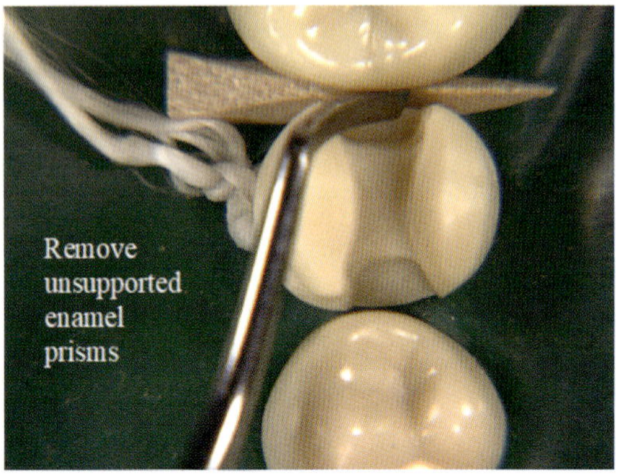

Unsupported prisms can be removed from the gingival floor using the appropriate end of the gingival margin trimmer.

A wooden wedge can be inserted to protect the soft tissues and the rubber dam at this stage.

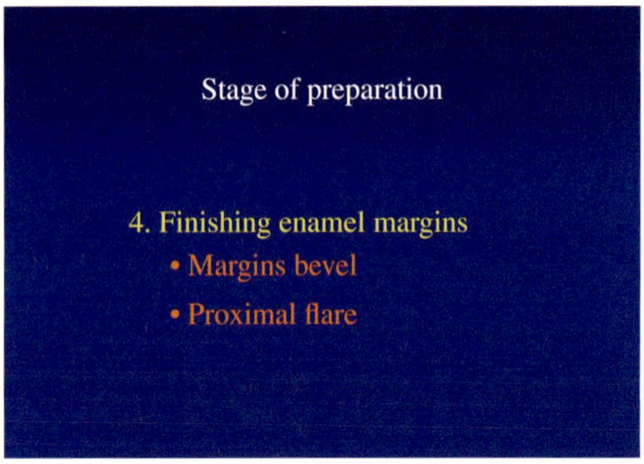

In the final stage of the preparation, the margins are bevelled to provide a thin area of cast gold alloy at the margins. This can be burnished to perfect the marginal seal.

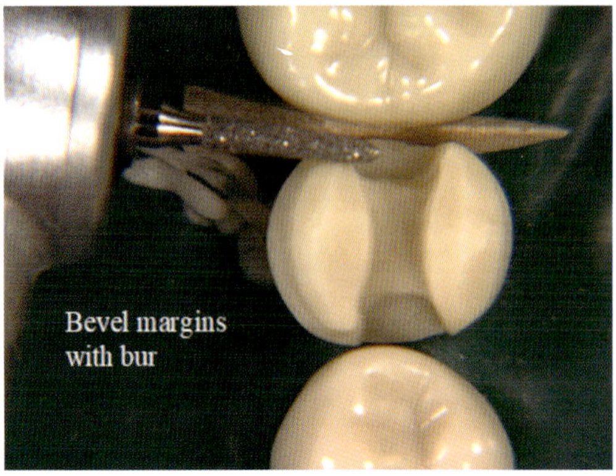

The most commonly used bur to prepare the marginal bevel and proximal flare is the torpedo shaped chamfer finishing bur.

This bur has the torpedo shape commonly used to prepare a chamfer finish.

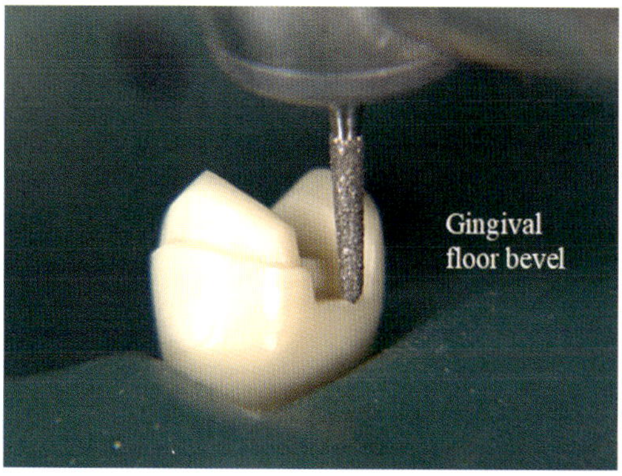

When the tip of this bur is used along the gingival margin of the box, a chamfer finish will result.

This view shows the tip of the bur resting on the enamel at the margin of the box floor.

To protect the rubber dam and the gingival tissues a wooden wedge is usually left in place.

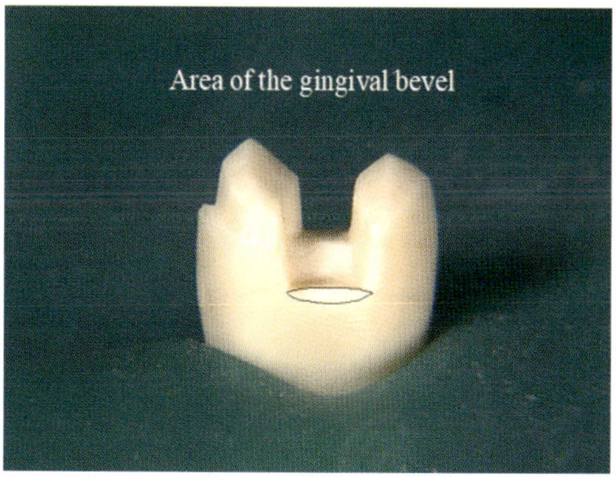

This view shows the elliptic shaped bevel created along the gingival floor.

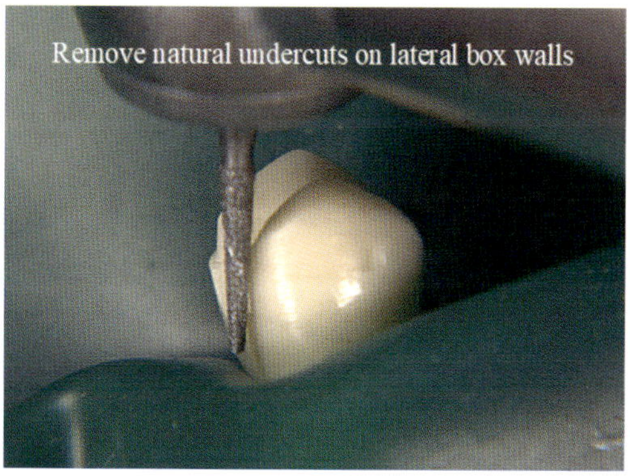

The lateral walls of the box should now be addressed. It can be seen that a natural undercut would be created by bevelling this surface below the most bulbous part of the tooth.

To avoid this, a greater reduction of the enamel is required in the area of the bulbous part of the tooth. This can be reduced to a thinner edge in the more undercut areas.

This is a difficult concept to grasp.

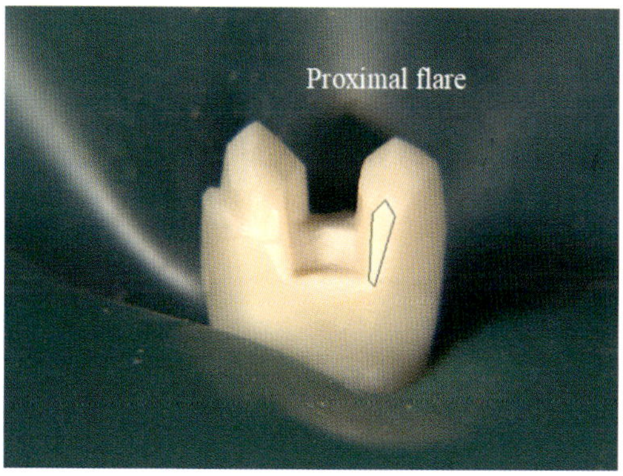

The proximal flare has been created here with a wider part more coronally where the tooth shape flares out.

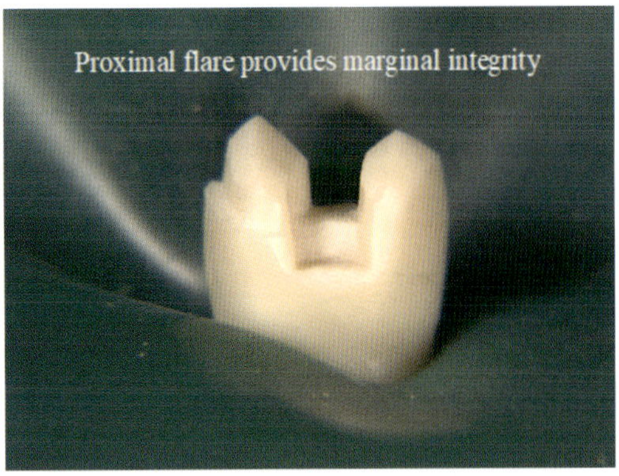

The function of the proximal flares and the marginal bevel is to improve the marginal integrity of the restoration.

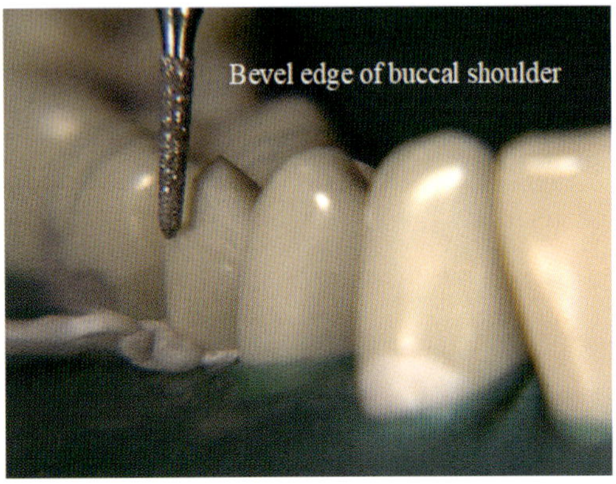

Problems are encountered when attempting to cast gold alloy to a shoulder with sharp line angles.

To avoid this, a bevel should be placed along the length of the buccal shoulder of the half enamel preparation.

The tip of the 877 bur can be used for this stage.

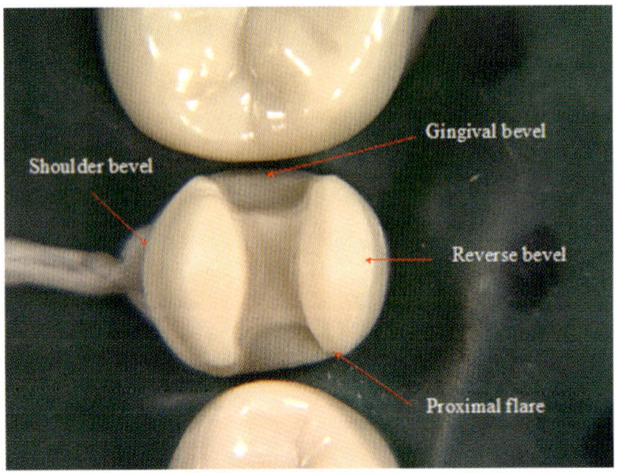

The entire margin of the preparation should now consist of a bevel finish:

- Gingival floor
- Proximal flare
- Half enamel prep bevel
- Reverse bevel

Full Gold Crown

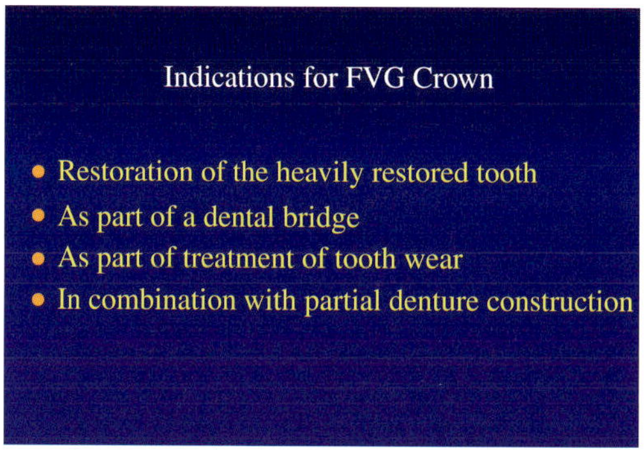

One of the main indication for the provision of a FVG crown is to restore the heavily filled posterior tooth where appearance is not important but function is vital.

It is also a useful restoration where the shape of a natural crown requires recontouring, as in the treatment of tooth wear and where removable partial dentures are being provided. In the latter case, occlusal rest and guide planes can be incorporated into the design.

This is also a useful restoration for a tooth that is to form one of the retainers of a fixed conventional bridge.

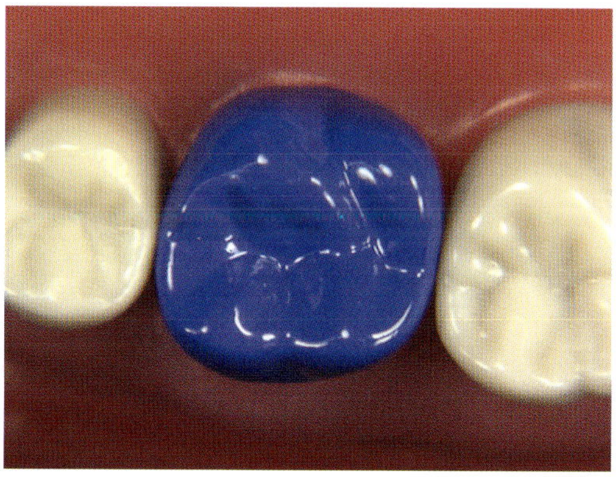

The first permanent maxillary molar tooth has been coloured to help visualisation of the stages of the preparation of the FVG crown.

Note that this tooth has a large oblique ridge that joins the disto-buccal cusp to the large mesio-palatal cusp.

In the maxillary arch the palatal cusps are the functional cusps.

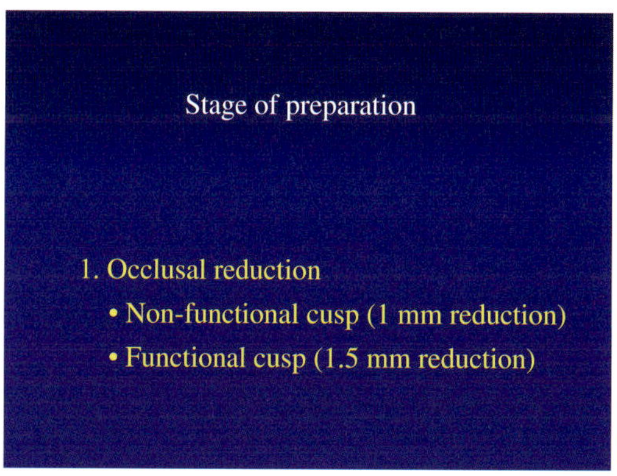

In the first stage of the preparation, the occlusal surface of the tooth is reduced evenly over the anatomical contour to retain cusp tips and slopes.

The depth of the reduction depends on the function that the cusps are expected to take.

1 mm reduction is advocated for the buccal non-functional cusps while 1.5 mm is recommended for the functional palatal cusps.

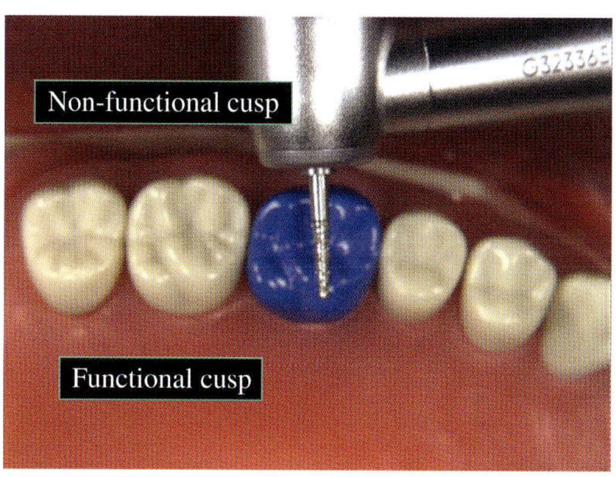

In the maxillary molar tooth the palatal cusp is the functional one that occludes with the lower tooth, and the buccal cusp is the non-functional one.

Note that the bur used for this preparation will be a medium tapered fissure that is diamond coated. The size of this bur is ideal for the bulk cutting of extra-coronal restorations.

As before, it is used with a water spray to help cool the tooth structure during preparation and keep the bur clean of cut debris.

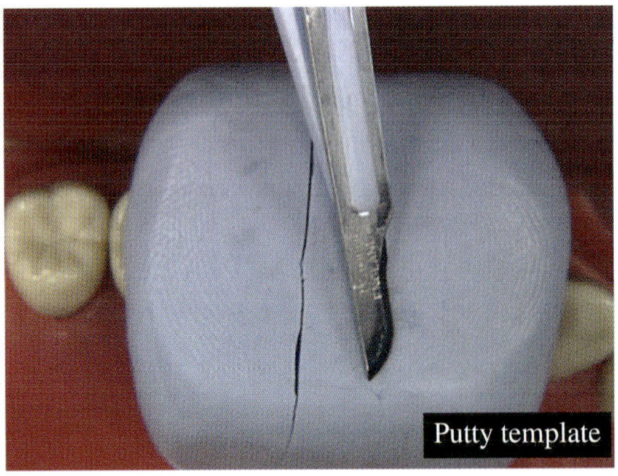

In this slide sequence an impression putty template will be used to demonstrate the amount of tooth preparation.

Some addition cured silicone putty has been formed over the tooth surface and onto the adjacent teeth.

When polymerised, it is sectioned using a scalpel.

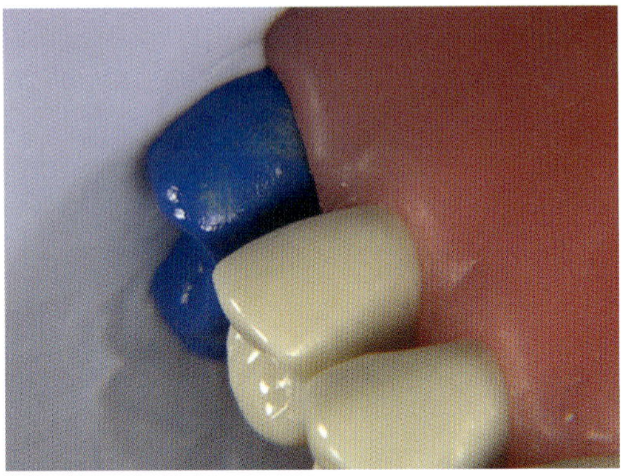

In this view the sectioned putty template can be seen lying over the distal half of the unprepared tooth.

Once the tooth is prepared in stages, the amount of tooth reduction will be seen clearly.

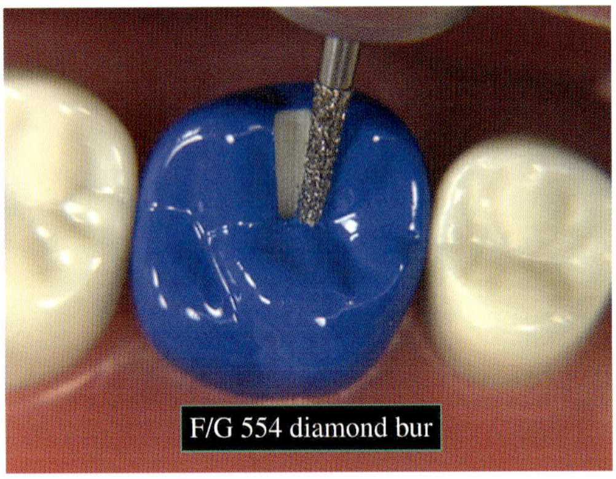

To indicate the desired amount of occlusal reduction, the 554 bur should be cut into the full width into the buccal fissure of the occlusal surface, as seen here.

The bur is approximately 1 mm at its tip.

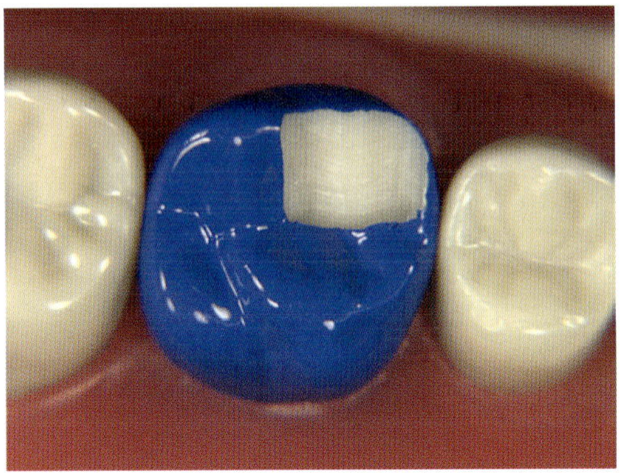

The initial depth of cut is continued along the occlusal surface following the cusp slopes and ridges to reproduce the gross anatomical contour but without its surface detail.

This is sometimes known as 'plain cusp contour'.

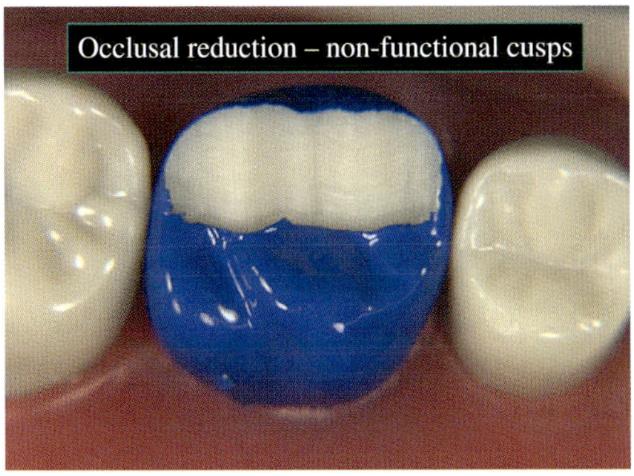

The non-functional cusp reduction of 1 mm is continued towards the other marginal ridge. Using this anatomical reduction will ensure that adequate tooth reduction is achieved evenly and minimally.

To ensure that the adjacent tooth is not traumatised during the cutting procedure, small areas of marginal ridge may be left at this stage because they will be removed safely at a later stage.

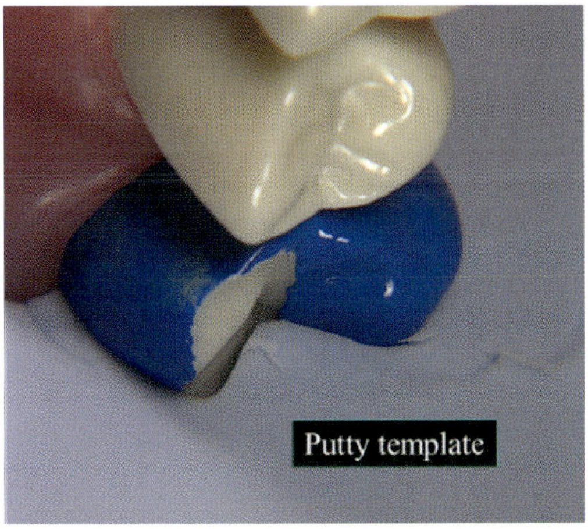

When the putty template is replaced, the amount of tooth reduction can be seen clearly.

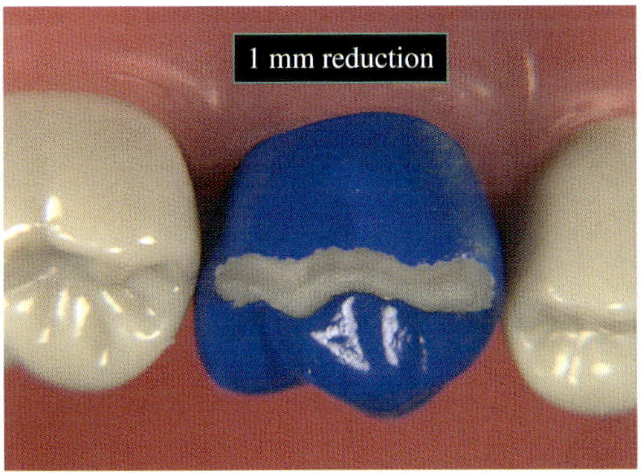

From the buccal view, the 1 mm occlusal reduction of the buccal side of the occlusal surface can be seen clearly.

There will be a step between the unprepared functional cusps and the prepared non-functional reduction.

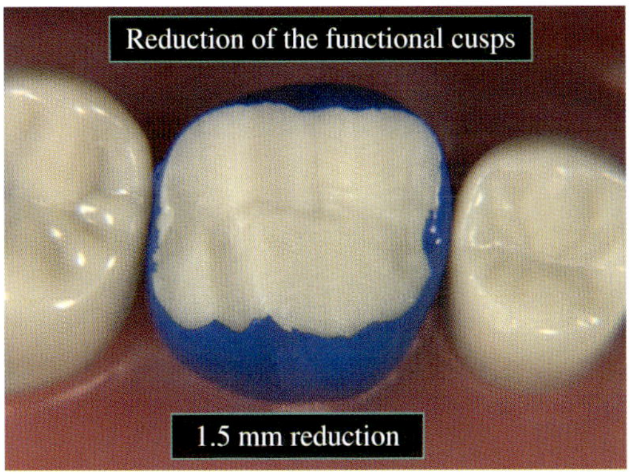

The reduction is then continued on the functional side of the occlusal surface by removing a depth of 1.5 mm.

The gross anatomy should be preserved where possible because this will give structural rigidity to the final casting and ensure an even thickness of gold.

The latter will give a more accurate casting because it will minimise the possibility of porosity in the thicker layers.

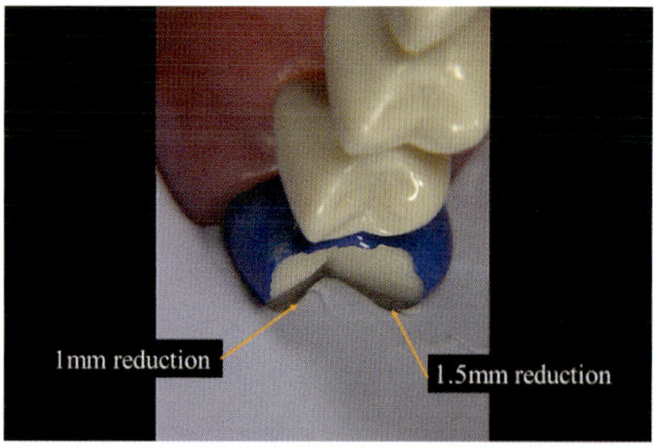

When the putty template is replaced the reduction can be checked again.

Note the reduction of the occlusal surface results in the loss of position of the original cusp tips because they move downwards and outwards during the preparation of the occlusal surface.

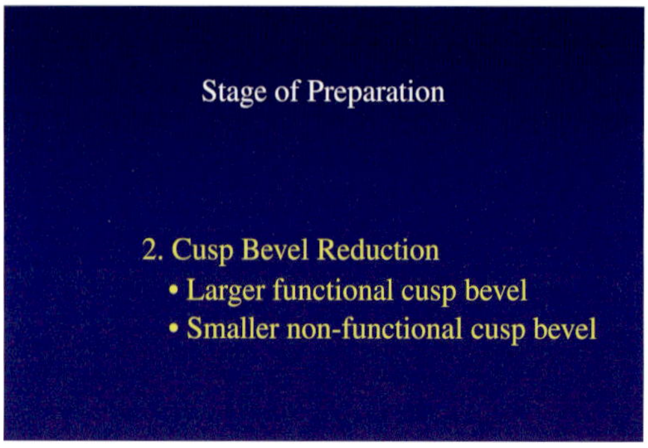

Using the same bur, the functional cusp bevel is placed to a depth of approximately 1.5 mm.

The angulation of the bevel is about 45° to the long axis of the tooth and should mirror the angle of the cusp slopes of the opposing mandibular molar tooth.

A shallower non-functional cusp bevel should also be prepared.

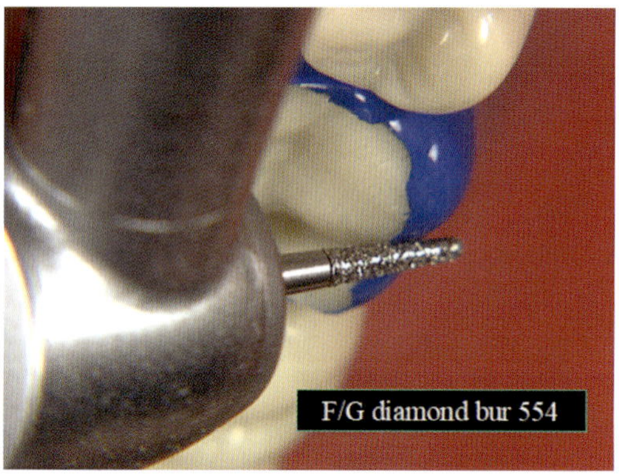

The F/G 554 bur shown here is held at 45° to the long vertical axis of the tooth in the production of this bevel.

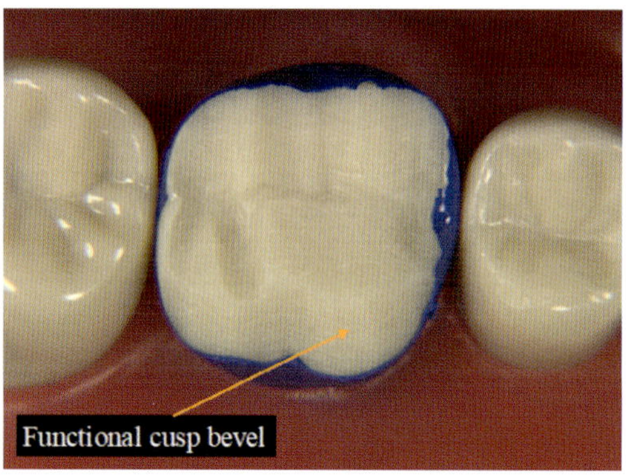

Here is the completed view of this stage of the preparation.

Note that the reduction continues not just along the palatal surface but also round towards the approximal tooth surfaces, stopping just short of the contact areas.

In this way, iatrogenic damage to the adjacent tooth will be avoided.

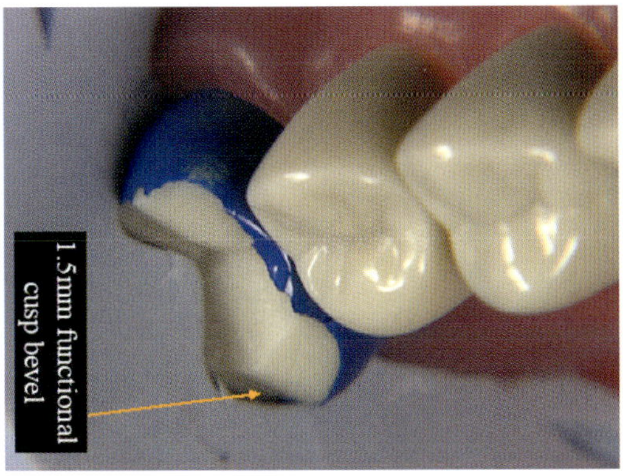

The amount of reduction is demonstrated clearly in this slide.

The reduced cusp tip has been re-created immediately under its original position.

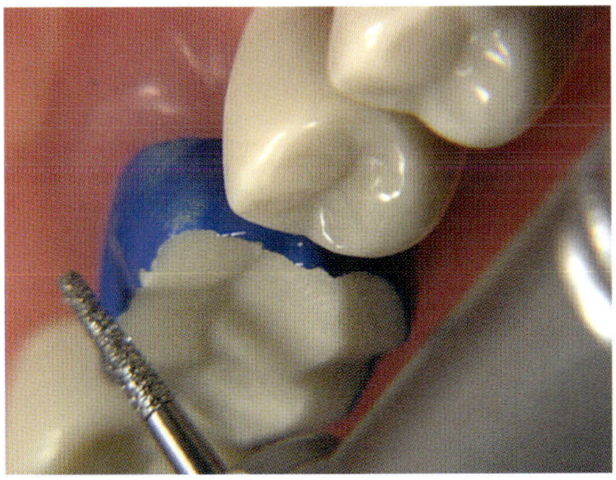

A bevel is now placed on the non-functional cusp.

This is achieved in a similar manner to that of the previous functional bevel 0 using a 45° angulation to the long vertical axis of the tooth.

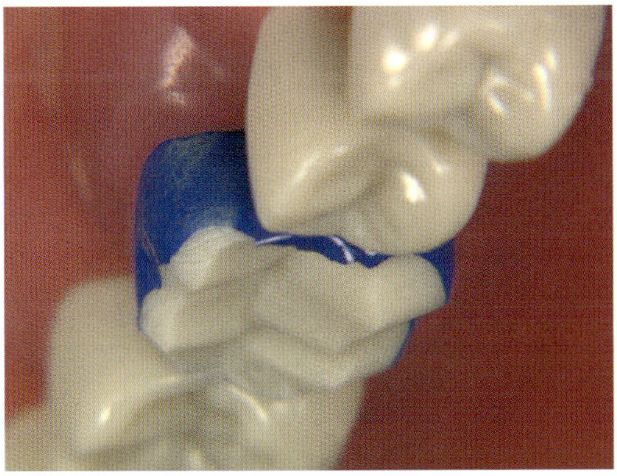

This non-functional bevel is more shallow than that placed on the functional cusp.

No more than 1 mm should be removed from this tooth surface.

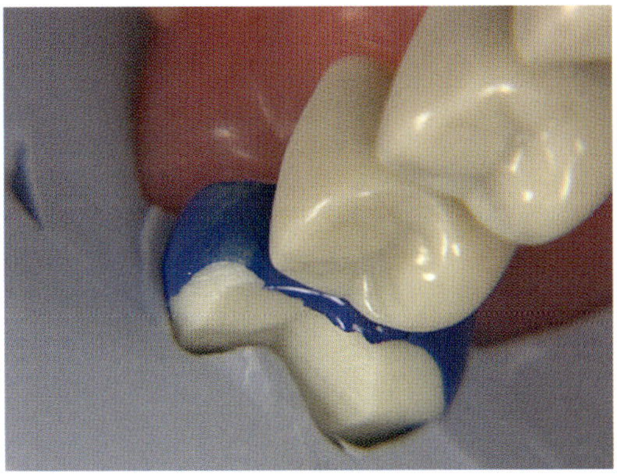

The reduced cusp tip is again re-created under the original position of the cusp.

On initial occlusal reduction the occlusal table is made wider, but, following placement of the bevels, the width is once again narrowed to the original dimensions.

At this stage the patient would be asked to bring the teeth together, and a visual check would be made for the clearance between the upper and lower teeth. The amount of clearance can be verified by the use of some green occlusal indicator wax.

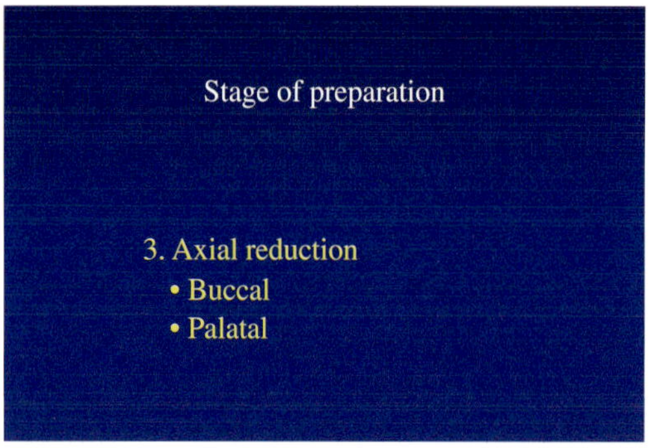

In the next stage of preparation, the buccal and palatal axial surfaces of the tooth will be reduced to produce surfaces that are almost parallel and have a taper towards the occlusal surface not exceeding 5° on each wall – making a convergence angle of less than 10° in total.

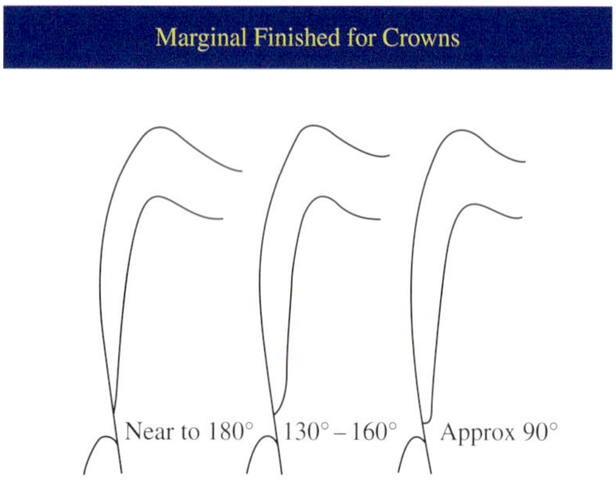

The marginal finish lines possible include those shown:

- A knife edge finish line (~180°) is difficult to see and the casting may be distorted during finishing. It has the advantage of close adaptation to the tooth surface.
- A butt joint (90°) will be seen clearly and the casting will not distort, but gold alloy does not cast well to this type of marginal finish.
- A 135° chamfer finish is a good compromise that will be seen readily, and the casting will resist distortion and have a reasonable adaptation to the finish line at the tooth margin.

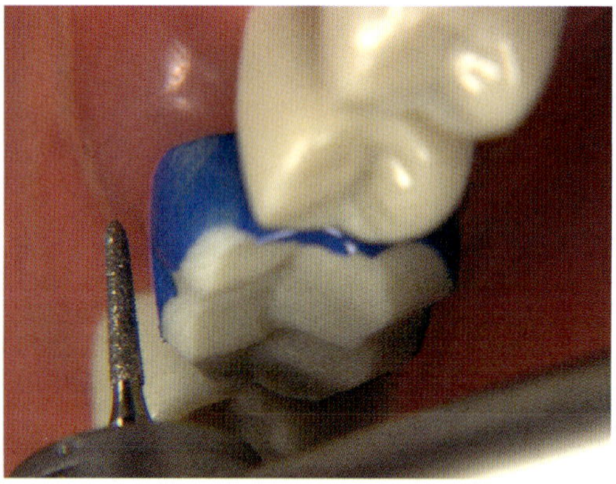

A torpedo shaped diamond bur can be used to produce the correct finish at the margin.

To prepare the axial surfaces, the bur should be held in line with the long axis of the tooth and the tip placed just above the gingival margin to allow the finish margin to be placed in an area that is readily cleansableby the patient.

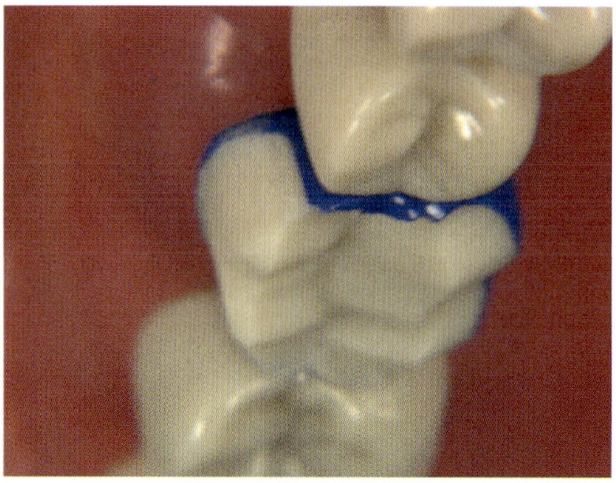

A torpedo-shaped diamond bur can be used to produce the correct finish at the margin.

To prepare the axial surfaces the bur should be held in line with the long axis of the tooth and the tip placed just above the gingival margin to allow the finish margin to be placed in an area that is readily cleansableby the patient.

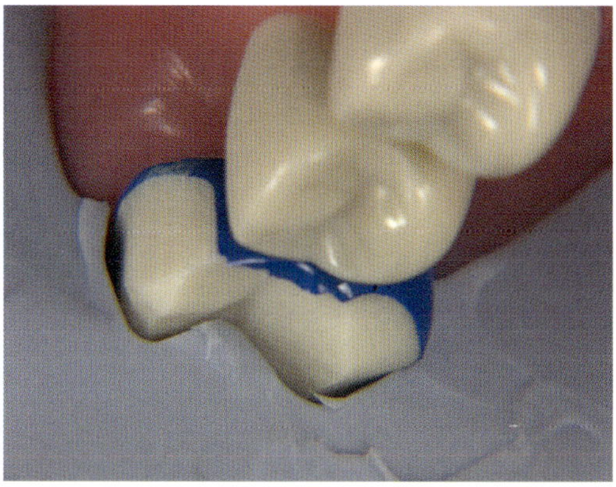

With the template in place, the amount of tooth reduction can be seen to be about 1 mm in this case. This will provide adequate thickness of cast alloy for rigidity.

Note that the two stages of reduction have been preserved where the small buccal bevel and the axial reduction are differentiated clearly.

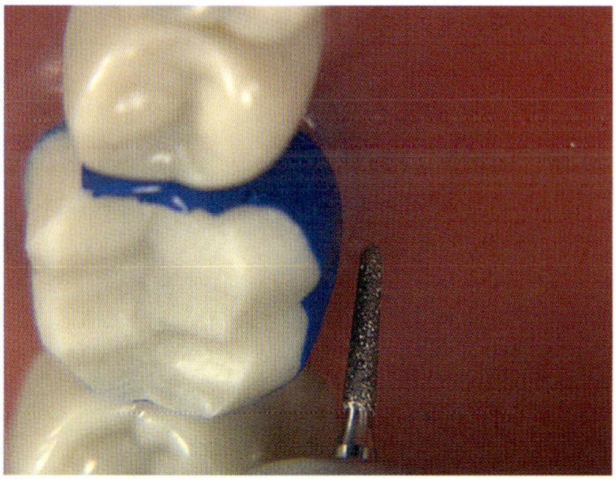

The reduction of the palatal surface is then carried out in a similar manner.

The bur must be held parallel to its alignment for the cut on the buccal side to allow these two axial reductions to have a convergence angle not exceeding 10°.

If this convergence angle is exceeded, retention of the restoration will be adversely affected.

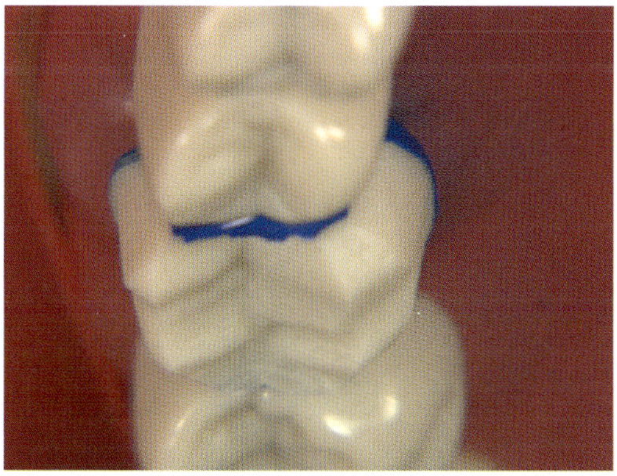

This view shows the anatomical reduction of the occlusal surface, the functional and non-functional bevels, and the prepared axial walls.

The tooth structure at the contact areas has been left undisturbed even on the marginal ridge on the occlusal surface.

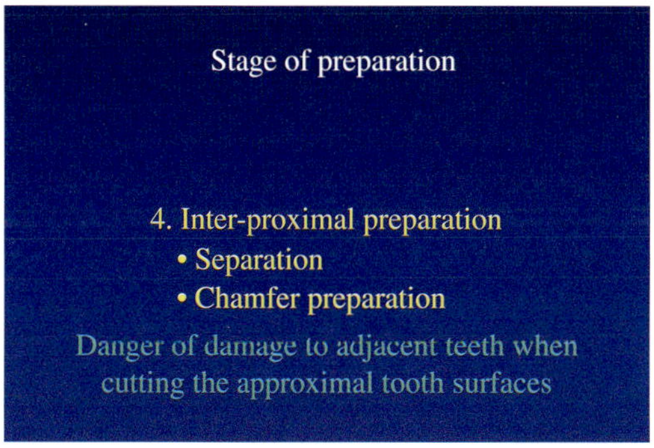

In the next stage of the preparation the interproximal surfaces will be prepared in two stages to minimise the risk of damage to the adjacent teeth.

Initially, the teeth will be separated using a long, narrow, tapered bur.

This will then be followed by the usual marginal finish for gold restorations – a 135° chamfer.

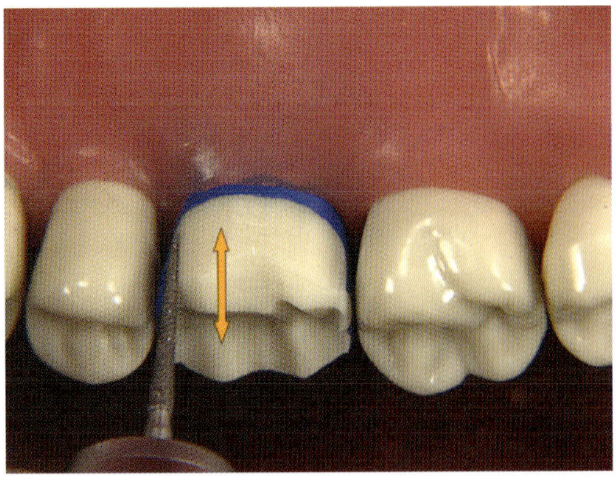

The fine tapered diamond bur can be used with a vertical sawing action, but care should be exercised to avoid not only damage to the adjacent tooth surface but also to the underlying gingival papilla.

The interproximal surface in this view is bulbous, and the aim of this stage is to remove that bulbosity and produce a vertical flat surface keeping the bur within the tooth substance at all times.

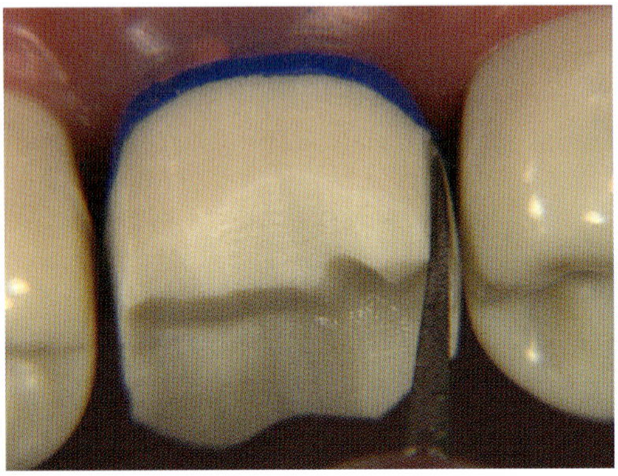

In this view the angulationof the bur can be seen along with its accommodation within the tooth substance.

The gentle sawing action has just commenced, and, at the same time, gentle pressure is exerted towards the other tooth surface.

The sawing action is required to:

- Improve the cutting efficiency of the small diameter bur
- Improve the view as the cut is made.

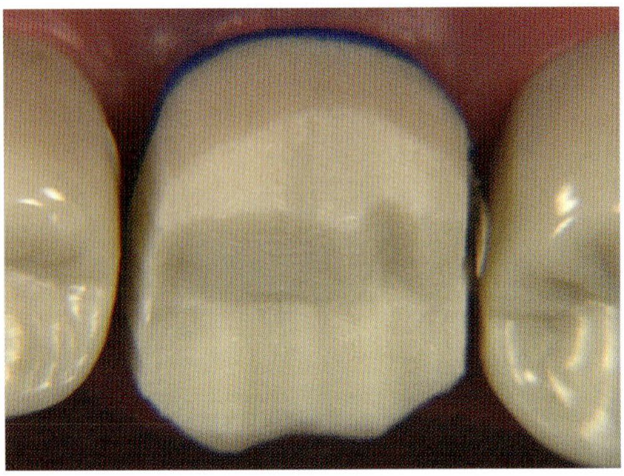

This action has been completed on one side of the tooth, and on the other side, a small piece of tooth structure remains against the contact area.

This is the ideal situation, This small fragment can be readily removed using an excavator. The operator can then be sure in the knowledge that the adjacent tooth surface has not been damaged.

To create sufficient space further surface reduction and finishing can now be done.

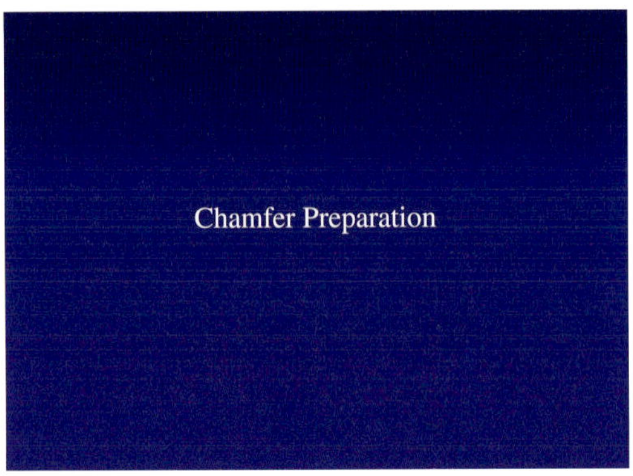

The finish line approximallycan now be adjusted to form a chamfer.

The initial stage of separation provides the space into which the torpedo shaped bur can be placed.

If this bur does not fit within the space created, the fine separating bur should be used carefully with a lateral sweeping action to increase the interproximal separation.

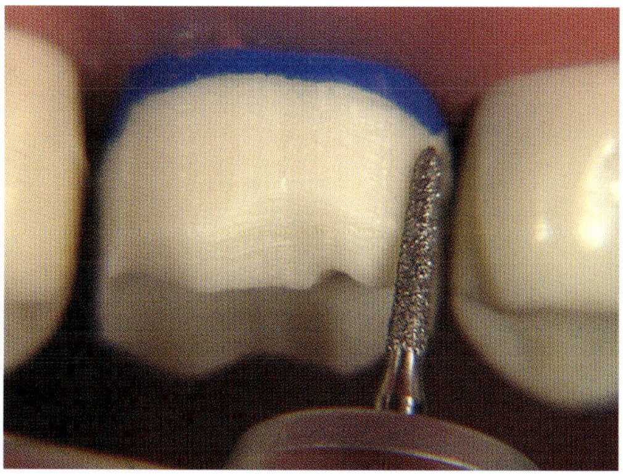

The bur is shown here ready to make the cut.

It is again important that the bur is held in line with the long axis of the tooth so that mesial and distal surfaces are as near parallel as possible but without undercuts.

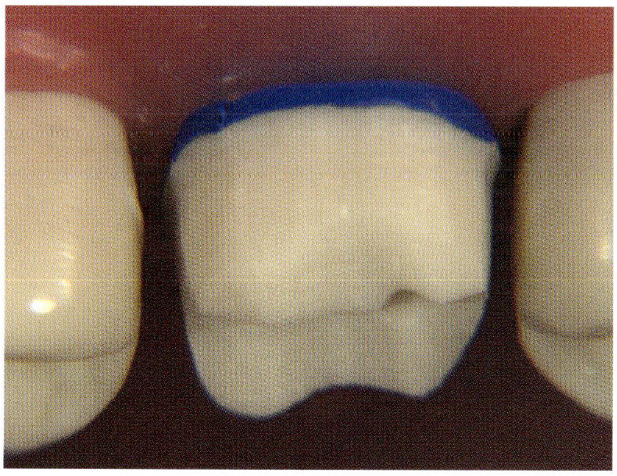

In this view the occlusally convergent surfaces can be viewed.

The shape of the chamfer line is also well illustrated in this view.

A common problem is for proximal surfaces to be under-prepared, forcing the technician to over-contour this surface on the crown.

Another common error is to produce a scallop shape at the junction of the proximal and the other axial surfaces. This can be avoided by paying particular attention to rounding off the preparation at the 'corner'.

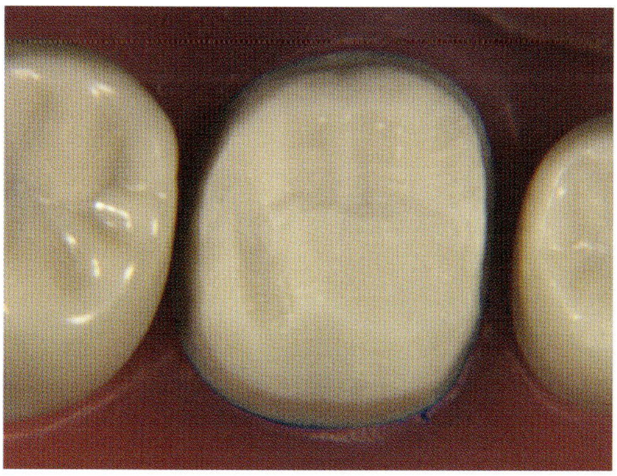

From an occlusal direction the operator should now be able to look down the walls of the preparation – using only one eye – and be able to see the entire marginal finish.

Undercuts should be suspected if the margins cannot be seen using monocular vision.

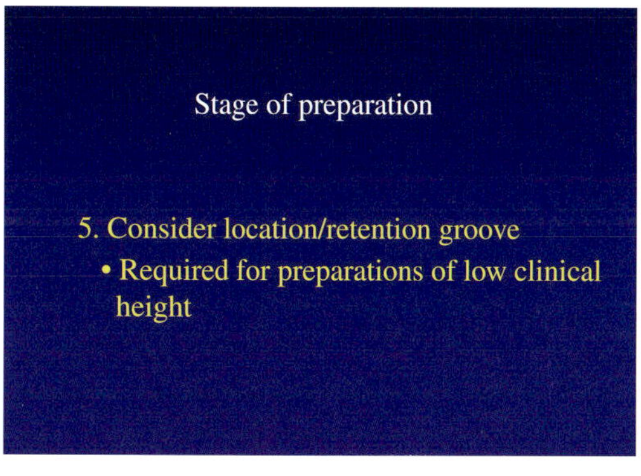

In the penultimate stage of the preparation consideration should be given to the amount of retention offered by the preparation.

Retention can be improved by incorporating a retention groove into the design.

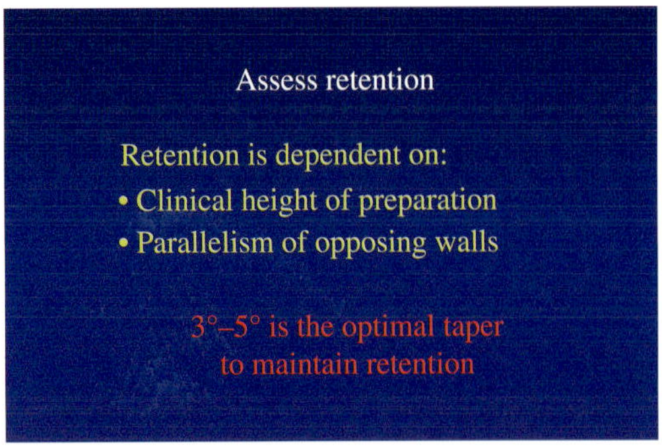

Retention is dependent on the clinical height and taper on the walls of the preparation.

Exceeding a 5° taper results in a significant loss of retention.

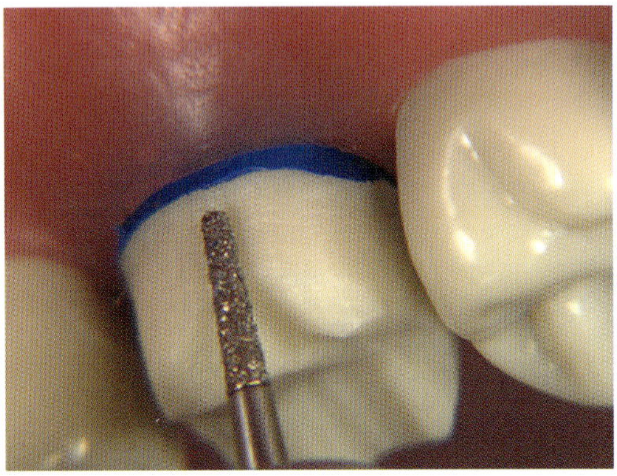

If required, this groove may be prepared using a short tapered crown bur.

The extent of the groove should be to within 0.5 mm of the chamfer.

Generally, these are placed at the area of the palatal fissure in maxillary molar teeth and at the area of the buccal fissure in the corresponding mandibular tooth.

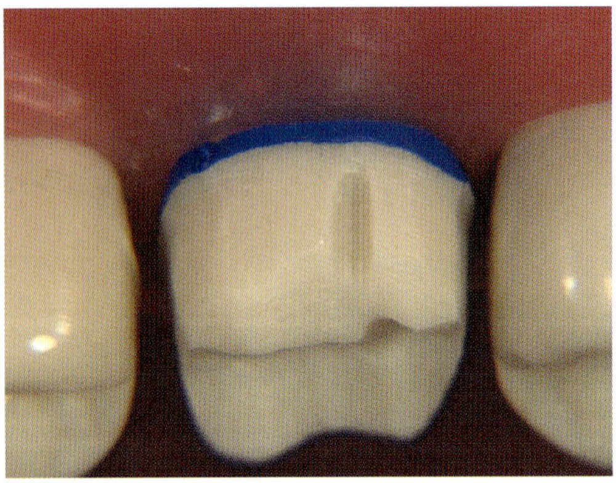

This view shows the groove at the area of the palatal fissure. Note that:

- The depth of the groove is the same as the radius of the bur and
- The groove has been prepared in the long axis of the crown preparation in line with the path of withdrawal of the crown

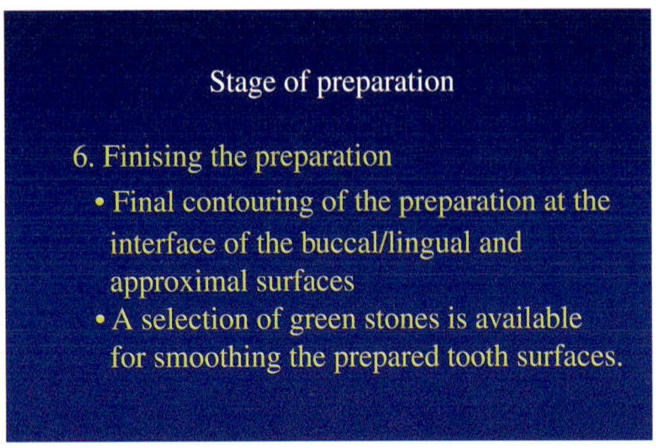

In the final stage of the preparation, the contour is refined and the walls smoothed.

Smooth walls are needed to prevent drag on the impression with subsequent distortion, and it may also be more difficult to seat the cast crown onto a rough preparation.

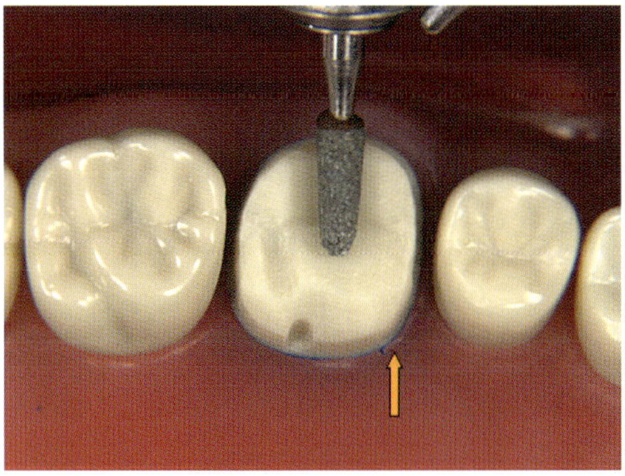

A selection of green stones may be used for the smoothing of the preparation.

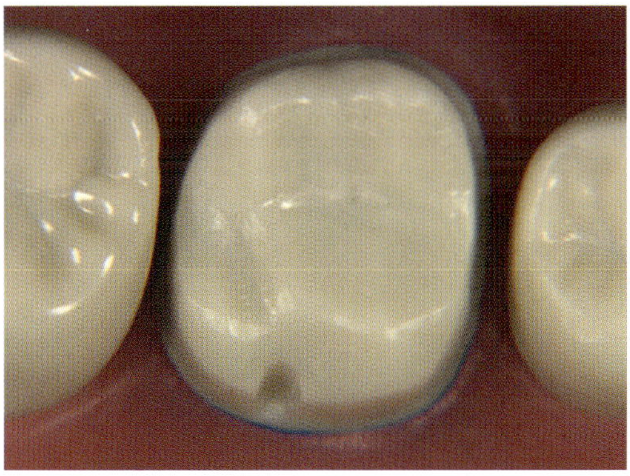

These should be able to remove most of the rough surface that would interfere with the intimate contact of the cast crown.

It is not desirable to have a perfectly smooth surface because this would result in poorer retention of the final restoration.

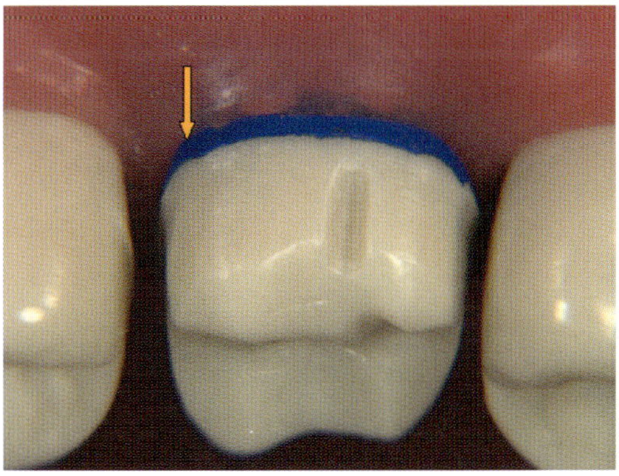

When the preparation is complete pay particular attention to the corners to ensure that scalloping has been avoided.

Removing a veneer from the clinical crown is a radical procedure and can be performed in the mistaken belief that it will protect the tooth from any subsequent caries. If the cause of the caries is not brought under control, the disease is likely to produce caries at the margin of the crown and herald the failure of the tooth and the restoration.

A cast full coverage crown will function well in protecting cusps weakened by extensive caries.

A Clinical Case of Porcelain Onlay

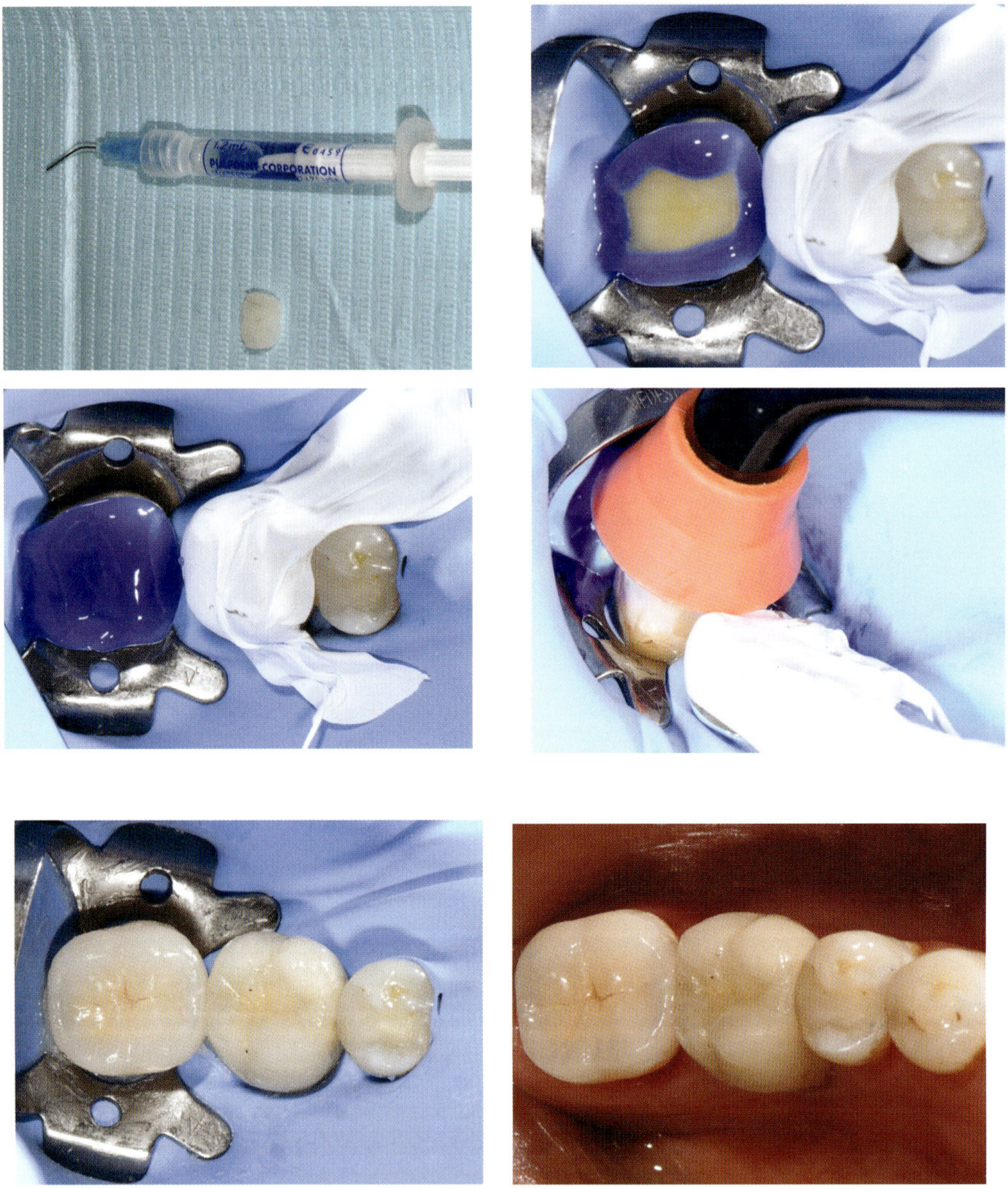

This sequence shows the restoration of a mandibular second molar tooth using a porcelain onlay.
Source: Printed by Kind Permission of Dr Osama Alkhatib.

Further Reading

Jacobsen, P.H. (2008). *Restorative Dentistry: An Integrated Approach*. Wiley Blackwell.
Qualtrough, A.J.E. (2005). *Principles of Operative Dentistry*. Wiley Blackwell.
Shillingburg, H.T. *Fundamentals of Fixed Prosthodontics*. Quintessence Publishing Co., Inc.
Smith, B.G.N. and Howe, L.C. (2013). *Planning and Making Crowns and Bridges*. CRC Press.
Walmsley, A.D. (2007). *Restorative Dentistry*. Churchill Livingstone.

10

Porcelain Fused to Metal and All-Ceramic Crowns

As new materials and techniques have been developed, the indication for providing crowns has reduced. The indications for providing a crown on a tooth remain in contemporary dental practice, but the operator must remember that a great deal of tooth substance is lost in this procedure. More conservative procedures should be considered before deciding to provide a full coverage crown. The indications are not definitive and are subjective in each case.

Indications include

- Replacement crown
- Protection of a root filled tooth
- Broken down and worn teeth
- Poor appearance
- Cracked teeth
- Realignment of teeth

The choice between a porcelain fused to metal (PFM) crown and an all-ceramic restoration is often determined by the cost and the availability of space for the tooth preparation. The main contraindications for the more expensive all-ceramic crown are signs of bruxism and tooth wear as fracture may occur or damage to the opposing dentition (see Figure 10.1).

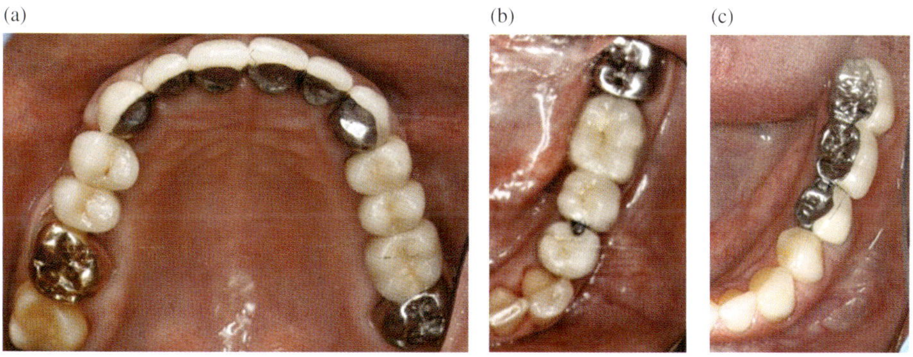

Figure 10.1 (a) The above patient has undergone extensive rehabilitation with the provision of PFM restorations. Porcelain has been used on the occlusal surfaces of the premolar teeth and UL6. (b) An occlusal rest has been incorporated into the distal aspect of the PFM on LL4 to provide support for a denture. When porcelain is placed occlusally, a greater amount of tooth reduction is required but the appearance is improved. (c) The PFM crowns shown here have bonding alloy on the occlusal surfaces. This surface can be adjusted and polished more easily compared to a porcelain surface. *Source:* Printed by kind permission of Dr M. Siddiqui.

A Practical Approach to Operative Dentistry, First Edition. Gordon B. Gray and Alaa H. Daud.

Companion website: www.wiley.com/go/gray/operative-dentistry

The original ceramic material was known as *feldspathic porcelain* and was made from silicone and aluminium dioxides with additions of fluxes made from boron, potassium, sodium, magnesium, and lithium oxides. This brittle material was improved by the creation of *aluminous porcelain*. This was achieved by the addition of crystalline alumina that increased the flexural and tensile strength of the porcelain to help it resist cracking or fracture when subjected to high occlusal loads

In a PFM crown, porcelain is added to surfaces of the inner metal coping that would be seen. These layers are applied starting with a dense opaque layer to mask the dark colour of the cast metal coping. Further layers of aesthetic porcelain are then added to replace the dentine and enamel and return the shape and shade of the missing tooth structure. In recent years there has been a reduction in use of the PFM crown as the popularity of the all-ceramic or metal-free crown has increased. The core of the all-ceramic crown is not made of metal but is often a dense and opaque material, such as zirconia, that requires masking with layers of dentine and enamel porcelains.

The all-ceramic or metal -free crown can be manufactured in a number of ways:

- Computer aided design/computer aided manufacturing (CAD/CAM)
- Castable or pressed ceramics
- Conventional

In some ***CAD/CAM systems***, a stone die is sent to the laboratory and scanned optically before being digitised. This is then sent to a milling centre, where a computer controlled milling machine produces a coping of high strength. The coping is usually 0.4 or 0.6 mm in thickness. It is then returned to the original laboratory, where conventional porcelain is added to the surface. The coping is a very accurate fit, and the marginal gap of these restorations is excellent.

There is another CAD/CAM system that can be used at the chairside. This is known as the Cerec system, in which an optical impression of the preparation is recorded in the mouth. This can be a crown, veneer, or inlay/onlay. The Cerec system has its own computer controlled milling machine that can produce a restoration from a block of ceramic. The latter can be homogenous or from a block with different layers of coloured ceramic. Milling takes about 15 minutes, and the restoration can be luted after this time. Alternatively, a technician can characterise by staining and glazing the surface.

If the Cerec system has been used to mill a coping, conventional ceramics can be added to the surface in a similar manner to the laboratory milled coping (see Figure 10.2).

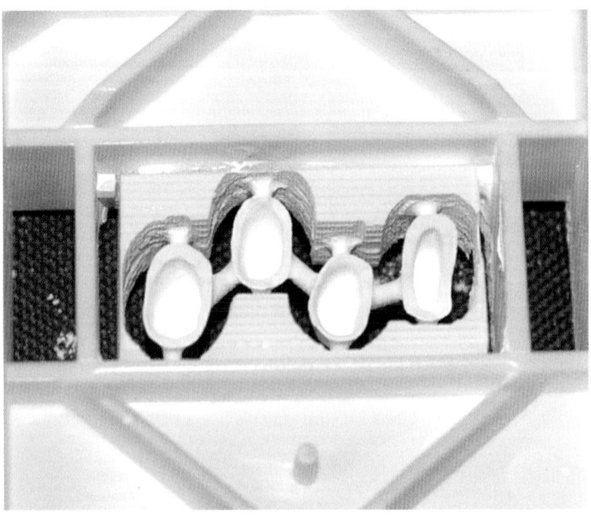

Figure 10.2 Multiple copings can be milled at the same time from a block of material. These are then heat treated to improve the compressive and tensile strength of the material.

When a ***castable ceramic*** is used, such as the Empress System from Ivoclar Vivadent, the technician waxes up the crown on a stone die. The bulk of the crown is made from a molten ingot of ceramic in a similar way to casting gold alloy using the lost wax technique. The surface of this cast ceramic can be characterised with low fusing porcelains.

In a ***conventional porcelain*** crown, such as the In-Ceram crown from Vita, the crown will consist of two distinct layers. The inner core provides the strength, but in this case, the layer is thick, and, although covered by a thin layer of conventional low fusing porcelain, the overall appearance can be compromised by the opaque and thick core.

Compare the look of the all-ceramic crowns in Figure 10.3.

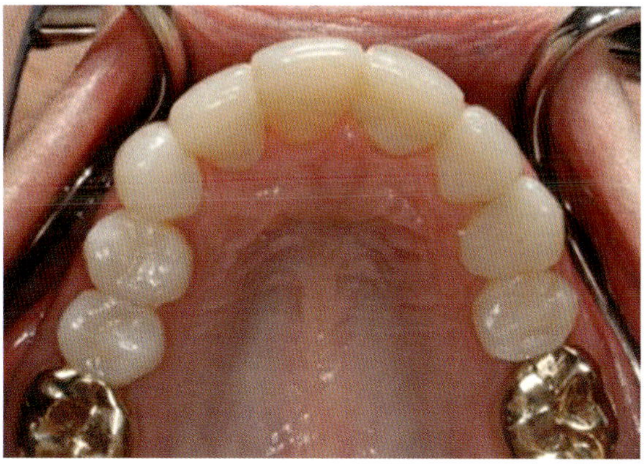

Figure 10.3 This patient has all-ceramic crowns placed on maxillary anterior and premolar teeth. The appearance is of a high order. *Source:* Printed by kind permission of Dr M. Siddiqui.

PFM Crown

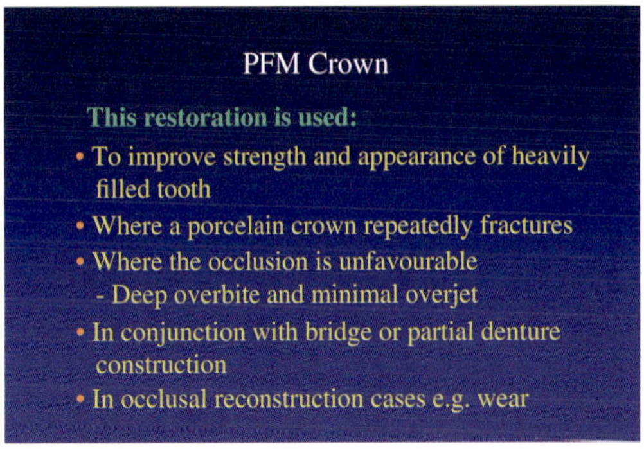

In the majority of cases, a PFM crown is placed to improve the appearance and function of heavily filled teeth.
Where a PJC is present anteriorly and repeatedly fractures, a metal backed crown would be indicated.
PFM preparation may also be indicated to provide patients with a conventional bridge or to provide guide planes, occlusal rests, and the correct degree of undercut for partial denture design.
In complicated cases where patient's teeth show marked signs of wear, they may be restored by crowning all standing teeth to re-establish the correct clinical height.

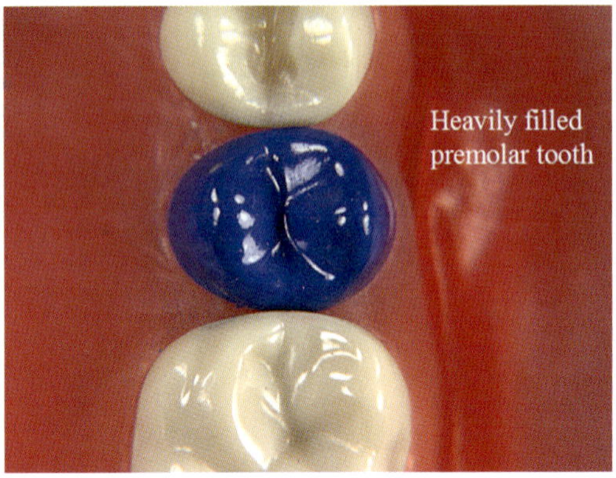

This maxillary second premolar tooth has been shaded in blue to allow easy identification of prepared surfaces. It should be assumed in this exercise that the tooth has been restored with a pinned MODB amalgam similar to the exercise previously performed in the course.

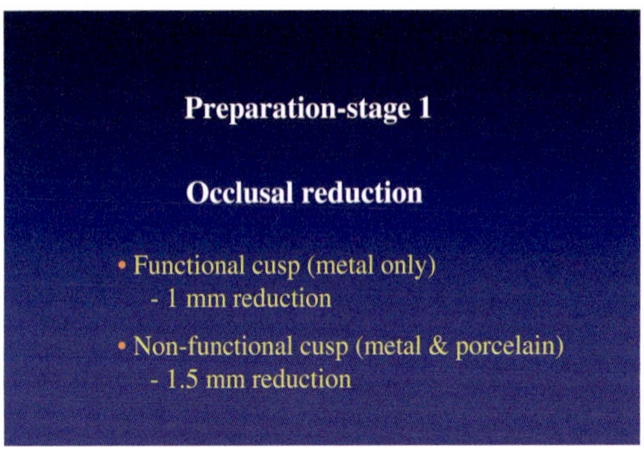

In the first stage of the procedure, the occlusal surface will be reduced in an anatomical fashion.
As the properties of the bonding alloy are superior to those of the type 4 gold alloy used in the gold crown, the functional cusp need only be reduced by 1 mm.
The non-functional buccal cusp should have a greater reduction of 1.5 mm to allow coverage with a layer of bonding alloy covered by porcelain.

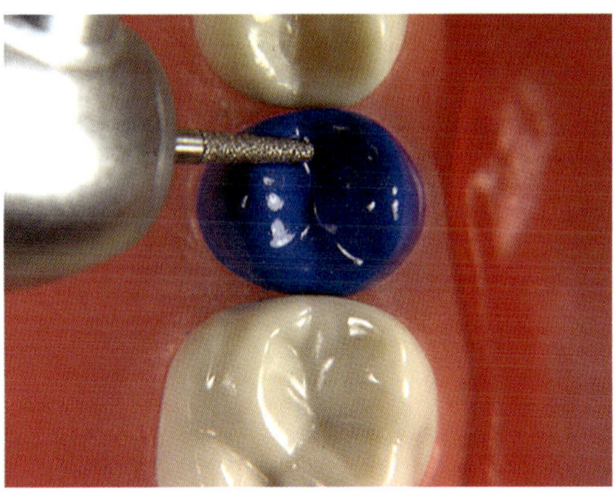

Friction grip diamond coated burs are efficient at abrading the tooth structure and reducing it but require an adequate water spray to cool the tooth and keep the bur free from clogging.
The tapered crown bur should be selected for this part of the procedure.

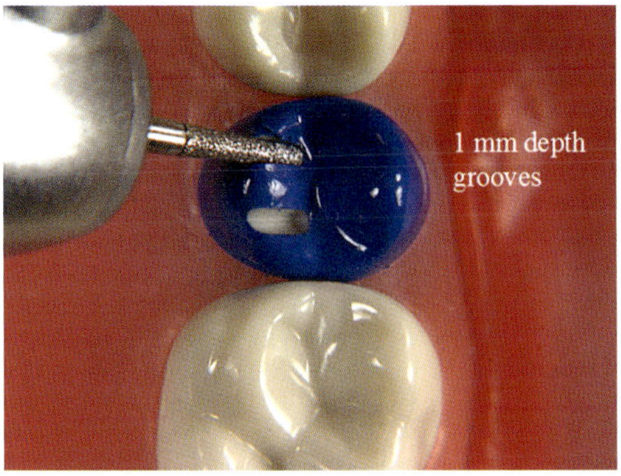

Placing depth grooves allows students to visualise the amount of reduction required.

In the functional palatal cusp, two depth grooves are usually prepared: one to either side of the cuspal ridge.

As the diameter of the tapered crown bur is 1 mm it should be sunk into the groove to its full width.

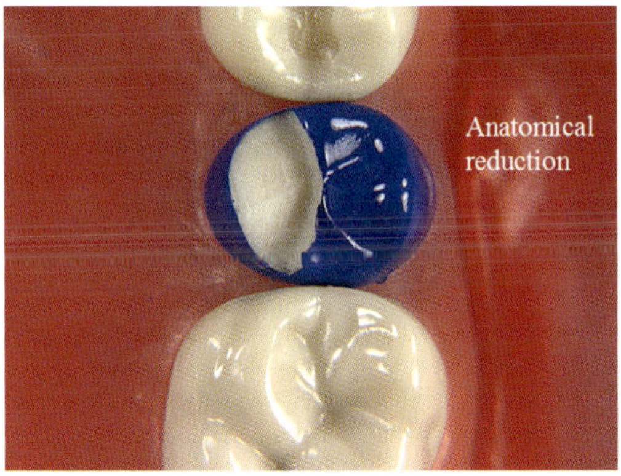

Reducing the tooth structure between the grooves should remove the correct amount of tooth structure. The preparation should then be continued towards the marginal ridges of the tooth, ensuring that damage does not occur to the adjacent teeth.

Preparation should be in an anatomical fashion so that the reduced cusp resembles that of the ideal cusp shape.

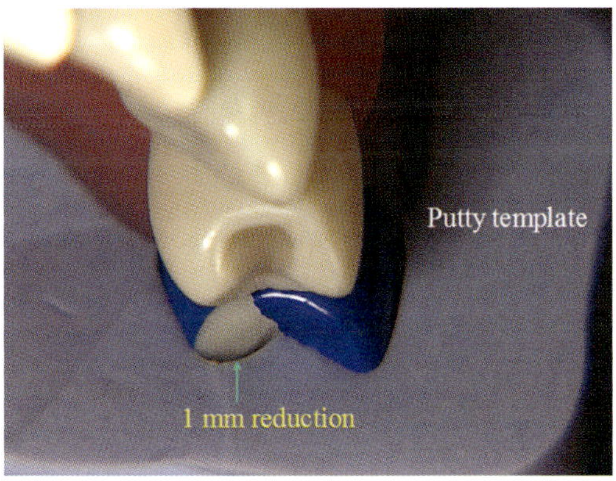

Where a template has been made from silicone putty, this may be tried and the amount of reduction viewed directly.

With this technique, however, the assumption is made that the existing anatomical form of the heavily restored tooth is ideal. Frequently heavily filled teeth are not restored back into the correct anatomical form and function.

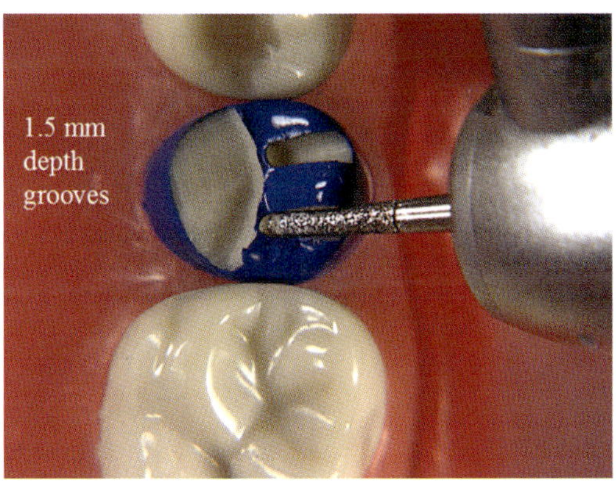

Depth grooves are now placed in the non-functional buccal cusp. These should be 1.5 mm in depth to allow for the placement of porcelain in addition to the metal surface.

Two grooves are usually sufficient to allow the operator to orientate the reduction appropriately.

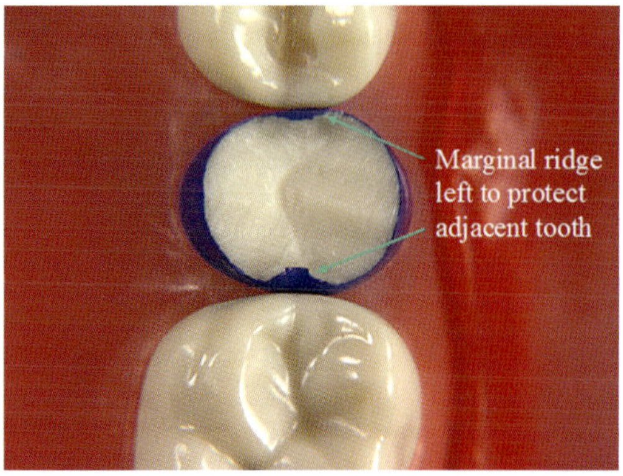

Marginal ridge may be left unprepard at this stage rather than risk damage to the adjacent teeth.
In the later stages of the preparation these areas will be adjusted.

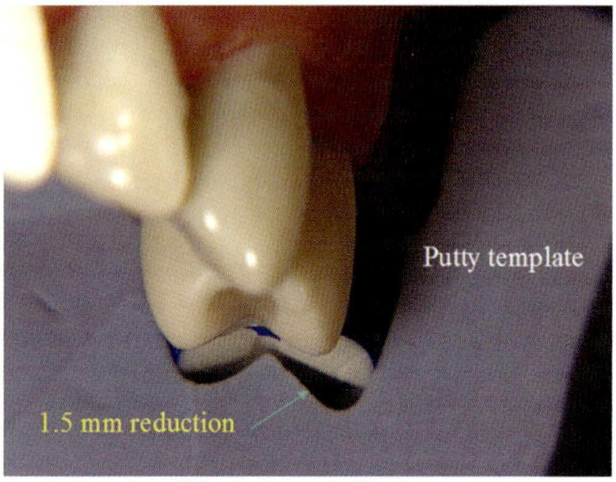

Check the amount of reduction with the putty template where this has been used.
It is not always necessary to use templates. Experienced operators should not need to use this method because clinical experience will guide their preparation.
The template is being used predominantly for presentation purposes in this sequence of slides.

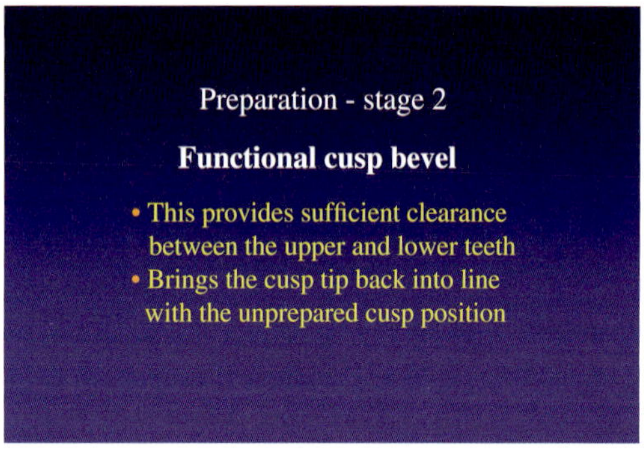

As the occlusal surface is reduced anatomically, the reduced cusp tip comes to lie at a lower level, but also it becomes more peripherally placed. By placing a bevel on the functional cusp, the tooth is reduced to provide clearance for the restorative material. In addition, the tip of the reduced cusp is brought back into line below original position.

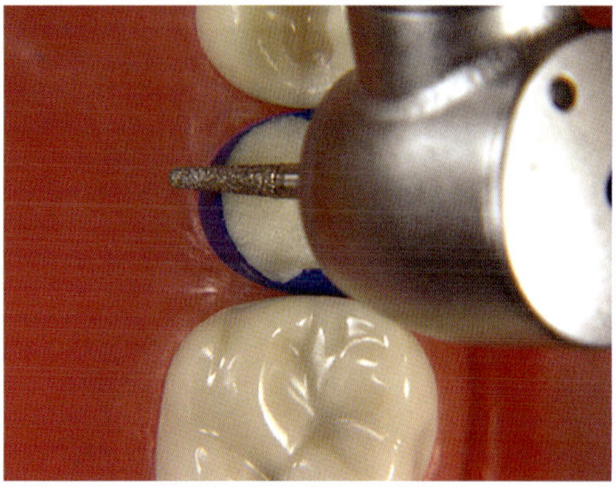

The tapered crown bur can be used for this stage of the preparation. The bur is held at 45° to the occlusal surface to effect the correct angle of preparation.

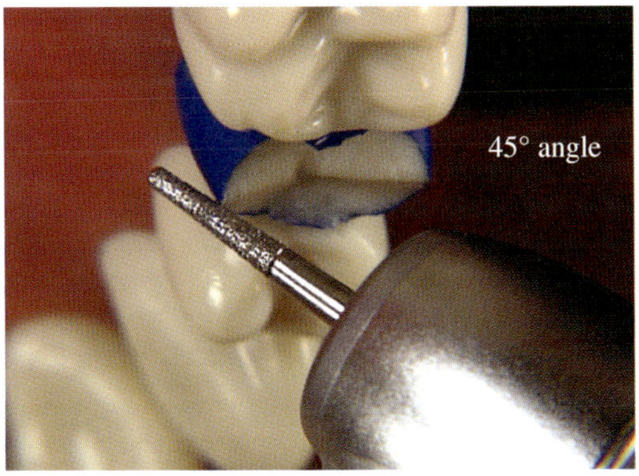

This angle should be approximately parallel to the slope of the lingual cusp of the lower tooth that occludes with this surface.

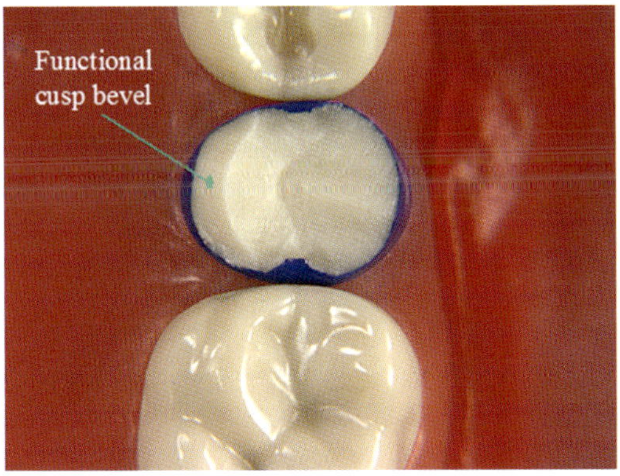

The functional bevel that is produced is carried around the palatal cusp but stops just short of the contact areas.
Note that it should not be a flat plane in only one direction.

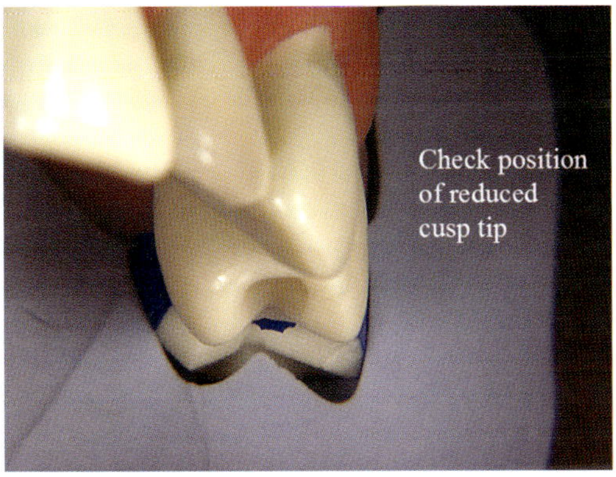

The putty template may be used to check that the reduction of this surface is also of about 1 mm.
Do not worry that it is less than this value where the functional bevel meets onto the unprepared palatal surface. This will be altered at a later stage of the preparation.

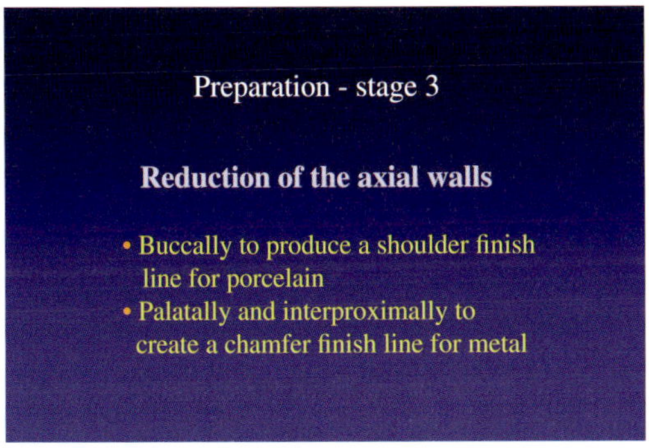

In the third stage of crown preparation, the axial walls are prepared. Initially the buccal and palatal surfaces will be prepared.
The buccal surface will be covered with a layer of metal and porcelain and, therefore, needs a shoulder preparation gingivally and a reduction of at least 1.3 mm.
The palatal surface will be covered in metal alloy only and requires substantially less reduction with a margin prepared to a 135° chamfer.

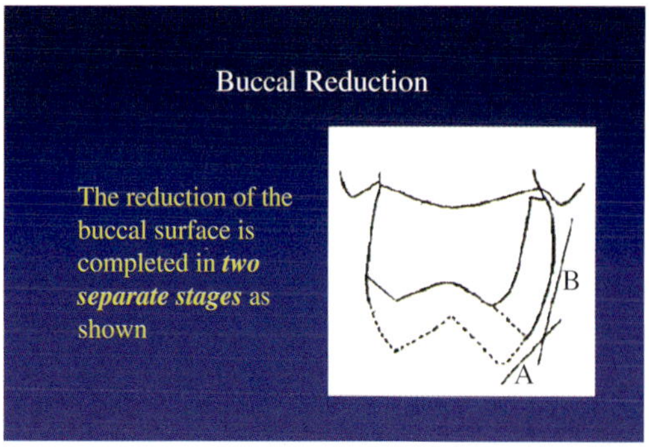

As the buccal surface of the natural crown is bulbous, the reduction of this surface requires a reduction is two separate stages as shown in the accompanying diagram.

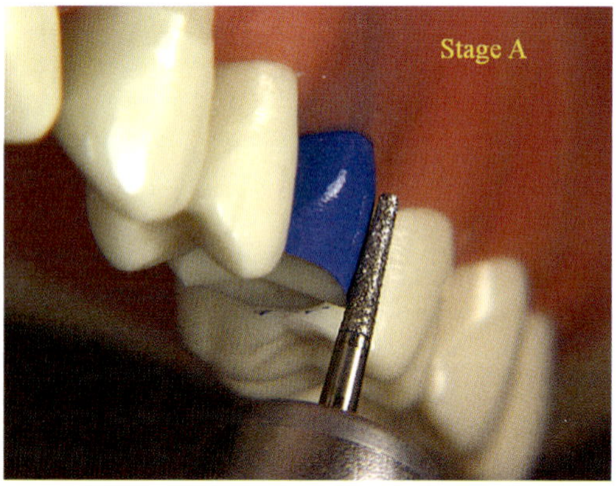

The first stage of the reduction will be accomplished using the tapered crown bur held parallel to the occlusal third of the buccal surface.

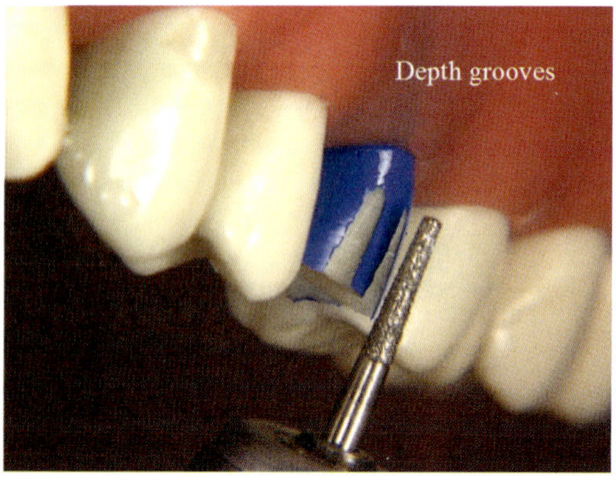

Depth grooves may be placed to just slightly greater than the diameter of the bur.

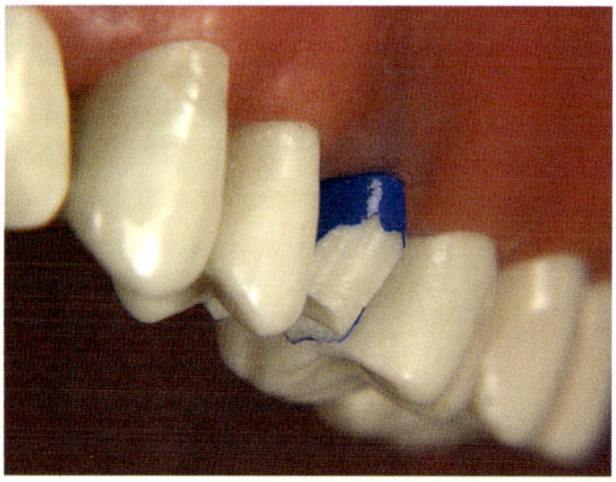

The reduction of this surface is then made following the contour of the crown.
As this is prepared, the effective cusp tip is brought back into line with the original position of the unprepared occlusal surface -similar to the functional bevel placed on the palatal side.

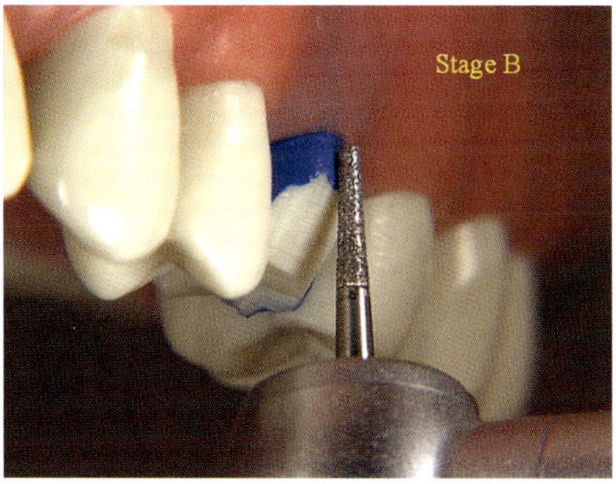

The second stage of the buccal reduction is then commenced.
The preparation of the gingival part of the crown prep is made parallel to the long axis of the tooth.

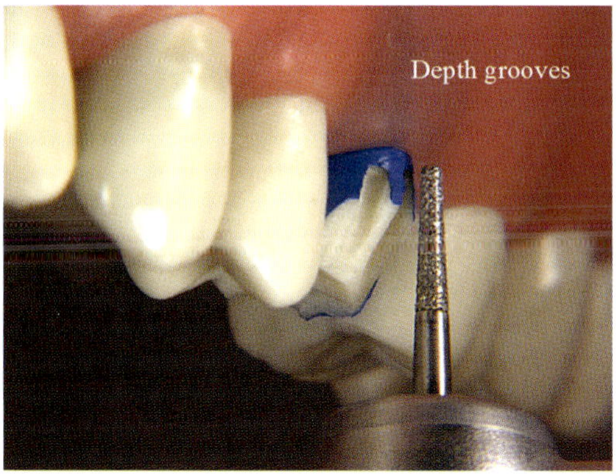

Depth grooves can be made as before to guide inexperienced operators as to the required depth of preparation.
The gingival extent of these grooves should be to a position just above gingival margin.

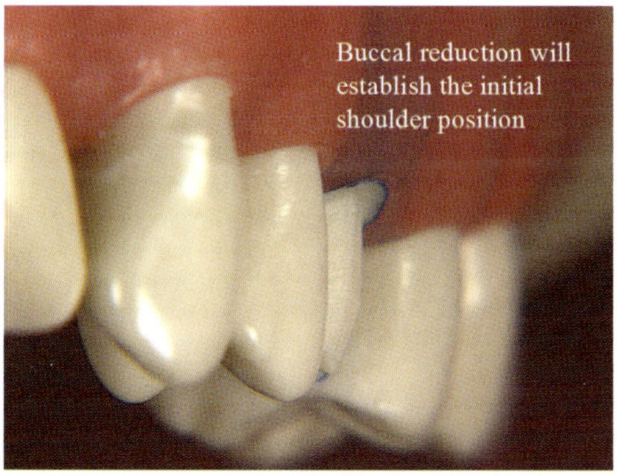

The reduction should follow the contour of the tooth and establish the buccal shoulder of the crown.
In this case a shoulder should be prepared and positioned on the gingival margin.
Margin placement depends on the appearance required. Where the lip line is high, the margin should be placed at or just within the gingival crevice. Where the margin is not seen, the shoulder may be left supragingivally where the patient may maintain good plaque control.

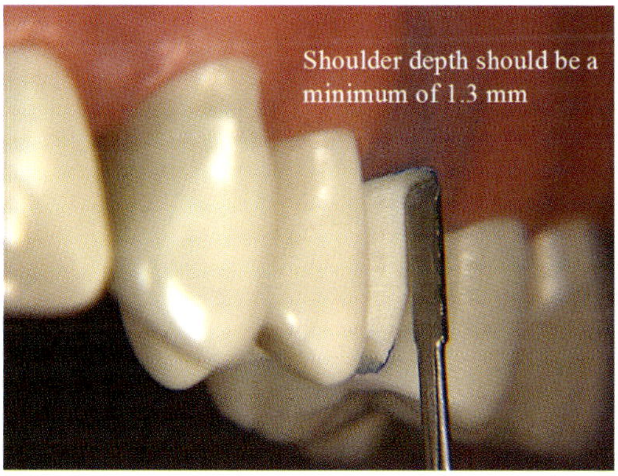

The width of the shoulder should be assessed.
The minimum depth should be 1.3 mm Assessment using a hand instrument of known blade width is easiest.
The enamel chisel shown has a width of 1.5 mm
If insufficient depth is provided, the final crown will invariably be over-contoured to allow for the opaque layer and the increments of dentine and enamel porcelain.

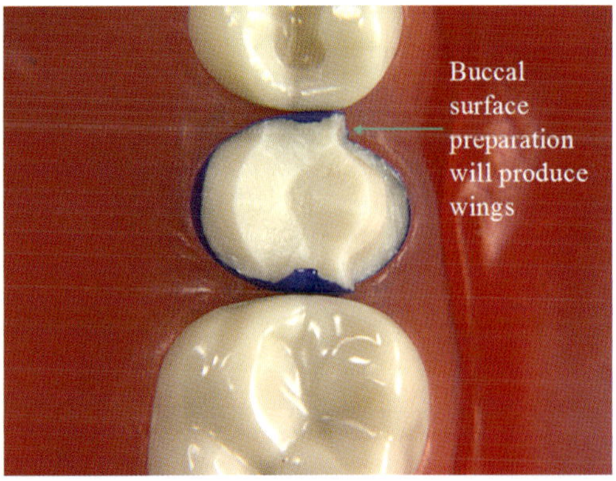

By following the contour of the buccal surface of the tooth, the reduction will produce wings on the mesial and distal surfaces of the teeth.

The position of these wings will be adjusted at a later stage.

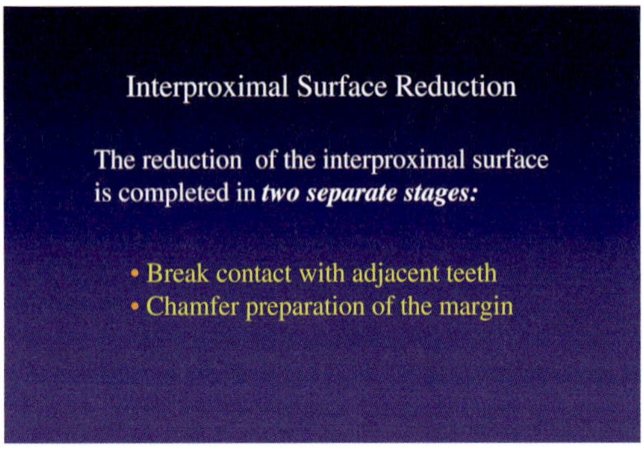

The interproximal surface must be prepared initially by breaking the contact in such a manner that the adjacent teeth do not get damaged.

Once this has been done, the mesial and distal surfaces can be prepared and the marginal finish placed at the appropriate level.

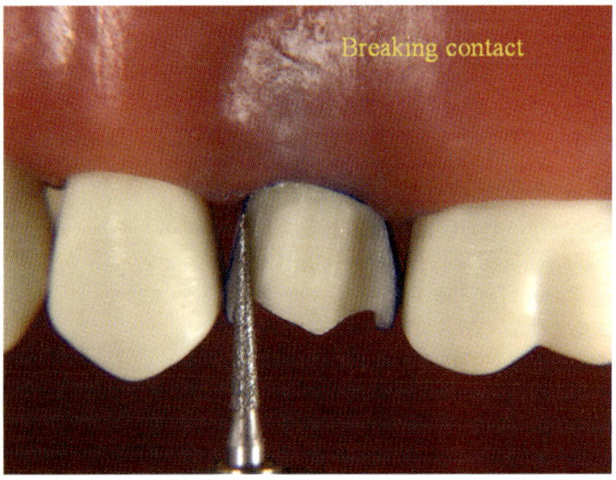

The contacts are broken using the fine tapered crown bur. A short sawing action is used with the bur at this stage to improve its cutting efficiency.
The motion should be in a controlled occluso-gingival direction.

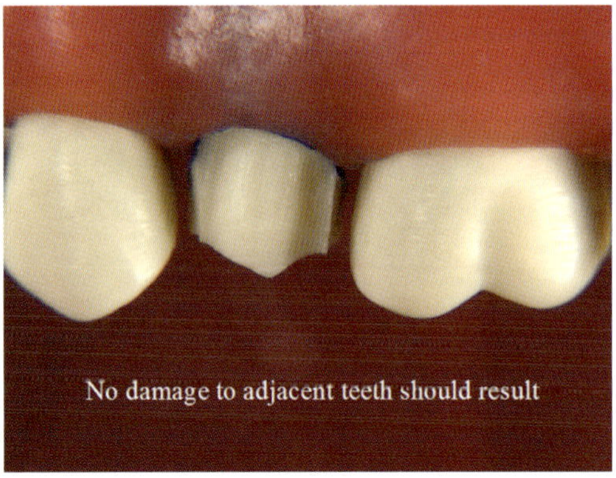

It is vitally important to avoid damage to the adjacent teeth while breaking the contacts.

Damage at this stage will result in roughening or gouging of the adjacent surfaces and will predispose to caries.

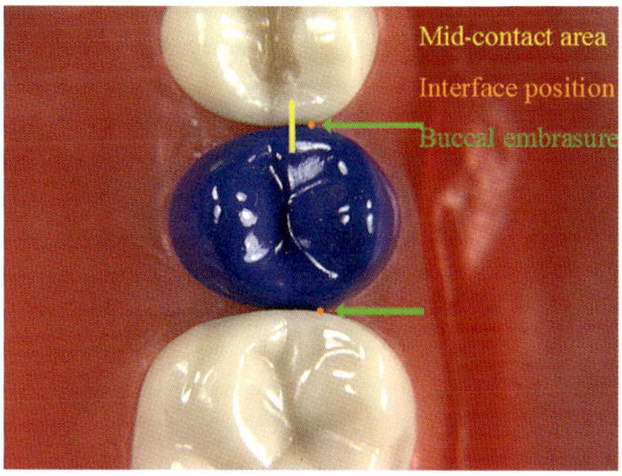

Before preparing the marginal finish interproximally, the position of the wings must be finalised.
Mesially, it is important that the appearance is not marred by the metal of the crown.
The buccal shoulder should be wrapped round into the mesial surface to a position that lies mid-way between the buccal embrasure on the midpoint of the contact area.
On the distal surface appearance is not so critical, so the shoulder finish can be placed at the buccal embrasure point marked here with orange dots.

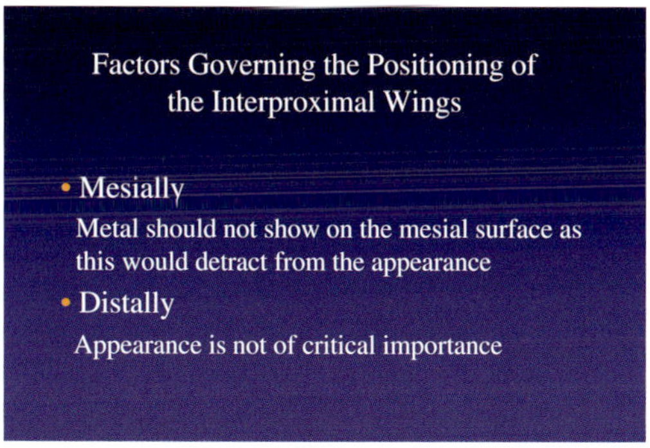

The factors governing the positoning of the wings are related to the appearance. Mesially this is much more critical than on the distal surface, where vision is more limited.

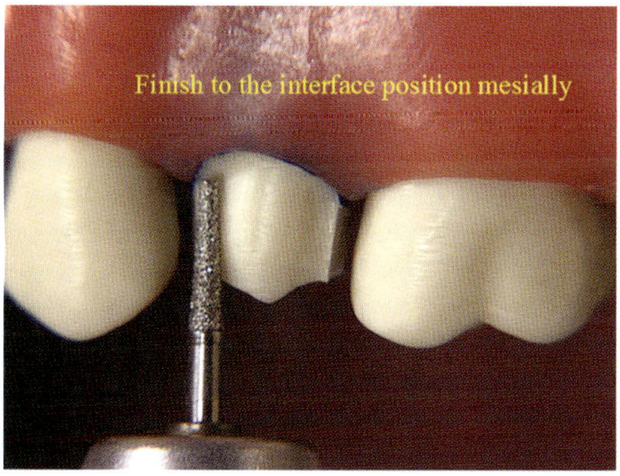

The buccal shoulder is adjusted accordingly and the wings placed to the appropriate position.

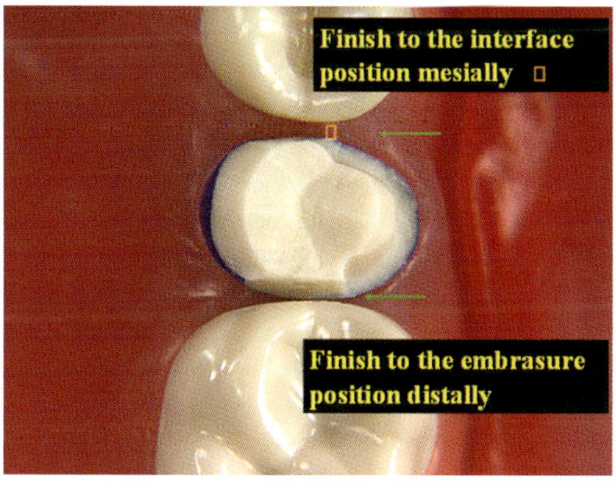

This occlusal view shows the further preparation of the mesial tooth surface to produce a wing that is further towards the palatal surface compared to the corresponding wing on the distal surface.

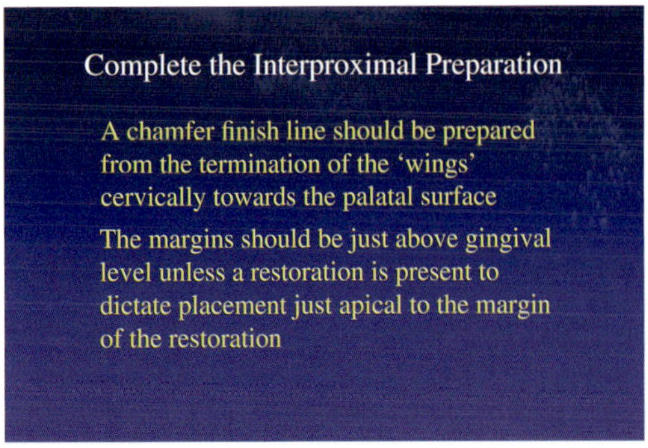

The interproximal surfaces can now be prepared further.
A chamfer finish line should be prepared from the edge of the shoulder and led towards the palatal surface.

This would normally be positioned just above gingival level to help maintain good plaque control.

Where there is a restoration present, the margin should be placed just cervical to the margin of the filling.

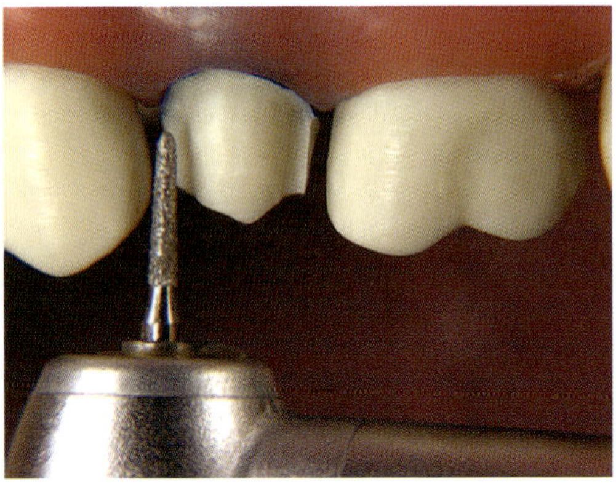

The torpedo shaped chamfer bur with the tapered shape tip should be used to produce a 135° chamfer finish on the approximal surfaces.

This bur should fit readily into the space created by breaking the contact points with the adjacent teeth.

If this is not the case, return to the thin separating bur to widen the space a little more.

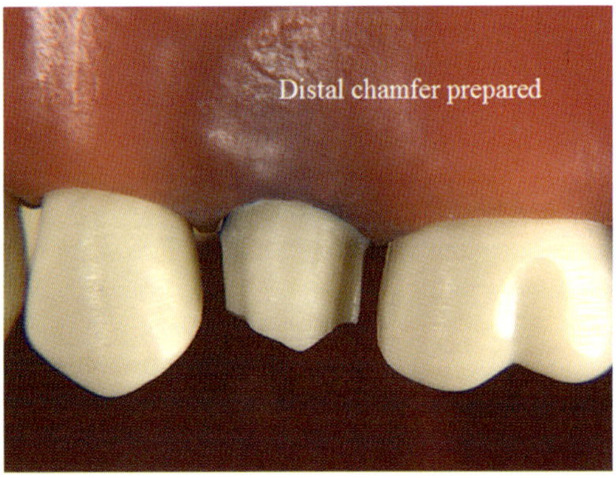

The chamfer margin has now been prepared on the distal surface. Note also that the preparation has been up-righted to lie parallel to the long axis of the tooth.
The taper of the preparation should not exceed 5° if excellent retention of the final restoration is to be maintained.

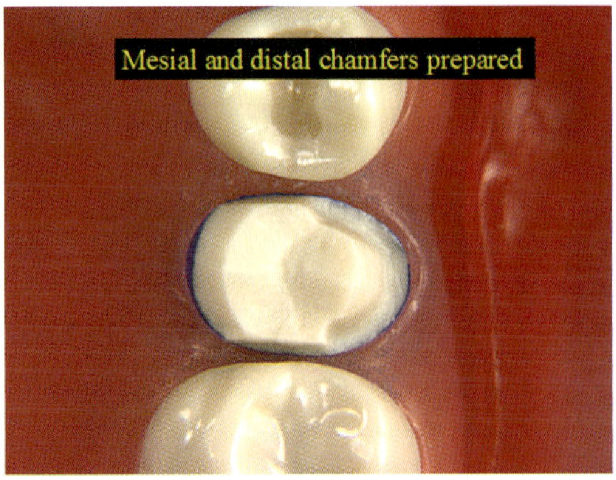

The mesial surface is prepared in a similar manner so that the mesial and distal walls of the preparation are almost parallel with only a slight convergence.

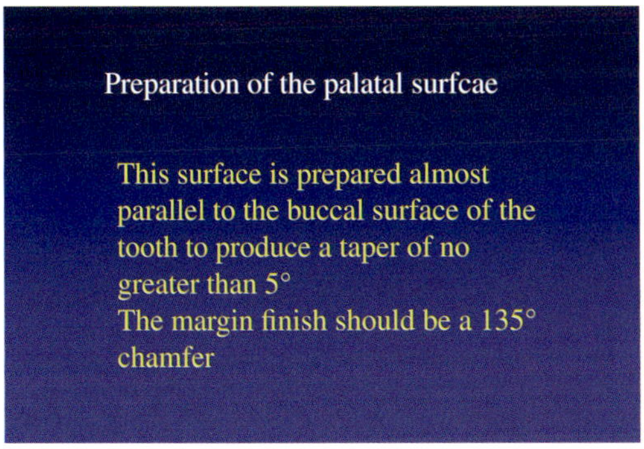

The last stage of the axial reduction is to prepare the palatal surface. This surface should be cut parallel to he buccal stage 2 reduction.
As metal will be present only at the margin of this surface, a chamfer finish is required.

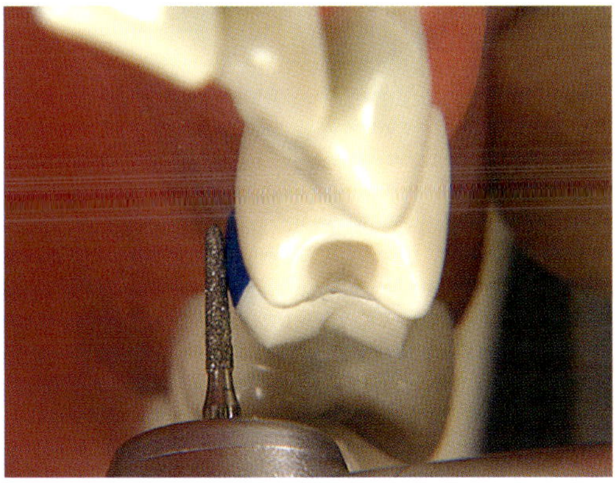

The chamfer preparation bur is held parallel to the long axis of the tooth and to the buccal surface preparation.

This should be carefully visualised before continuing.
Preparation of this surface should follow the contour of the tooth and merge into the chamfer finish lines prepared on the approximal tooth surfaces.

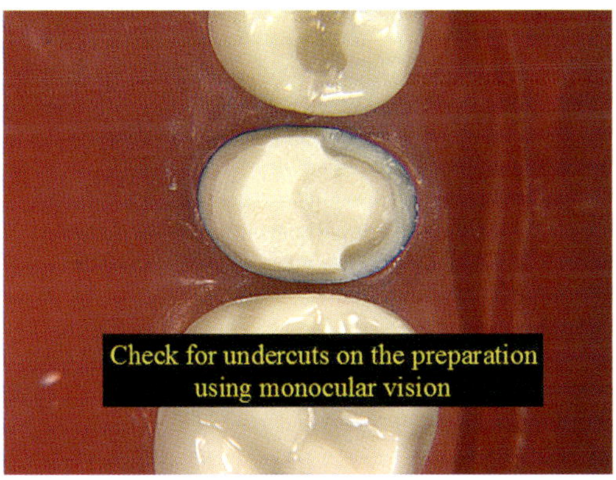

When this stage of the preparation has been completed, a mirror should be used to look from the occlusal surface towards the finished margins. It should not be possible to detect undercuts when monocular vision is used.

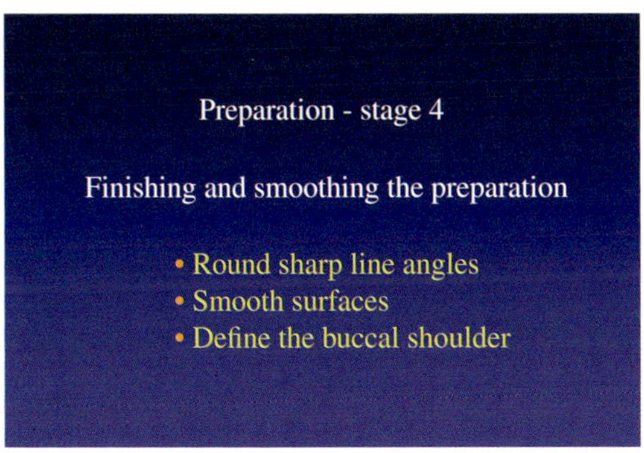

In the final stages of the preparation, surfaces and line angles are smoothed using:
- Superfine diamond burs
- Multi-fluted tungsten carbide burs
- Green stones

At this stage the shoulder should be smoothed and refined also.

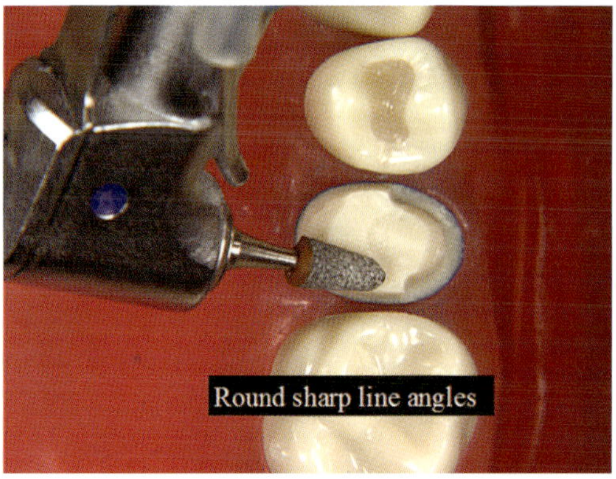

In this view the sharp line angles between the occlusal and functional bevel are being smoothed using a L/G green stone.
The disadvantage of using stones is the vibration that the patient experiences during preparation. However, slow-speed preparation provides the operator with good control of cutting.

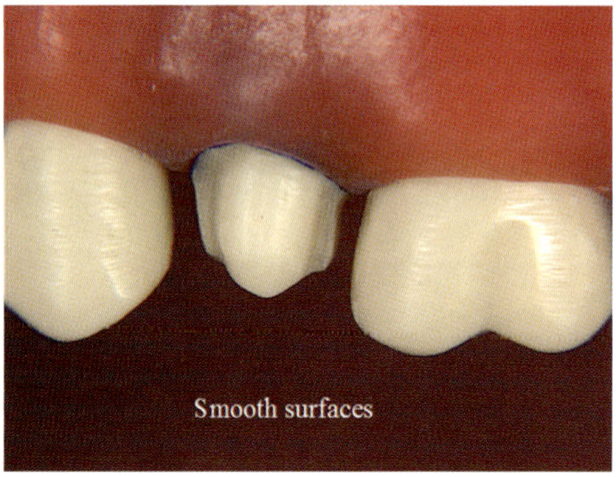

Surfaces should then be smoothed in a similar manner to eradicate the rough surface produced when preparing with diamond burs.
Smooth surfaces reduce drag on the impression material on removal from the mouth and also produce a smooth surface on the die that facilitates the technical procedures.

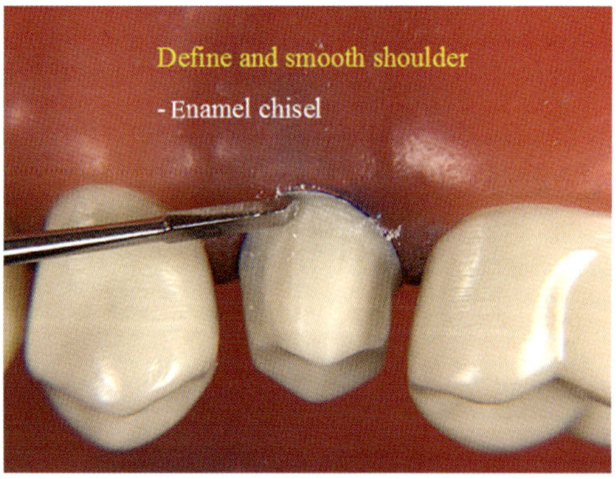

One of the instruments that can be used to define the shoulder is an enamel chisel. This will remove any small areas of unsupported enamel along the edge of the preparation.
It is important that a good finger rest is used at this stage because it is easy for the instrument to slip. This would result in tissue trauma and make isolation problematic.
Shoulder files may be used as an alternative to the straight enamel chisel. There is less likelihood of tissue damage using this designated instrument.

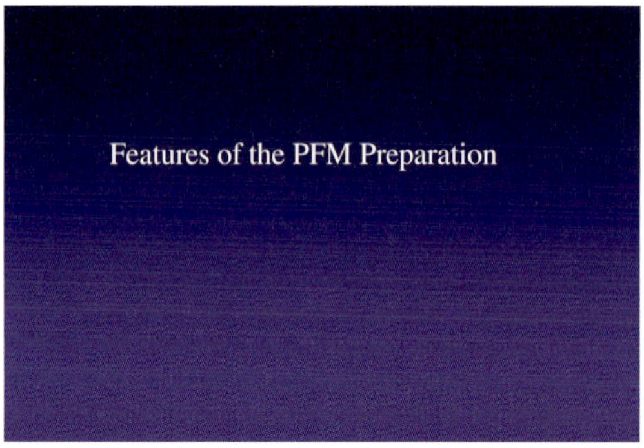

Let us now review the main features of the porcelain fused to metal crown.

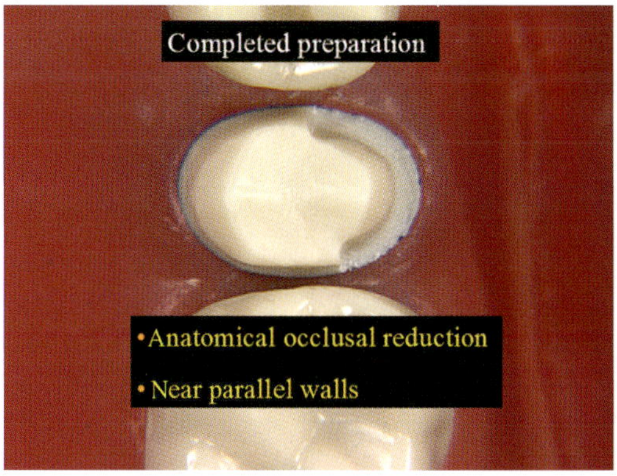

The occlusal reduction should be completed in an anatomical fashion so that the cusp tips and slopes are still recognisable.
A small taper of no more that 5° should be incorporated in the axial reduction. Monocular vision in the dental mirror should allow the operator to see down all axial surfaces to the marginal finish.

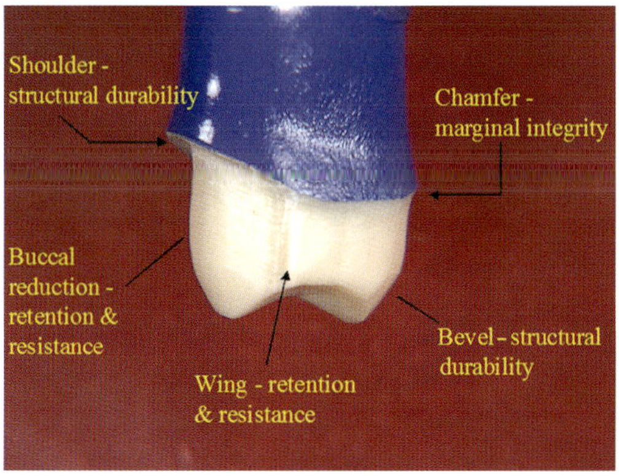

For structural durability of the restoration:
the shoulder should be of the correct width of >1.3 mm and the functional cusp bevel correctly angled.
For resistance and retention:
near parallelism of the buccal and palatal axial reduction is required. The wings on the approximal surface also aid in the resistance form.

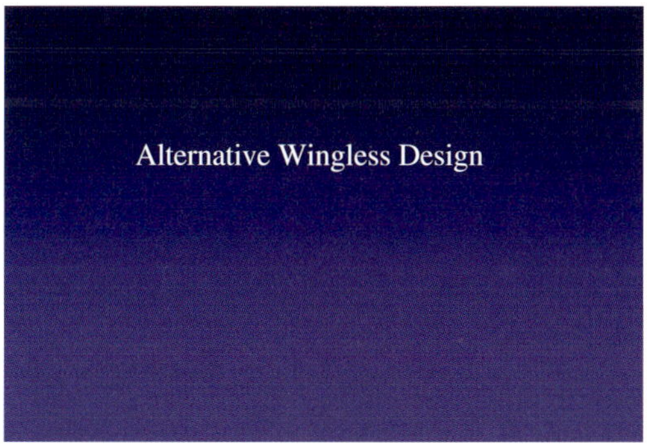

The wings that are created when the buccal reduction merges with the approximal surface preparation may aid with resistance form of the restoration, but they can also be a potential source of undercut if both do not lie in the same non-undercut plane.
For this reason some authorities advocate that they should be removed and the preparation smoothed gradually from a shoulder to a chamfer finish.

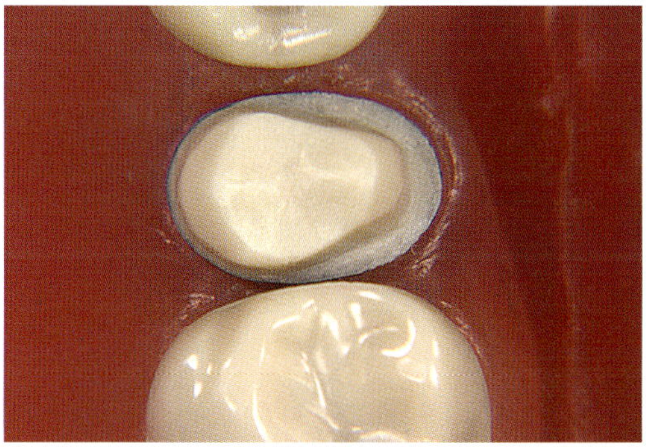

The disadvantage of this style of preparation is that it removes even more tooth structure from what is already a radical reduction.

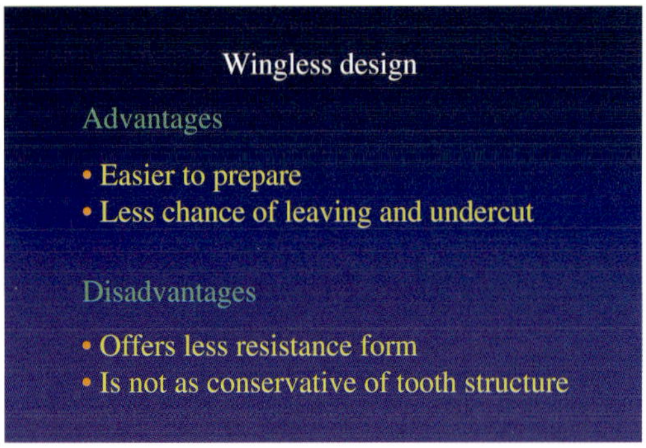

Here is a summary of the relative merits of the wingless preparation.

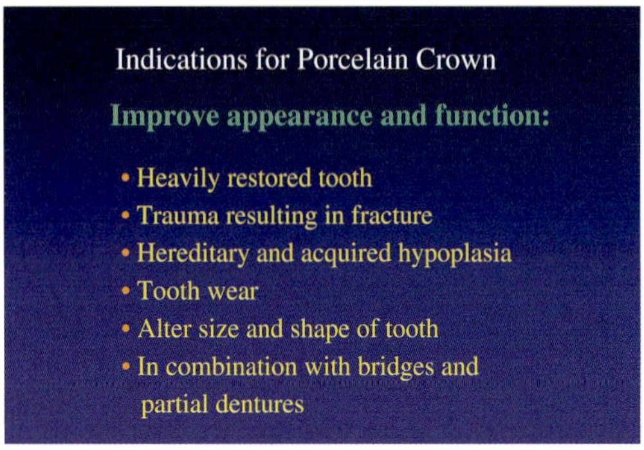

Most of the indications for the all-ceramic crown are concerned with improving the appearance of anterior teeth. Today, many of these improvements can be achieved using a porcelain or composite veneer that is less destructive of remaining natural tooth structure. A range of indications are shown in the accompanying slide.

All-Ceramic Crown

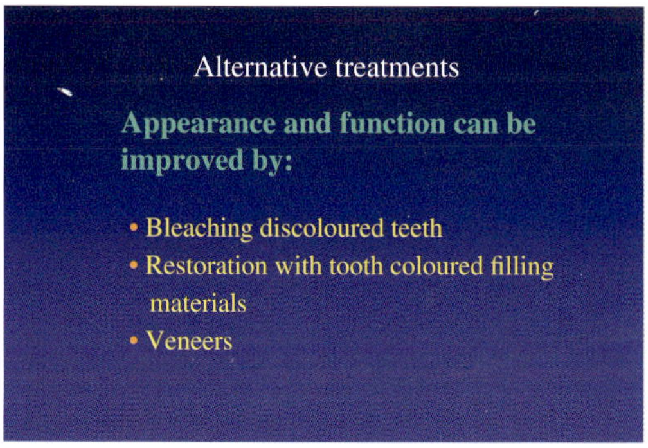

Less destructive treatment options are available rather than a PJC.

Internal or 'walking bleaching' may be completed following root canal treatment, and external bleaching is again allowed using carbamine peroxide in specially constructed trays.

Replacement composite restorations may achive an acceptable improvement, but it should be that these will gradually stain and yellow with age.

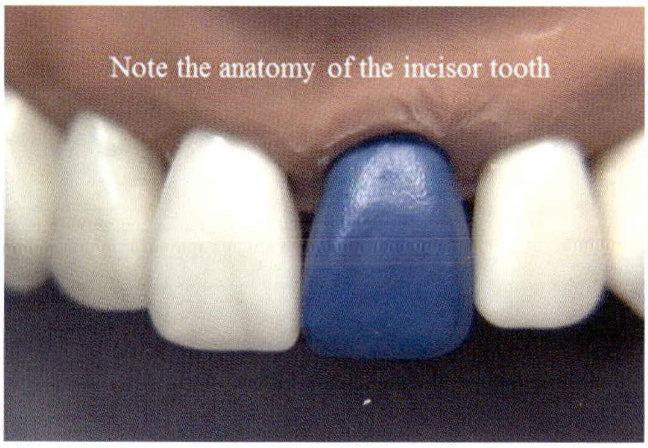

The central incisor tooth in this sequence has been coloured blue to allow the various stages of preparation to be seen more readily.

Maxillary incisors are described as being shovel shaped. The tooth fans out from the cervical margin towards the incisal edge.

On the palatal surface the cingulum is quite pronounced and the mesial and distal marginal ridges run from the cingulum towards the incisal edge.

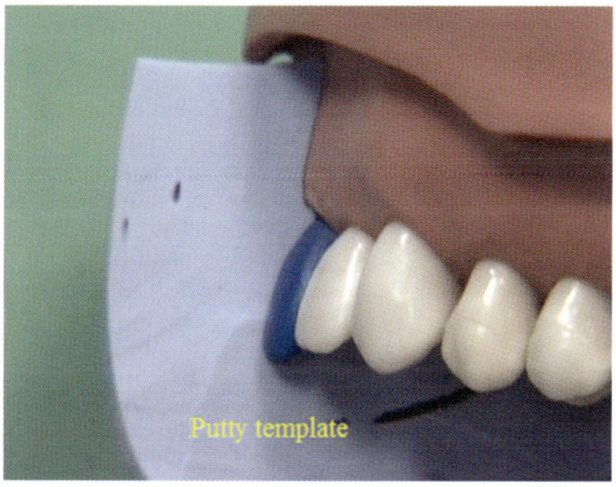

The central incisor tooth in this sequence has been coloured blue to allow the various stages of preparation to be seen more readily.

When the incisor surface is viewed from the side, it can be seen that the labial profile is slightly curved.

When the labial surface is prepared along its long axis, the amount of reduction between the putty template and the dentine surface will be evident.

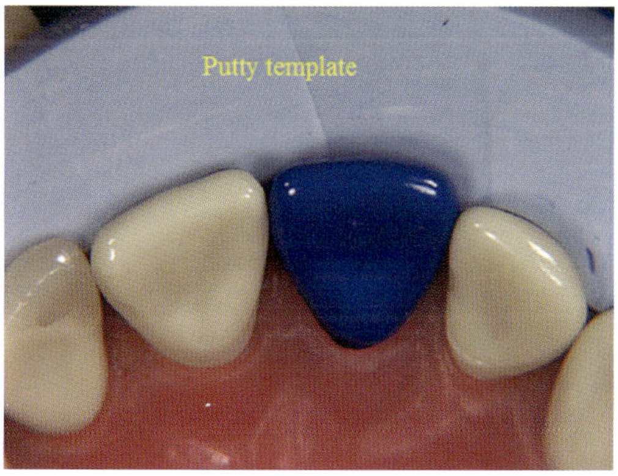

Sometimes the template may be sectioned in a mesio-distal direction so that students may see that sufficient tooth structure has been removed from the labial surface.

Generally, it is more useful to section the template in an inciso-gingival direction.

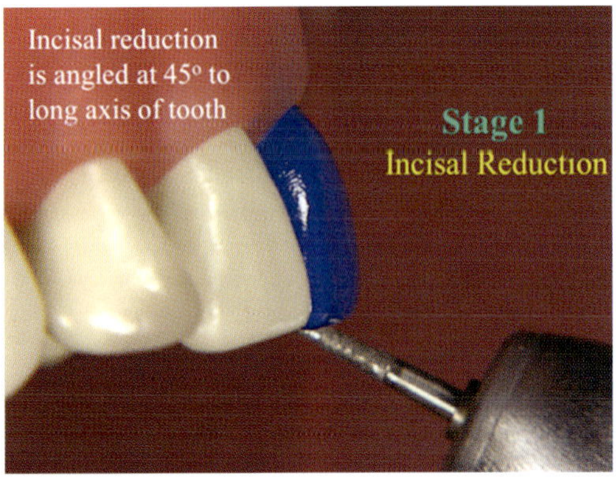

In the first stage of the preparation, the incisal edge is reduced.

It should be noted that this is completed with an inciso-palatal angle of 45° so that this reduced surface lies perpendicular to the forces of mastication.

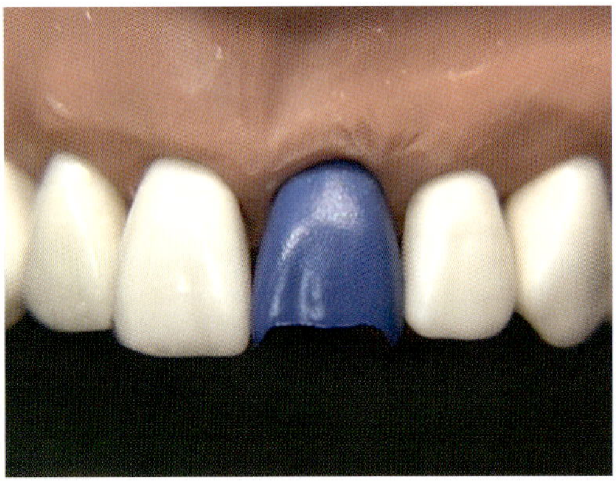

There is some debate as to the correct amount of reduction. Reports vary from 1 to 2 mm reduction. Increasing the amount of incisal reduction beyond 2 mm has been reported to increase the incidence of labial surface fracture in the final restoration.

Generally, a quarter of the clinical height of the crown is removed but the incisal corners are left unprepared to avoid damage to the adjacent teeth.

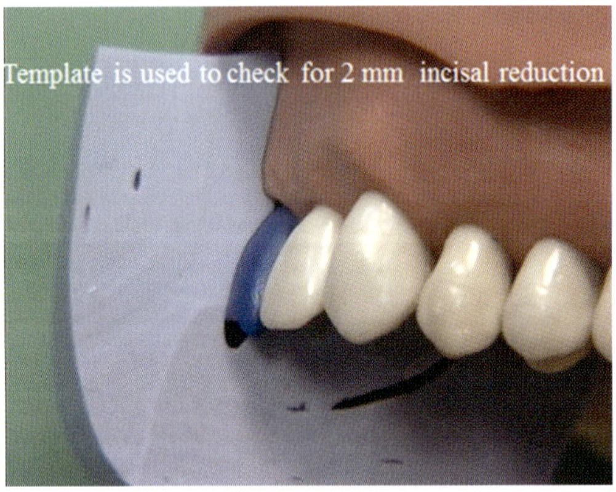

When the template is replaced on the tooth the amount of reduction can be seen.

It is also important at this stage to observe carefully the angle of the cut surface to ensure that is at 45° to the long axis of the tooth.

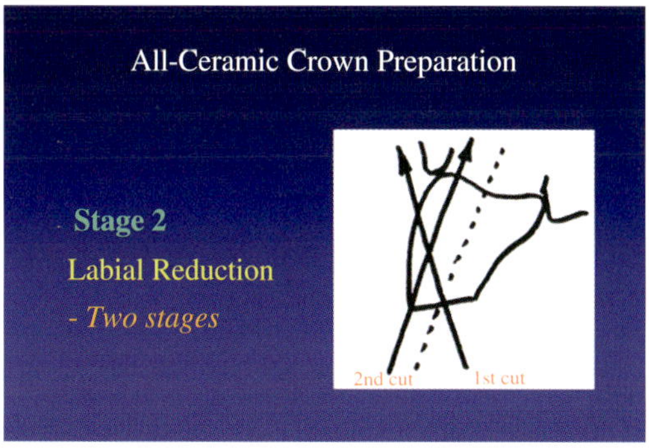

In the second stage of the preparation the labial surface of the incisor will be prepared in two distinct planes. This avoids the cutting of an over-tapered preparation.
It will be remembered that retention of the final crown relies predominantly on two factors:
• Clinical height
• Minimal taper

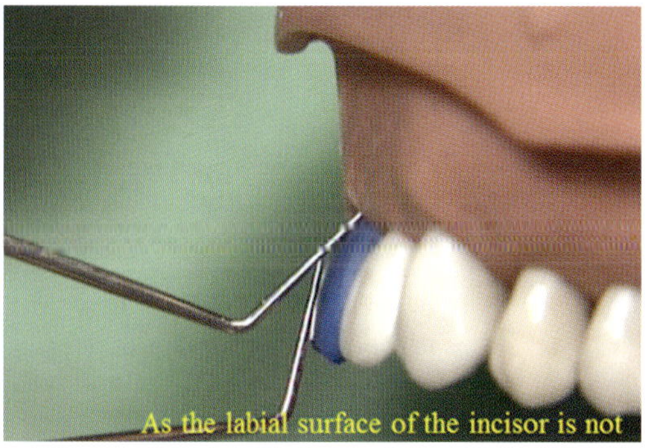

Two probes have been placed parallel to the labial surface of the incisor tooth.
These show the marked curvature of this surface and the necessity to prepare it in two distinct planes.

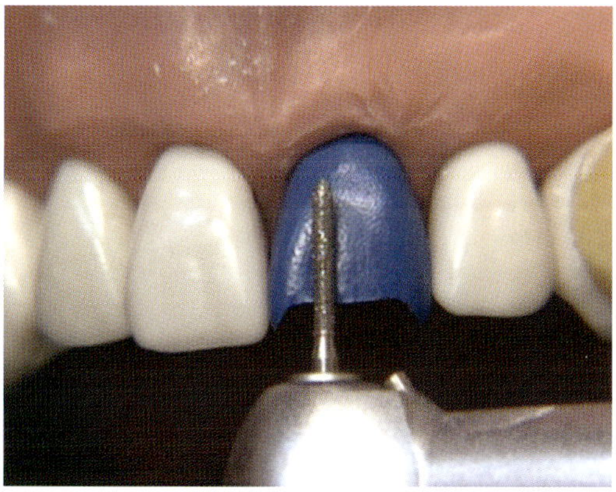

The slightly longer dome tipped crown bur may be used to prepare depth grooves to aid preparation. This bur is 1 mm in diameter.
Some operators feel that this is an inadvisable practice as remnants of the grooves may remain on the finished preparation surface.
When grooves are used the bur must be held parallel to the more incisal labial plane and, for the second cut, the bur should be in the long axis of the tooth.

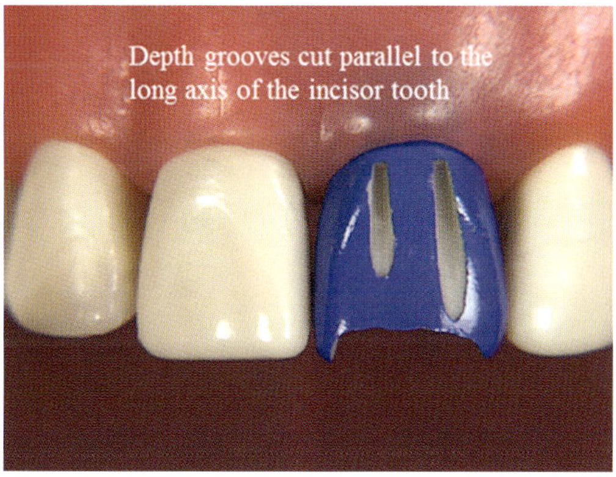

In this view the depth grooves have been prepared parallel to the long axis of the tooth and rest in the gingival part of the preparation.
The known diameter of the tip of the crown bur can be used to gauge the depth of the cut.

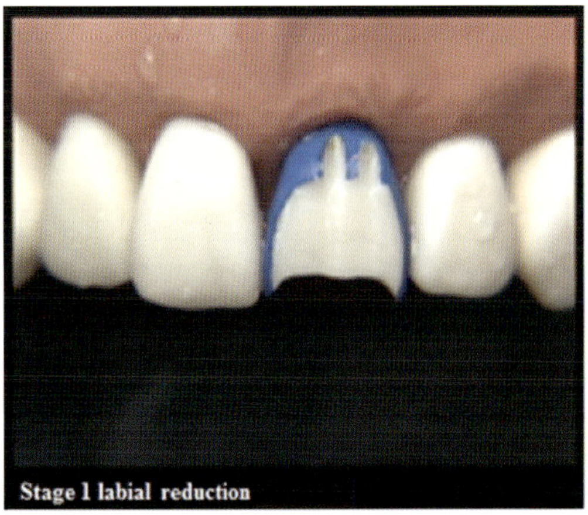

The incisal cut is made first of all.
The tooth structure is removed to the bottom of the grooves in the incisal region of the crown.
The grooves in the long axis of the tooth will still remain as grooves at this stage.

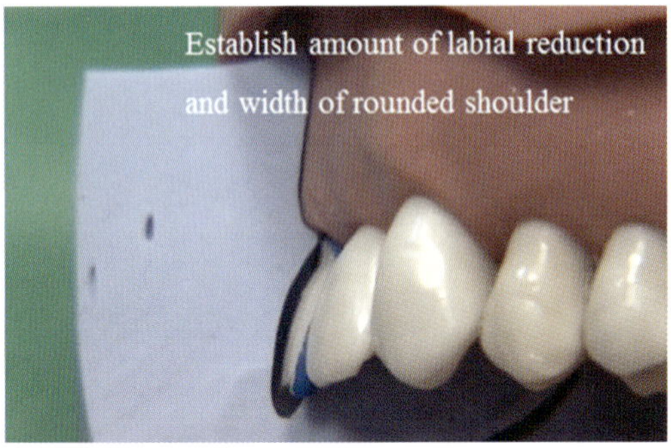

After the second cut is made, the template can be tried on to acertain the amount of labial tooth reduction completed.
If insufficient reduction has been made, the technician will either:

* Overbulk the labial surface making it unnecessarily bulbous, or
* Make the crown with a thin labial surface and poorer appearance. This is the result of insufficient dentine and enamel porcelain covering the core material.

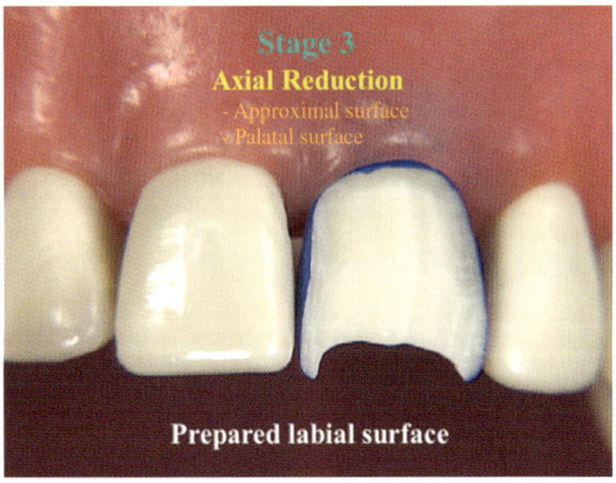

This is the start point for this stage of the procedure where the labial face has been reduced in its two phases.
In the axial reduction stage, the approximal tooth surfaces will be reduced and the palatal surface will then be prepared to produce a rounded shoulder that runs all the way around the preparation

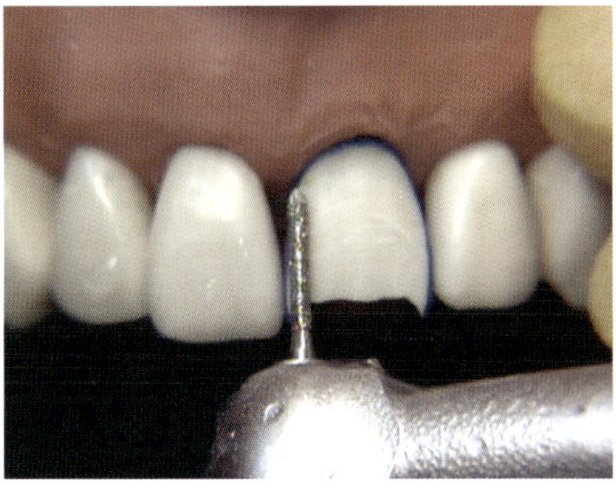

The dome tipped crown bur can be used to cut through between the teeth and create a rounded shoulder of 1 mm width.
The bur should be held upright and the cut made within the bulk of the tooth structure to avoid damage to the adjacent tooth.

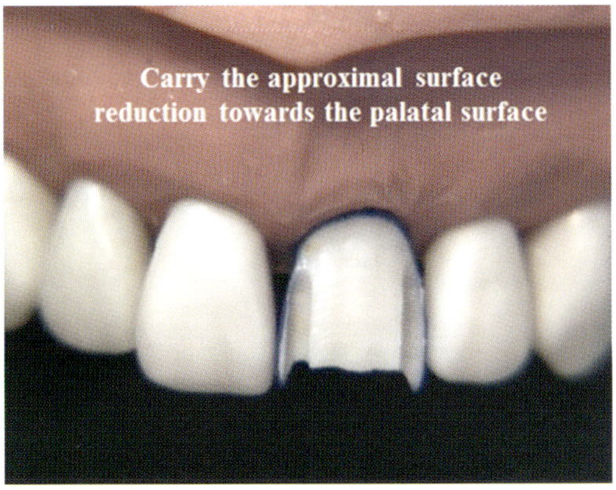

This view shows the thin area of tooth structure that remains adjacent to the neighbouring teeth. Note the upright cut surface.
If retention is not to be compromised all axial surfaces should diverge with no more than a 3°–6° angle

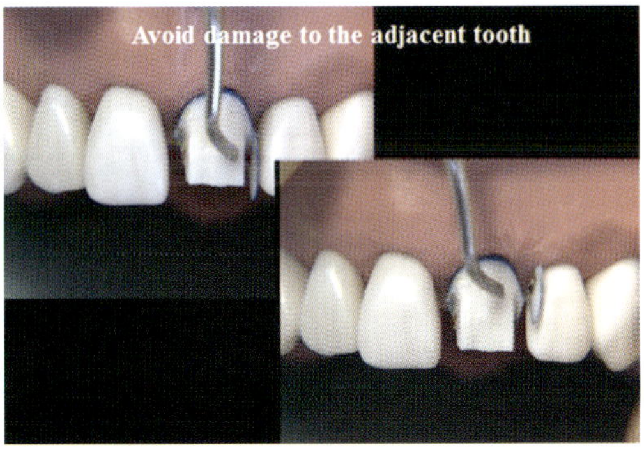

The thin fragile area of tooth can then be fractured away using an instrument. This avoids damage to the adjacent teeth.

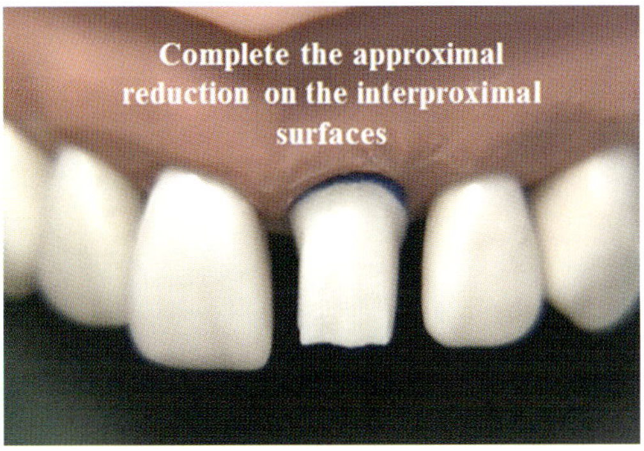

The same preparation is then made on the other approximal surface so that the rounded shoulder is confluent from the labial surface onto both the mesial and distal tooth surfaces.
Similarly, the shoulder finish should be made just above gingival level at this stage. The shoulder should rise and fall as it follows the position of the dental papilla through the approximal surfaces.

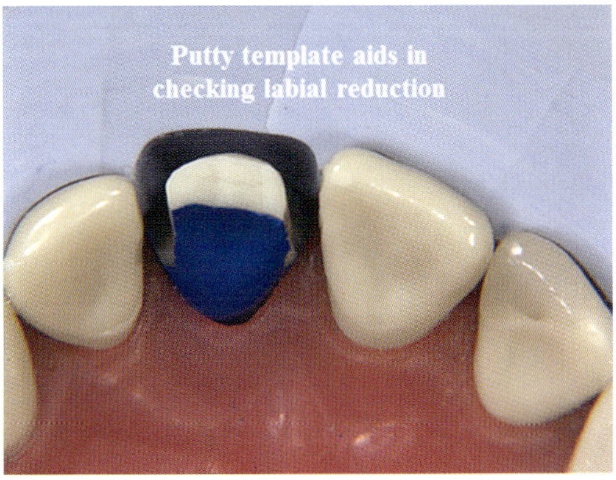

Check for the correct amount of labial reduction using the labial template.
Do not be tempted to proceed if this stage is not correctly completed.

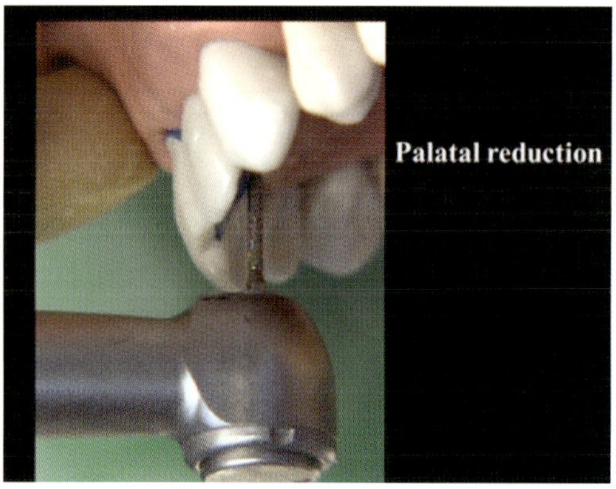

The palatal reduction can now be completed using the crown bur by continuing from the approximal surface reduction.
It is important that this surface is reduced to be almost parallel to the gingival part of the labial reduction.
In this way, maximal retention will be achieved. Note that the bur is being held parallel to this plane before the preparation is completed.

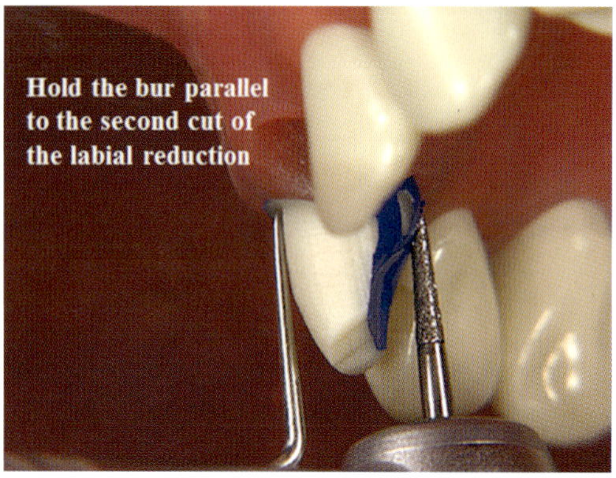

Parallel the bur with the labial surface and hold it in this alignment during all cutting procedures involving the palatal surface.

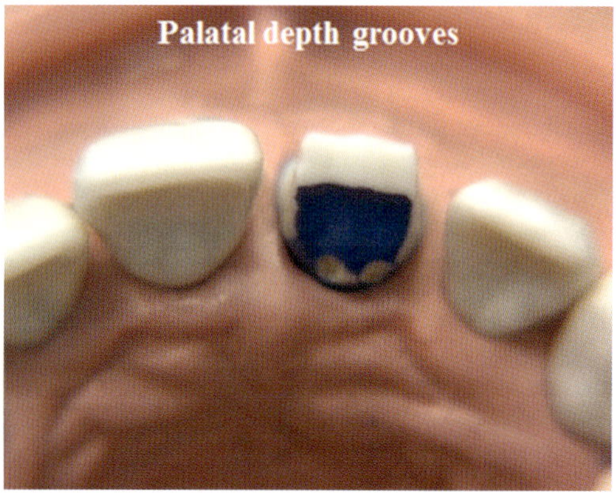

Depth grooves in this surface may help to ensure sufficient depth of preparation.

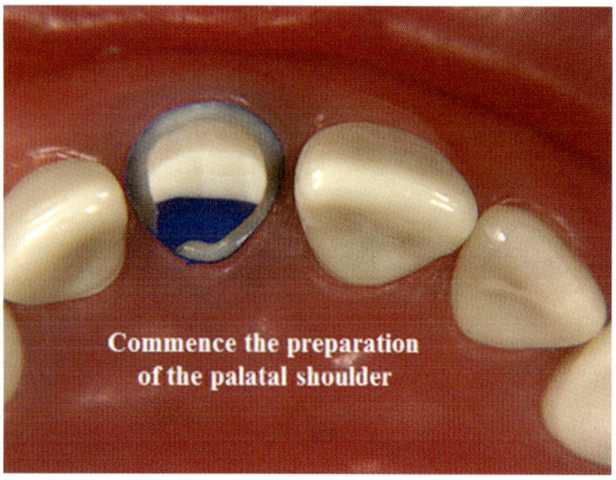

The palatal shoulder preparation is commenced by cutting from the palatal extent of the approximal surface reduction.
With the bur held upright, the first of the depth grooves is incorporated.

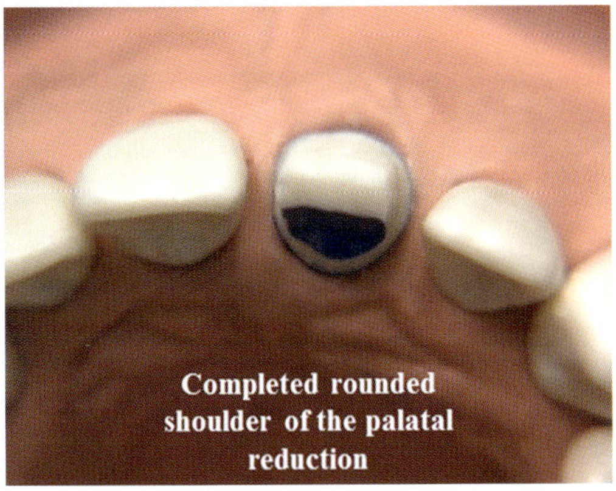

Eventually the shoulder should be taken all the way round to join up with the other approximal preparation.

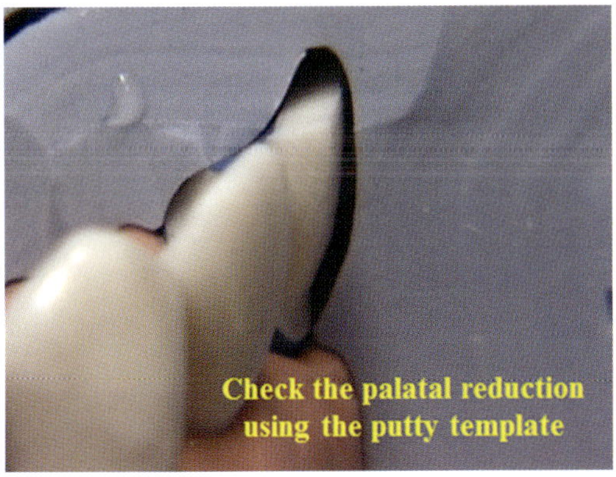

The amount of palatal reduction can be checked by replacing the template.

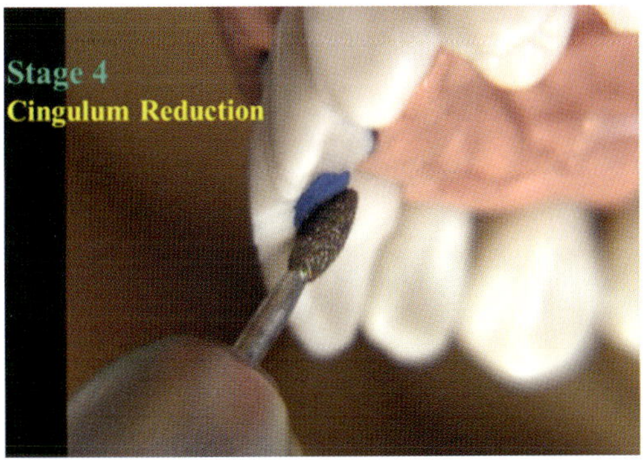

To continue the palatal reduction, the remaining tooth structure is reduced in the palatal concavity to allow for a 1 mm thickness of porcelain.
The bur used is egg or rugby ball shaped. This slide shows how it adapts well into the concave palatal surface.
Using this rotary cutting instrument it should be possible to get maximum reduction in the middle of this surface where clearance is needed from the opposing mandibular incisors.

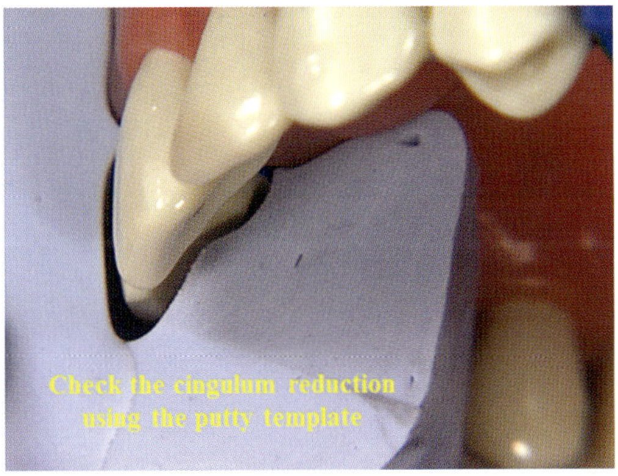

The distinctly curved cingulum reduction provides a more horizontal and vertical area. This adds to the resistance and retention form of the restoration while reducing stress within the ceramic material of the crown.

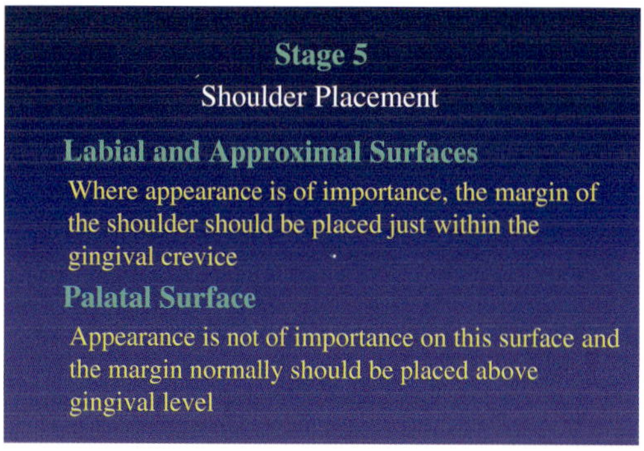

Where the lip line is such that the margin of the tooth cannot be seen during smiling, the shoulder can be placed at gingival level so that plaque control is easier. If the margin can be seen, then it should be palced just within the gingival crevice.

On the palatal side where the shoulder margin cannot be seen, placement above gingival level is advocated for ease of cleaning and for professional inspection/review. This ensures that the crown is fully seated and free from marginal defects.

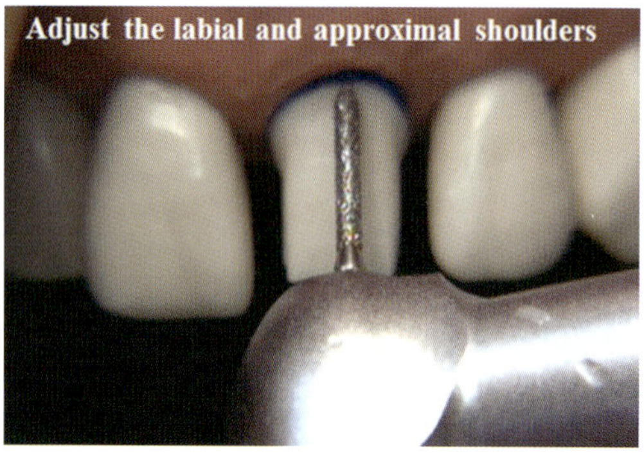

In this slide sequence the margin will be taken to lie at the gingival margin.

In the phantom head jaw the labial shoulder should be placed just above the gingival margin taking care not to damage the gingival mask.

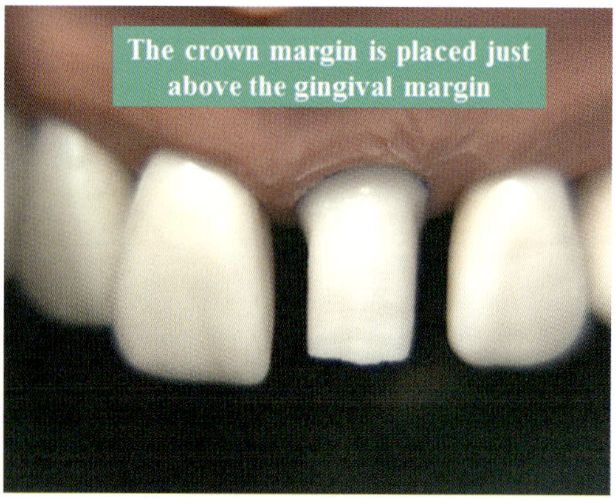

This view shows the finished shoulder and its proximity to the gingival margin.

It is important that the shoulder is smooth and free from sharp line angles as it goes over the papilla on the approximal surfaces.

Leaving sharp line angles leads to a wedging effect and fracture of the crown.

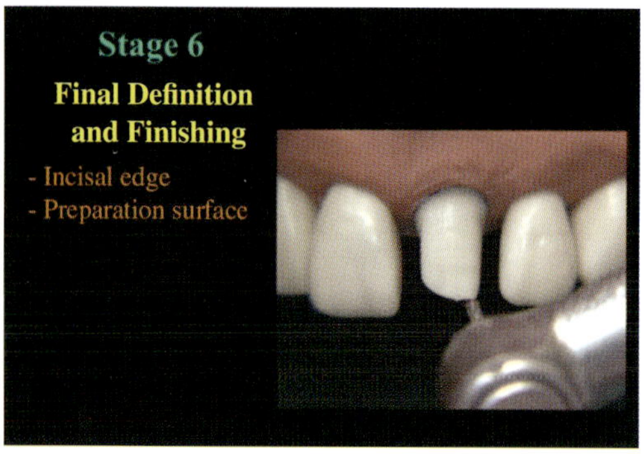

In the final stage, definition and smoothness should be perfected. A smooth surface is required to prevent dragging of the impression and provide a surface that will allow a close fit for the crown.

The incisal edge of the preparation is rounded using the domed crown bur held at an angle towards the palatal surface.

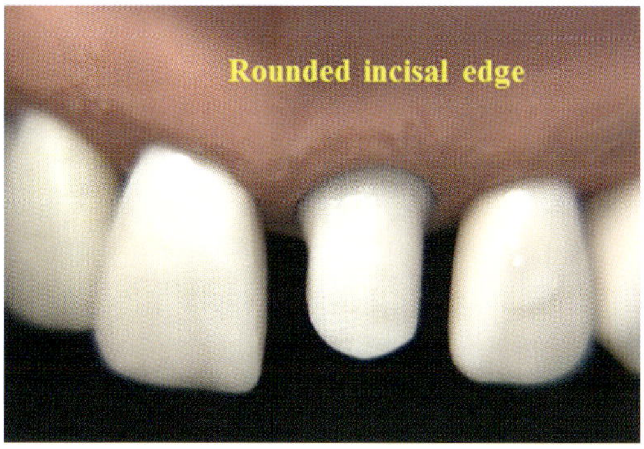

In this view, the rounded nature of the incisal edge can be seen directly from the labial surface. The sharp edges on the labial and palatal aspects should be rounded to avoid line angles.

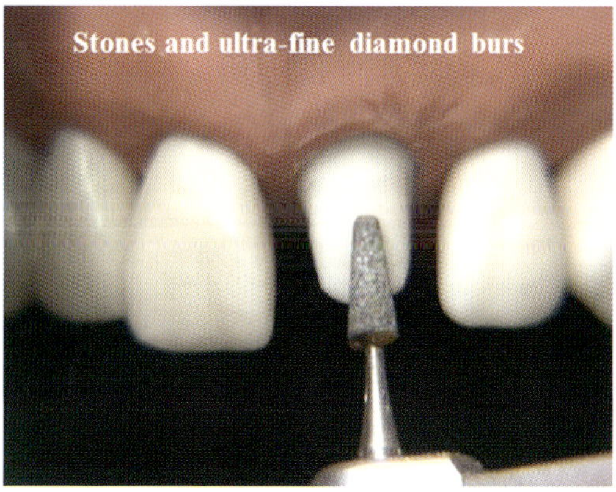

A range of ultra-fine diamond burs are available in a variety of shapes. These leave the surface much smoother than can be created with the normal variety of industrial diamond coated burs.

Green stones are also useful in achieving a smooth surface and give good control at slow speed for the operator, but they do create a lot of vibration for the patient.

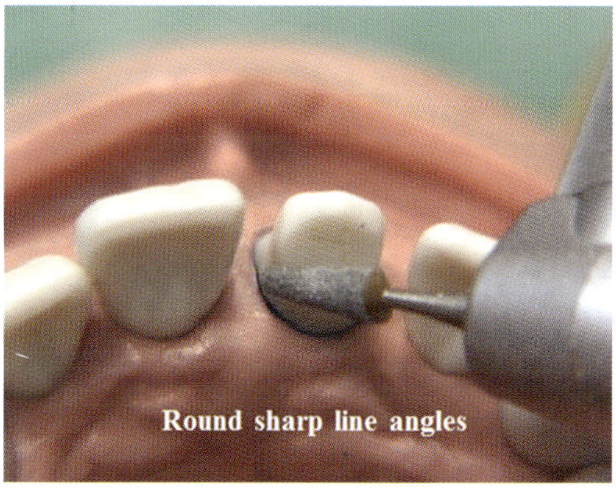

Green stones are particularly useful to round the sharp line angles on the preparation.

Sharp line angles would be areas of stress concentration and should be avoided in preparations for ceramic restorations.

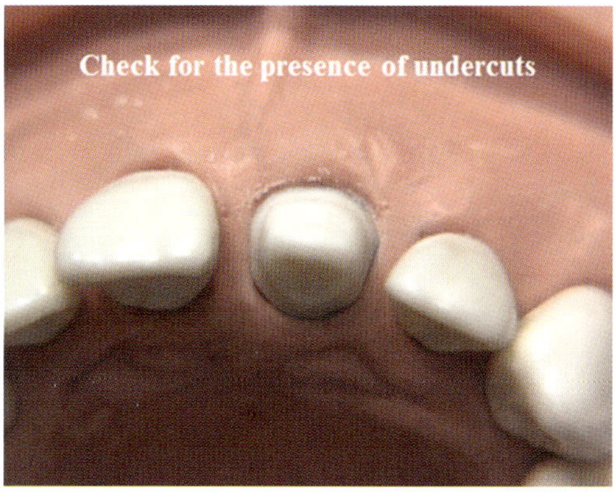

Check for undercuts using monocular vision.

Mesial/distal and labial/palatal surfaces should be carefully viewed. Even slight undercuts may result in a failure of the ceramic crown to seat during the try-in stage of its fracture.

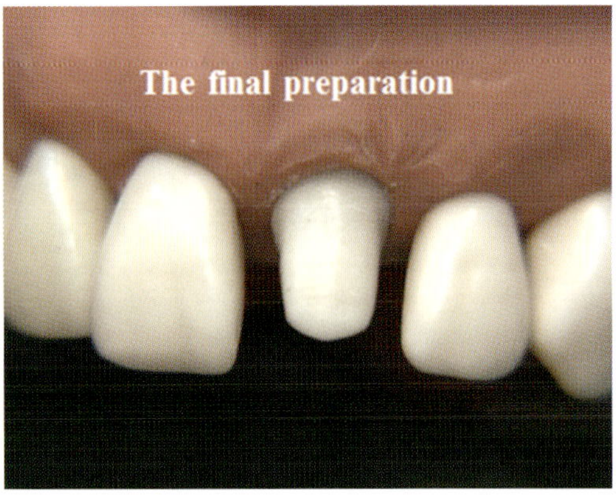

This labial view shows the final preparation after finishing...

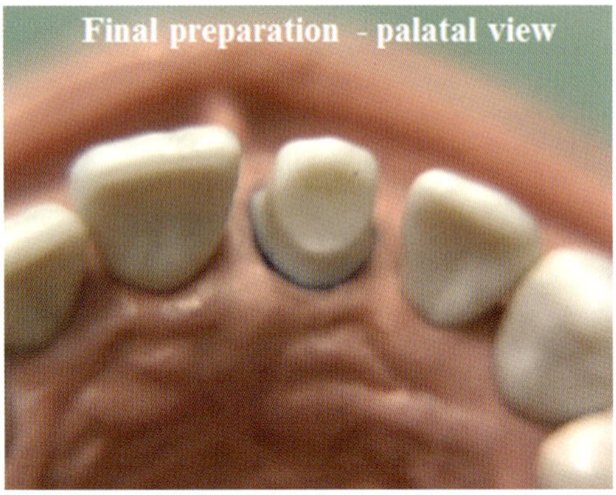

... and the clearly defined palatal view with obvious palatal and cingulum reductions but with rounded line angles between them.

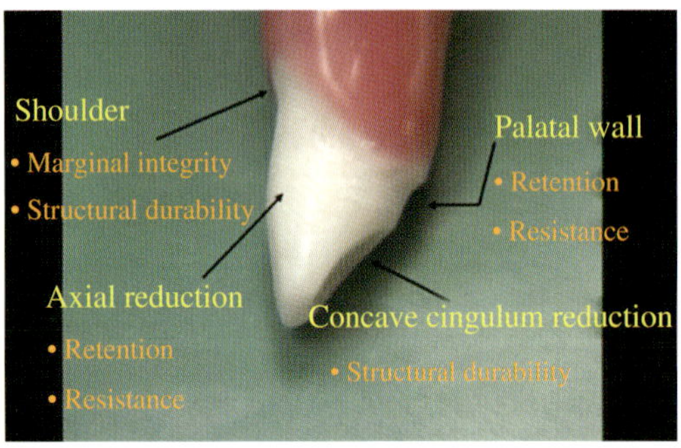

The function of the various parts of the preparation:
Rounded shoulder provides marginal integrity and structural durability.
Axial reduction provides resistance and retention form to the restoration.
The concave cingulum reduction provides needed inter-occlusal clearance and structural durability.

Clinical Sequence for All-Ceramic Crown

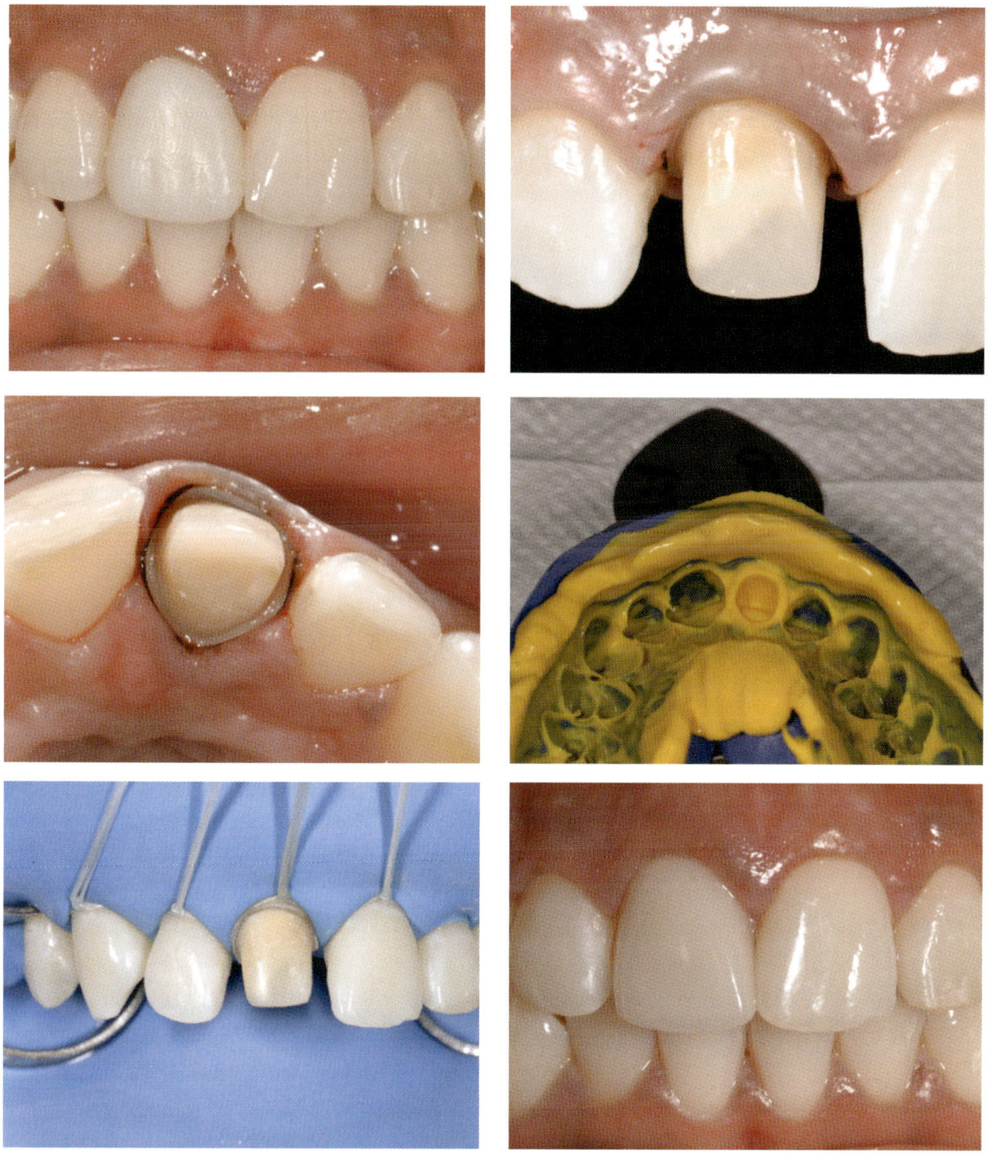

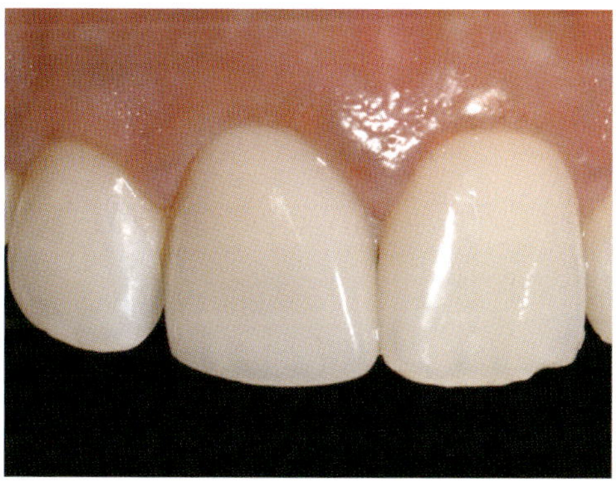

Clinical sequence for replacing an anterior crown with an all-ceramic restoration

Source: Printed by permission of Dr Osama Alkhatib.

Further Reading

Bajraktarova-Valjakova, E., Korunoska-Stevkovska, V., Kapusevska, B. et al. (2018). Contemporary dental ceramic materials, a review: chemical composition, physical and mechanical properties, indications for use. *Open Access Macedonian Journal of Medical Sciences* 6: 1742–1755.

Pjetursson, B.E., Sailer, I., Makarov, N.A. et al. (2015). All-ceramic or metal-ceramic tooth-supported fixed dental prostheses (FDPs)? A systematic review of the survival and complication rates. Part II: multiple-unit FDPs. *Dental Materials* 31: 624–639.

Shenai, A., Ganapathy, D. & Gounder, R (2019). All ceramic systems in dentistry. *Drug Intervention Today* 14: 1035–1041.

Index

a

A Practical Approach to Operative Dentistry, First Edition. Gordon B. Gray and Alaa H. Daud.

Companion website: www.wiley.com/go/gray/operative-dentistry

b

c

n

o

p